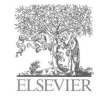
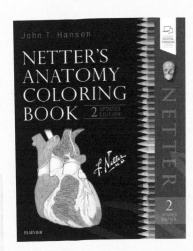
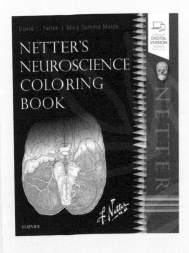

NETTER'S PHYSIOLOGY COLORING BOOK

SUSAN E. MULRONEY, PhD
Professor of Pharmacology and Physiology
Director, Special Master's Program
Georgetown University Medical Center

ADAM K. MYERS, PhD
Professor of Pharmacology and Physiology
Associate Dean and Assistant Vice President, Special Graduate Programs
Georgetown University Medical Center

ARTISTS
Art based on the works of the **Frank H. Netter, MD**, collection
www.netterimages.com

Modified for coloring by
Dragonfly Media Group

ELSEVIER

Elsevier
1600 John F. Kennedy Blvd.
Ste 1600
Philadelphia, PA 19103-2899

NETTER'S PHYSIOLOGY COLORING BOOK   ISBN: 978-0-323-69463-6
Copyright © 2022 by Elsevier, Inc. All rights reserved.

Publisher: Elyse O'Grady
Content Strategist: Marybeth Thiel
Publishing Services Manager: Catherine Jackson
Senior Project Manager/Specialist: Carrie Stetz
Design Direction: Patrick Ferguson

Printed in China

Last digit is the print number: 9   8   7   6   5   4   3

Working together
to grow libraries in
developing countries

www.elsevier.com • www.bookaid.org

Dedication

To the thousands of students we have worked with over the years who have gone on to become skilled and caring physicians, dentists, nurses, other health professionals, and scientists. Their dedication, hard work, and success have inspired us to be the best educators we can be and give us confidence in the future of healthcare and medicine.

Preface

Welcome to *Netter's Physiology Coloring Book.* Our purpose is to provide an interactive method for reinforcing physiologic principles and mechanisms. Physiology can be a challenging subject because by nature it is integrative, building on material from many fields, including basic biology, physics, and chemistry. Reading text, performing specific coloring tasks and other exercises, and then answering review questions will help clarify and reinforce major principles of human physiology. Working through this coloring book in conjunction with the textbook *Netter's Essential Physiology* will greatly enrich your understanding of human physiology.

About the Authors

SUSAN E. MULRONEY, PhD, and **ADAM K. MYERS, PhD,** authors of the second edition of both *Netter's Essential Physiology* and the associated study tool, *Netter's Essential Physiology Flash Cards*, are faculty at Georgetown University in Washington, DC. They are also co-authors of a series of original research papers on the use of educational technology and flipped learning in biomedical education.

Dr. Mulroney is Professor of Pharmacology and Physiology and Director of the highly acclaimed Physiology Special Master's Program at Georgetown University Medical Center. She lectures to medical and graduate students in multiple areas of human physiology, including renal, gastrointestinal, and endocrine physiology. Dr. Mulroney has received numerous teaching awards, including the 2015 Arthur C. Guyton Physiology Educator of the Year Award from the American Physiological Society. Her research focuses on renal development and sex differences in renal disease.

Dr. Myers is Professor of Pharmacology and Physiology and Associate Dean and Assistant Vice President for Special Graduate Programs at Georgetown University Medical Center. He is co-director of the Health and the Public Interest Master's Program at Georgetown and has developed and directed other innovative graduate programs over the years. Dr. Myers has won many teaching awards and has extensive experience in educational program development and administration as well as implementation of new educational technologies. He has authored numerous original research papers in the field of cardiovascular physiology.

About the Artists

Frank H. Netter, MD

Frank H. Netter was born in 1906 in New York City. He studied art at the Art Student's League and the National Academy of Design before entering medical school at New York University, where he received his MD degree in 1931. During his student years, Dr. Netter's notebook sketches attracted the attention of the medical faculty and other physicians, allowing him to augment his income by illustrating articles and textbooks. He continued illustrating as a sideline after establishing a surgical practice in 1933, but he ultimately opted to give up his practice in favor of a full-time commitment to art. After serving in the United States Army during World War II, Dr. Netter began his long collaboration with the CIBA Pharmaceutical Company (now Novartis Pharmaceuticals). This 45-year partnership resulted in the production of the extraordinary collection of medical art so familiar to physicians and other medical professionals worldwide.

In 2005 Elsevier purchased the Netter collection and all publications from Icon Learning Systems. There are now more than 50 publications featuring the art of Dr. Netter available through Elsevier.

Dr. Netter's works are among the finest examples of the use of illustration in the teaching of medical concepts. The 13-book *Netter Collection of Medical Illustrations,* which includes the greater part of the more than 20,000 paintings created by Dr. Netter, became and remains one of the most famous medical works ever published. *Netter's Atlas of Human Anatomy,* first published in 1989, presents the anatomic paintings from the Netter collection. Now translated into 16 languages, it is the anatomy atlas of choice among medical and health professions students all over the world.

The Netter illustrations are appreciated not only for their aesthetic qualities but also, more important, for their intellectual content. As Dr. Netter wrote in 1949, "clarification of a subject is the aim and goal of illustration. No matter how beautifully painted, how delicately and subtly rendered a subject may be, it is of little value as a medical illustration if it does not serve to make clear some medical point." Dr. Netter's planning, conception, point of view, and approach are what informed his paintings and what make them so intellectually valuable.

Frank H. Netter, MD, physician and artist, died in 1991.

Learn more about the physician-artist whose work has inspired the Netter reference collection: https://netterimages.com/artist-frank-h-netter.html

Carlos A.G. Machado, MD

Carlos Machado was chosen by Novartis to be Dr. Netter's successor. He continues to be the main artist who contributes to the Netter collection of medical illustrations.

Self-taught in medical illustration, cardiologist Dr. Carlos Machado has contributed meticulous updates to some of Dr. Netter's original plates. He has created many paintings in the style of Dr. Netter as an extension of the Netter collection. Dr. Machado's photorealistic expertise and his keen insight into the physician-patient relationship inform his vivid and unforgettable visual style. His dedication to researching each topic and subject he paints places him among today's premier medical illustrators.

Learn more about Dr. Machado's background and see more of his art at: https://netterimages.com/artist-carlos-a-g-machado.html

Contents

Chapter 1 Cell Physiology and Homeostasis

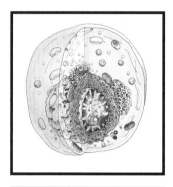

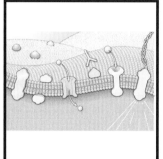

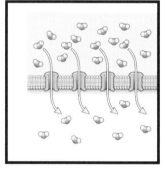

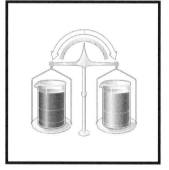

Cells are the basic structural and functional units of living organisms. Although intracellular organelles can differ depending on the cell type, in general, cells have common components that perform basic functions such as protein synthesis; cellular respiration; lipid synthesis; and production, packaging, and excretion of various materials. All of the components are surrounded by the semifluid **cytosol** and the **cell membrane.**

Important Structures

- The **nucleus,** where genetic information in the form of DNA, genes, and chromosomes is housed and controls cellular function and reproduction
- The **nucleolus,** within the nucleus, which initiates production of **ribosomes,** which are necessary for protein synthesis
- The **endoplasmic reticulum**, which comprises flattened tubular membranes or sacs. **Rough endoplasmic reticulum (RER)** is distinguished by ribosomes on the membranes and is integral in protein synthesis. **Smooth endoplasmic reticulum (SER)** does not have ribosomes and synthesizes lipids, including steroid hormones.
- The **Golgi apparatus**, which consists of fluid-filled sacs that process the synthesized proteins for use in other cellular organelles or transport from the cell via vesicles.
- **Vesicles,** which function in the secretion, import, storage, or processing of various materials. Vesicles may fuse to the cell membrane for **exocytosis** and secretion of the contents outside the cell. Conversely, **endocytosis** involves the cell membrane engulfing material outside the cell and fusing to produce a vesicle within the cell. Lysosomal vesicles contain enzymes that can break down unwanted material in the cell.
- **Mitochondria,** which are the metabolic engines of the cell. These organelles produce **adenosine triphosphate (ATP),** which is used as a source of chemical energy throughout the cell. The amount of mitochondria in cells gives you an idea of the metabolic demands of the cell.

LABEL the following cellular components:

- [ ] 1. Vesicle
- [ ] 2. Golgi apparatus
- [ ] 3. Nucleus
- [ ] 4. Nucleolus
- [ ] 5. RER
- [ ] 6. SER
- [ ] 7. Mitochondria
- [ ] 8. Cell membrane

COLOR and **LABEL** the components that have a primary role in:

- [ ] 1. Energy production: mitochondria (green)
- [ ] 2, 3, 4, 5. Protein synthesis: Golgi apparatus, nucleus, nucleolus, RER (yellow)
- [ ] 6, 7. Lipid synthesis: SER (red)

REVIEW ANSWERS

A. Mitochondria

B. Nucleolus, RER

C. Vesicles

D. Nucleus

Plate 1.1   **Cell Physiology and Homeostasis**

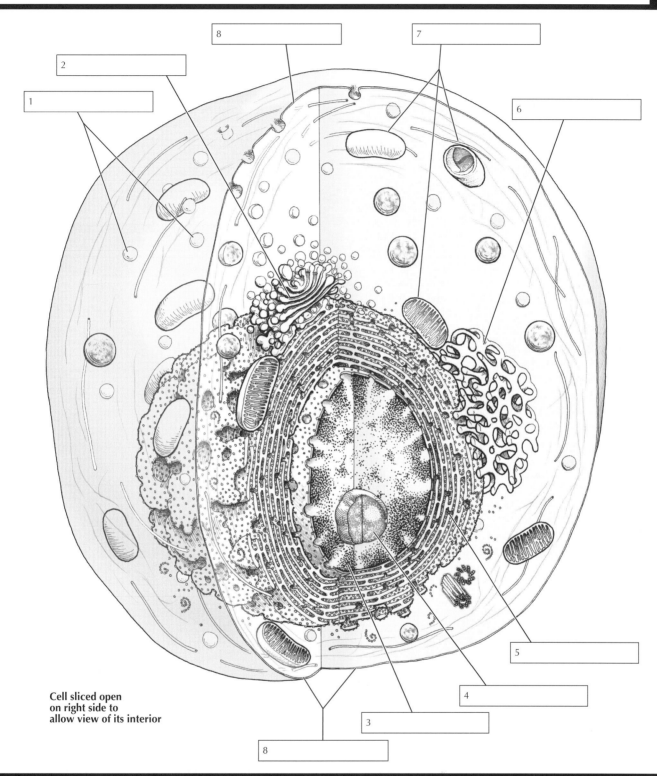

8

7

2

1

6

Cell sliced open
on right side to
allow view of its interior

5

4

3

8

REVIEW QUESTIONS

A. What organelle produces ATP to provide energy for cellular functions?

B. Ribosomes are produced in the _____ and, in association with the _____, synthesize proteins.

C. _____ can fuse with the cell membrane, resulting in secretion of contents through exocytosis.

D. Genetic information is housed in what organelle?

---

1 Cell Membrane

The cell membrane **(plasma membrane),** which separates the cell from its external environment, consists of a **lipid bilayer** made primarily of phospholipids, with varying amounts of glycolipids, cholesterol, and proteins. The lipid bilayer is positioned with the **hydrophobic** fatty acid tails of phospholipids oriented toward the middle of the membrane and the **hydrophilic** polar head groups oriented toward the extracellular or intracellular space. The **fluidity** of the membrane is largely a function of **short-chain and unsaturated fatty acids** incorporated within the phospholipids; incorporation of cholesterol into the lipid bilayer reduces fluidity. The oily, hydrophobic interior region makes the bilayer an effective barrier to fluid (on either side), with permeability that can diffuse through the lipids.

There are a variety of proteins associated with the lipid bilayer. These proteins function as **ion channels** (pores in the membrane), **ligand receptors, adhesion molecules** (for adhesion to **extracellular matrix** or other cells), and **cell recognition markers** (such as surface antigens). Transport across the membrane can involve passive or active mechanisms and is dictated by the membrane composition, concentration gradient of the solute, and availability of transport proteins. If membrane fluidity, protein concentration, or thickness is altered, transport processes can be impaired.

COLOR and **LABEL** each of the following membrane proteins:

- ☐ 1. Ion channel
- ☐ 2. Surface antigen (cell recognition marker)
- ☐ 3. Ligand receptor
- ☐ 4. Adhesion molecule

Notice which structures span the cell membrane (integral proteins) and those that are only peripheral proteins.

COLOR and **LABEL** each of the following molecules, using the same color as their associated membrane protein (colored in 1–4):

- ☐ 5. Ion
- ☐ 6. Antibody
- ☐ 7. Ligand
- ☐ 8. Extracellular matrix protein (e.g., collagen)

REVIEW ANSWERS

A. Lipid bilayer, hydrophilic

B. Proteins

C. Fluidity

Plate 1.2   **Cell Physiology and Homeostasis**

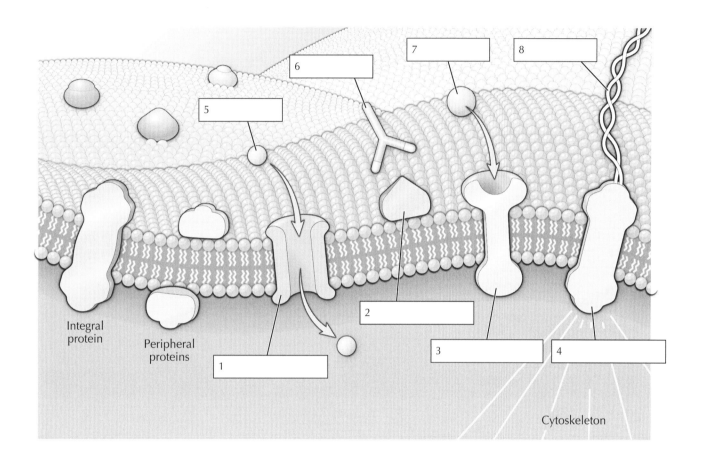

Integral protein

Peripheral proteins

Cytoskeleton

REVIEW QUESTIONS

A. The cell membrane is made of a _____, with the _____ head groups of each phospholipid layer on the outer surface of the membrane.

B. Movement of ions across the membrane, binding of specific ligands, and cellular adhesion are functions of _____ associated with the membrane.

C. Unsaturated and short-chain fatty acids confer the property of _____ to the membrane.

1 Diffusion

Homeostasis, the process of maintaining the internal environment, is a core concept in physiology. At the organismal level, the internal environment of our bodies is maintained in the face of environmental changes and stressors; at the cellular level, the intracellular environment must remain balanced for physiologic function as well.

While the cell membrane protects the internal environment of the cell and limits movement of solutes, particles, and water between the intracellular and extracellular compartments, it is also necessary that movement occur to bring in nutrients, remove unneeded elements, allow communication between inside and outside, and for a myriad of other purposes. The cell membrane can be modeled as a **semipermeable membrane** across which only some substances can freely pass. A number of transport processes permit such movement.

Passive transport is **energy independent** and occurs via **simple** or **facilitated diffusion. Diffusion** is the net movement of a dissolved substance from an area of high concentration to an area of low concentration.

Simple diffusion is the most basic type of transport across a membrane and is described by **Fick's law:**

$$J_i = D_i \times A \, (1/X) \times (C_1 - C_2)$$

where:
- J_i represents the net flux of substance *i*
- D_i is the coefficient of diffusion
- A is the area of the membrane
- X is the distance through the membrane
- $(C_1 - C_2)$ is the difference in concentration across the membrane

The rate of net flux (diffusion) is directly proportional to the surface area of the membrane and the difference in concentration of the molecule across the membrane. It is inversely proportional to the thickness of the membrane.

Facilitated diffusion occurs through specific channels or carrier proteins in the membrane. **Channels** consist of protein "pores" that allow a specific substance to pass through the hydrophobic region of the cell membrane. In the case of **carrier proteins,** the binding of a specific ligand to the protein results in translocation of the molecule across the membrane. Facilitated diffusion increases the rate of diffusion for a molecule but is subject to a **maximal rate of transport.** At higher concentrations, the carriers will be saturated, and the rate of transport will remain constant.

COLOR

☐ 1. Molecules on either side of the membrane (blue)

☐ 2. Arrows indicating net direction the molecules will move via diffusion through the membrane

REVIEW ANSWERS

A. Simple

B. Facilitated

C. Facilitated

D. No, energy expenditure is not needed for diffusion to occur, but diffusion does depend on the composition of the membrane and concentration gradient for the solute.

Plate 1.3   **Cell Physiology and Homeostasis**

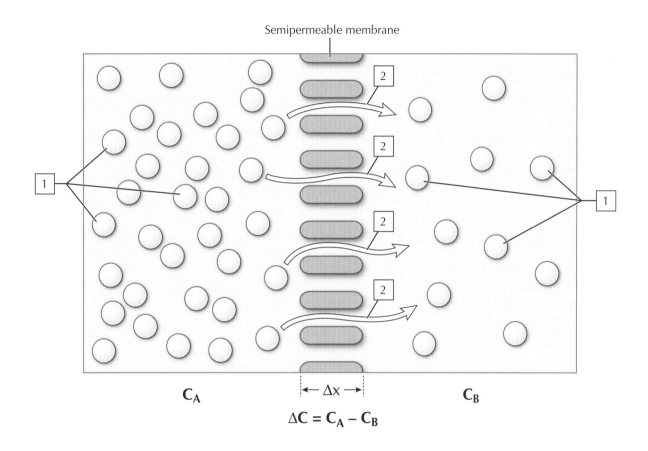

Semipermeable membrane

C_A

$\leftarrow \Delta x \rightarrow$

C_B

$$\Delta C = C_A - C_B$$

A. _____ diffusion occurs over all concentration gradients greater than zero at a rate linearly related to the size of the gradient.

B. _____ diffusion occurs through channels or carrier proteins.

C. Which type of diffusion is associated with a transport maximum?

D. Is expenditure of energy required for diffusion to occur?

The amount of solutes in the **intracellular fluid (ICF)** and **extracellular fluid (ECF)** is expressed in milliosmoles and concentration is expressed as the **osmolarity** of the fluid. In humans the osmolarity is ~290 milliosmoles/L (mOsm/L) throughout the body water (intra- and extracellular osmolarity is the same at steady state). This equilibrium is accomplished via osmosis.

In contrast to the movement of *solutes* by diffusion, **osmosis** is the movement (or diffusion) of *water* from an area of low solute concentration to an area of high solute concentration. The water movement occurs because of the **osmotic pressure** exerted by the concentration of solutes.

Osmotic pressure is equivalent to the **hydrostatic pressure** necessary to prevent movement of fluid through a semipermeable membrane by osmosis. This concept can be illustrated by using a U-shaped tube with different concentrations of solute on either side of an **ideal semipermeable membrane** (i.e., the membrane is permeable to water but is impermeable to solute).

Because of the unequal solute concentrations, fluid will move to the side of the tube with the higher solute concentration, against the gravitational force (hydrostatic pressure) that opposes it, until the hydrostatic pressure generated is equal to the osmotic pressure. (Do not confuse this with oncotic pressure, which specifically refers to osmotic pressure exerted by proteins!) In this example, at equilibrium, solute concentration is nearly equal on either side of the membrane, and the water level is unequal—the displacement of water is due to osmotic pressure. When this example is applied to the whole body, it should be clear that changes in ECF solute concentration will cause osmotic flow and could result in the swelling or shrinking of the cells (not desirable).

COLOR and LABEL

☐ 1. Osmotic pressure; note the unequal water levels in the U-tube on the right

☐ 2. Hydrostatic pressure

REVIEW ANSWERS

A. Water will move to the higher solute concentration, from ICF to ECF (and the cells will shrink).

B. For water to move into the cells, the osmolar concentration would have to be higher in the ICF than in the ECF.

Plate 1.4   *Cell Physiology and Homeostasis*

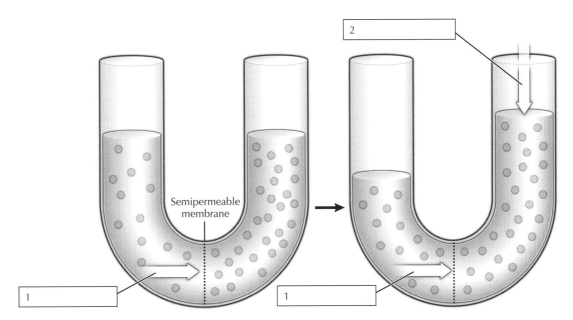

A. Initial state of unopposed osmotic pressure

B. Equilibrium state in which remaining osmotic pressure is opposed by equal and opposite hydrostatic pressure

REVIEW QUESTIONS

A. If the solute concentration is higher in the ECF than in the ICF, in which direction will water flow?

B. What conditions in the ECF would cause cells to swell?

Primary active transport involves the direct expenditure of energy derived from the conversion of ATP to **adenosine diphosphate (ADP)** to transport ions across the cell membrane.

Na$^+$/K$^+$ ATPase is the ubiquitous active transporter that expends energy in the form of ATP to drive Na$^+$ out of the cells and K$^+$ into the cells, establishing the essential intracellular and extracellular ion environments. Because three positive Na$^+$ ions are transported out of the cell while only two positive K$^+$ ions are transported into the cell, the pump is referred to as electrogenic. The concentration gradient established for Na$^+$ allows for sodium ion diffusion down its concentration gradient during various cellular processes, including secondary active transport (next topic).

Other examples of primary active transport include **H$^+$/K$^+$ ATPase, H$^+$ ATPase,** and **Ca^{2+} ATPase.** In each case, ATP is used to move an ion (or ions) against the concentration gradient.

Plate 1.5 illustrates Ca^{2+} ATPase primary active transport.

Clinical Note

Primary active transport is essential for fluid homeostasis (Na$^+$/K$^+$ ATPase), cellular signaling (Ca^{2+} ATPase), acid secretion (H$^+$/K$^+$ ATPase), and other functions. While blocking most of these transporters can cause serious, life-threatening effects, transporters can be targets for drug action, for example, in heart failure (Na$^+$/K$^+$ ATPase) and excess stomach acid secretion (H$^+$/K$^+$ ATPase).

REVIEW ANSWERS

A. Any of the following: Na$^+$/K$^+$ ATPase; H$^+$/K$^+$ ATPase; H$^+$ ATPase; Ca^{2+} ATPase

B. ATP to ADP

Plate 1.5 **Cell Physiology and Homeostasis**

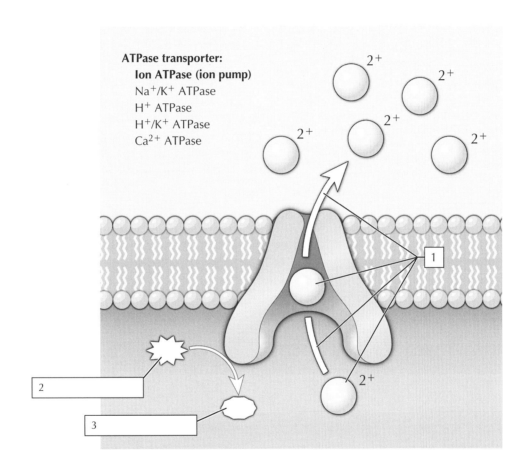

ATPase transporter:
Ion ATPase (ion pump)
Na^+/K^+ ATPase
H^+ ATPase
H^+/K^+ ATPase
Ca^{2+} ATPase

REVIEW QUESTIONS

A. Give two examples of primary active transport.

B. To transport ions against their concentration gradients, energy is derived from the conversion of _____ to _____.

Cellular Transport: Secondary Active Transport

Many substances are transported into or out of the cell via **secondary active transport** with Na⁺. This can be in the form of a **symport** (going the same direction) or an **antiport** (antiporters are also called *exchangers*, because when one ion or molecule goes in, another ion or molecule leaves the cell).

The Na⁺ concentration gradient is maintained by the **active Na⁺/K⁺ ATPase,** which produces a concentration gradient for Na⁺ to move into the cell through a specific symporter or antiporter (as described earlier), allowing simultaneous transport of another molecule into or out of the cell. The *active* portion of this process is the original transport of Na⁺ against its gradient by the Na⁺/K⁺ ATPase; the subsequent events are *secondary*.

A typical example of secondary active transport by symport is **Na⁺-glucose and Na⁺-galactose transport** across the intestinal epithelium. An example of antiport is **Na⁺/H⁺ exchange** that occurs in many cells, including renal and intestinal cells, in which Na⁺ enters the cells along its concentration gradient through the antiporter, while H⁺ leaves the cells. In both of these examples, the gradient for Na⁺ movement into the cell is established by the active transport of Na⁺ out of the cell by the Na⁺/K⁺ ATPase.

The Na⁺/K⁺ ATPase activity also results in **passive** diffusion of ions through channels: Na⁺ (down its concentration gradient), **Cl⁻** (following Na⁺ to preserve electroneutrality), and H₂O (following the osmotic pressure gradient).

Each panel illustrates primary active transport (the sodium pump), setting up a gradient for a type of secondary active transport.

COLOR and **LABEL** each example of secondary AT:

☐ 1. Sodium ions going *into the cell* through symport or antiport (yellow) to denote they are going down their concentration gradient

☐ 2. Ions or molecules going into the cell through symport with sodium (blue)

☐ 3. Ions or molecules leaving the cell through antiport with sodium (red)

☐ 4. Sodium ions going into the cell through a channel (yellow)

REVIEW ANSWERS

A. Na⁺

B. The Na⁺/K⁺ ATPase (primary active transport) sets up a concentration gradient for sodium to move from the high ECF concentration to the low ICF concentration.

Plate 1.6　　　　　**Cell Physiology and Homeostasis**

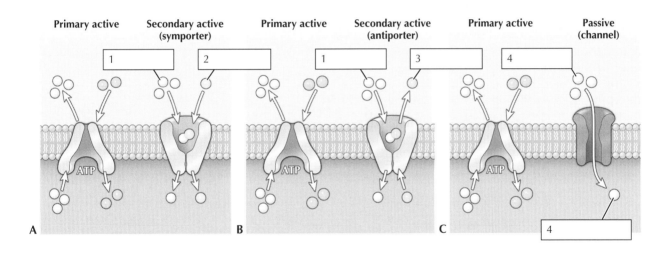

Primary active Secondary active (symporter) Primary active Secondary active (antiporter) Primary active Passive (channel)

A   B   C

1 Ion Channels

Movement of ions occurs through channels in addition to membrane carrier–mediated processes. **Ion channels** generally show high selectivity and allow specific ions to pass down their concentration gradient (e.g., Na^+, Cl^-, K^+, Ca^{2+}). Selectivity is based on the size of the ion, as well as its charge. **Gated channels** can **open** or **close** in response to different stimuli. Stimuli such as sound, light, mechanical stretch, chemicals, and voltage changes can affect the ion flux by controlling the gating systems.

Types of channels include the following:

- **Ligand-gated channels** are opened by the binding of a specific ligand, such as **acetylcholine (ACh)** or serotonin. Binding of the ligand to its receptor causes the channel to open, allowing ion movement. These are tetrameric or pentameric (four- or five-protein subunit) channels.
- **Voltage-gated channels** open in response to a **change in membrane voltage.** These channels are **ion specific** and are composed of several subunits, with transmembrane domains forming a pathway for ion flux through the membrane.
- **Gap junction channels** are formed between two adjacent cells and allow passage of **ions and small molecules** between the cells. A **hemichannel,** also called a **connexon,** from one cell is aligned with the hemichannel of another cell to create the gap junction. Each hemichannel is a hexameric array of six **connexin** subunits.

COLOR and LABEL

- ☐ 1. Open gate (green); to indicate molecules moving through the channel down their concentration gradient
- ☐ 2. Closed gate (red)

Clinical Note
Drugs that block specific ion channels have important clinical uses. For example, calcium channel blockers (such as nifedipine or verapamil) are used to treat cardiac arrhythmias and hypertension, whereas sodium channel blockers such as lidocaine are used for local anesthesia.

REVIEW ANSWERS

A. Ligand-gated and voltage-gated

B. Ligand-gated

C. Voltage

D. Ions and small molecules, cells

Plate 1.7

Cell Physiology and Homeostasis

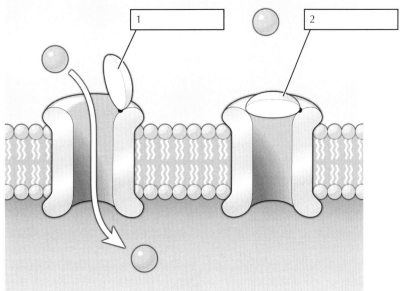

Channel
Na⁺ K⁺   Cl⁻
Ca²⁺ H₂O

1

2

REVIEW QUESTIONS

A. What are two types of gated channels?

B. Substances such as ACh or serotonin may bind to open a _____ channel.

C. Channels can open in response to a change in membrane _____.

D. Gap junctions allow _____ and _____ to pass between adjacent _____.

Plate 1.7

In addition to channels that allow ion flux, cell membranes can have specific water channels, or **aquaporins (AQPs),** that allow water to pass through the hydrophobic cell membrane following the **osmotic pressure gradient.** Aquaporins have a vital role in maintaining equal osmolarity between the intracellular and extracellular spaces.

Many types of AQPs have been identified. The channels can be constitutively expressed in the membranes, or their insertion into the membrane can be regulated (e.g., regulation of AQP-2 by antidiuretic hormone [ADH]). For example, **AQP-3** is always present in the *basolateral* membranes of renal collecting duct cells, whereas regulation of water flux from the renal tubule through the collecting duct cells is accomplished through the ADH-stimulated insertion of **AQP-2** into the *apical* (luminal) membranes.

COLOR

☐ 1. Fluid on side of membrane that has more water present relative to solute (blue)

☐ 2. Fluid on side of membrane that has less water present relative to solute (a different color, to reinforce that the water molecules move to the compartment with the higher solute concentration)

Clinical Note

In diabetes insipidus (a condition unrelated to diabetes mellitus), the patient suffers from extreme thirst and high production of urine. It can be caused by lack of ADH, lack of a renal response to ADH, and other causes. Defects in AQP genes are one cause of nephrogenic diabetes insipidus, a condition in which renal tubules fail to respond normally to ADH.

REVIEW ANSWERS

A. AQPs

B. AQP-3

C. AQPs allow water to pass through the cell membranes following the osmolar concentration gradient.

D. ADH

Plate 1.8   **Cell Physiology and Homeostasis**

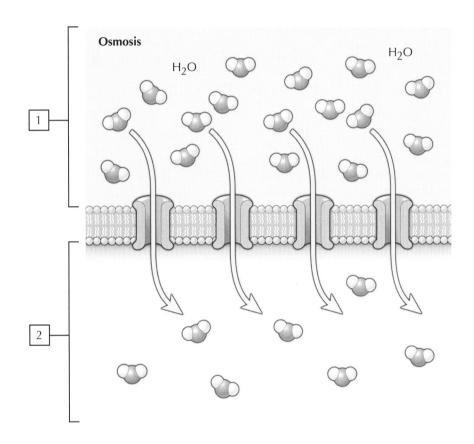

A. What are water channels called?

B. Which water channel is always found in the basolateral membrane of the renal collecting duct cells?

C. What is the function of water channels?

D. What hormone causes insertion of AQPs into the apical membrane of renal collecting duct cells?

The ability to maintain **constant internal environment** during changes in the external environment is termed **homeostasis.** Homeostasis is accomplished through integrated regulation of the internal environment by the multiple organ systems.

On the cellular level, homeostasis is made possible as a result of expandable semipermeable membranes that can accommodate small changes in osmolarity (solute concentration) via osmosis. However, for proper cellular function, the ICF, and thus osmolarity, must be kept under tight control. Plasma osmolarity is in equilibrium with the osmolarity of the ICF and **interstitial fluid (ISF);** therefore regulation of plasma osmolarity by the renal handling of water and electrolytes and central control of thirst are important keys to cell homeostasis.

On a minute-to-minute basis, the endocrine and sympathetic nervous systems work to regulate the amount of sodium and water retained by the kidneys, thus controlling plasma osmolarity (see Chapter 5, Renal Physiology). This integrated control is the key to fluid homeostasis. **Fluid intake** (water and food) and **output** (e.g., urine, feces) must be in **balance.** If fluid intake is greater than fluid output, plasma osmolarity will decrease, and the kidneys will **excrete** the excess fluid.

If fluid intake is less than fluid output, the organism develops a deficit of fluid, and plasma osmolarity will increase. In this situation, the thirst response will be activated, and the kidneys will retain fluid, producing **less urine.** This idea of balance is expanded upon in the following sections, and the integration of the endocrine, cardiovascular, and renal systems in regulation of fluid and electrolyte homeostasis is examined.

COLOR

☐ 1. Arrow on the left indicating that an excess of fluid and urine should increase urine output (green).

☐ 2. Arrow on the right indicating that there is a deficit of fluid and excretion needs to be reduced (and thirst stimulated) (red).

REVIEW ANSWERS

A. The plasma is the interface between the internal (cells) and external environment.

B. Excess fluid intake will decrease plasma osmolarity.

C. Increased plasma osmolarity. This will stimulate retention of fluids and reduced urine excretion. It will also stimulate thirst.

D. Increased urine output

E. Fluid retention, reduced urine output, and stimulation of thirst

Plate 1.9

Cell Physiology and Homeostasis

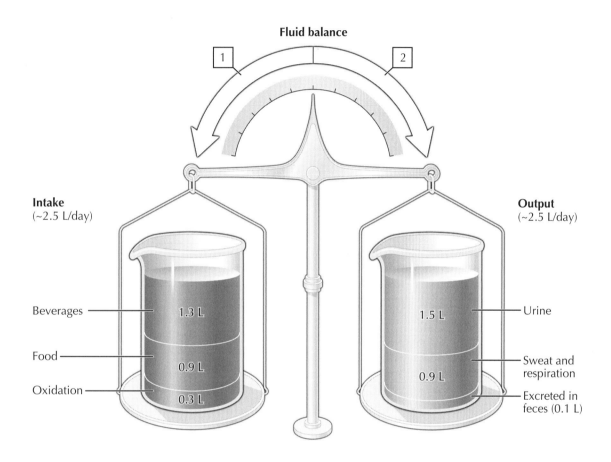

Fluid balance

| 1 | | 2 |

Intake
(~2.5 L/day)

Output
(~2.5 L/day)

Beverages — 1.3 L

Food — 0.9 L

Oxidation — 0.3 L

1.5 L — Urine

0.9 L — Sweat and respiration

Excreted in feces (0.1 L)

REVIEW QUESTIONS

A. What fluid compartment can be conceptualized as the interface between the internal and external environments?

B. An excess of fluid intake will have what effect on plasma osmolarity?

C. A reduction in fluid intake (or increase in fluid excretion) will have what effect on plasma osmolarity?

D. What effect does excess fluid ingestion have on urine excretion?

E. What effects does a deficit of fluid ingestion have on urine excretion?

1 Body Fluid Compartments

The typical adult body is approximately 60% water, which, in a 70-kg person, equals 42 liters (L), since 1 L of water weighs 1 kg.

The actual size of all the fluid compartments depends on a variety of factors, including the person's size and body mass index.

In a normal 70-kg adult:

- ICF constitutes two-thirds of the **total body water (TBW)** (28 L), and the ECF accounts for the other third of TBW (14 L).
  - ICF = $\frac{2}{3}$ TBW
  - ECF = $\frac{1}{3}$ TBW
- The ECF compartment is composed of the **plasma** (i.e., blood without red blood cells [RBCs]) and the ISF, which is the fluid that bathes cells (outside the vascular system), as well as the fluid in bone and connective tissue. Plasma constitutes one-fourth of ECF (3.5 L), and ISF constitutes the other three-fourths of ECF (10.5 L).
  - **Plasma volume (PV)** = $\frac{1}{4}$ ECF
  - ISF = $\frac{3}{4}$ ECF

The intracellular and extracellular compartments are separated by the cell membrane. Within the ECF, the plasma and ISF are separated by the endothelium and basement membranes of the capillaries. The ISF surrounds the cells and is in close contact with both the cells and the plasma.

The ICF has different solute concentrations than the ECF, primarily because of the Na^+/K^+ ATPase, which maintains an ECF high in Na^+ and an ICF high in K^+.

COLOR and **LABEL** the schematic representation of fluid compartments:

- ☐ 1. TBW
- ☐ 2. ICF
- ☐ 3. ECF
- ☐ 4. ISF
- ☐ 5. PV

COLOR and **LABEL** membrane barriers:

- ☐ 6. Cell membrane
- ☐ 7. Capillary wall (note the hatched line to represent the selective permeability of the capillary wall)

REVIEW ANSWERS

A. *40-kg person:*
TBW = 24 L
ICF = 16 L
ECF = 8 L (ISF = 6 L; PV = 2 L)
85-kg person:
TBW = 51 L
ICF = 34 L
ECF = 17 L (ISF = 12.75 L; PV = 4.25 L)

B. Plasma, ISF

C. ICF = $\frac{2}{3}$ TBW; ECF = $\frac{1}{3}$ TBW

Plate 1.10

Cell Physiology and Homeostasis

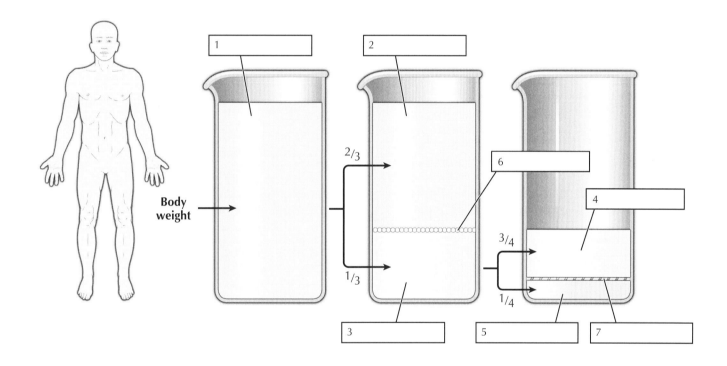

Body
weight

REVIEW QUESTIONS

A.   Determine the TBW, ICF, ECF, ISF, and PV in a 40-kg person and in an 85-kg person.

B.   The capillary wall separates _____ from _____.

C.   The ICF and ECF constitute what fraction of TBW?

The **indicator-dilution method** is used to determine the volume of fluid in the different fluid compartments. Indicators with volumes of distribution specific to particular compartments are used (see later). A known amount of the substance is infused into the bloodstream of the subject and allowed to disperse. A plasma sample is then obtained, and the concentration of indicator is determined. The compartment volume is then calculated using the following formula:

$$\text{Volume (in liters)} = \frac{\text{Amount of indicator injected (mg)}}{\text{Final concentration of indicator (mg/L)}}$$

- TBW can be determined by injecting **tritiated water,** which will diffuse and equilibrate through all compartments.
- ECF can be determined by injecting **inulin** (a large sugar molecule), which cannot cross cell membranes.
- PV can be determined by injecting **Evans blue dye,** which binds to plasma proteins (and thus does not get into the ISF).
- The ISF and ICF can be determined by extrapolation using the following formulas:

$$ICF = TBW - ECF$$

$$ISF = ECF - PV$$

Because **blood volume (BV)** equals the PV plus the volume of red blood cells, it can be calculated by the following formula:

$$BV = PV/(1 - \text{hematocrit})$$

(The **hematocrit [HCT]** is a measure of the volume percentage of RBCs in blood.)

COLOR and **LABEL** the fluid compartments in different colors (colors may overlap):

- ☐ 1.   TBW
- ☐ 2.   ECF
- ☐ 3.   PV
- ☐ 4.   ICF

COLOR and **LABEL** the arrows with the appropriate indicator used to measure the volume of fluid corresponding to the compartment(s) that the indicator can diffuse through, by using the same colors in 1–4:

- ☐ 5.   Evans blue dye
- ☐ 6.   Inulin
- ☐ 7.   Tritiated water

REVIEW ANSWERS

A.   ECF – PV = ISF, so inject inulin (for ECF) and Evans blue dye (for PV); ICF = TBW – ECF, so inject tritiated water (for TBW) and inulin (for ECF).

B.   You can directly determine the ECF using inulin (20 mg/1.67 mg/L = 12 L) and PV using Evans blue dye (0.5 mg/0.17 mg/L = 3 L). BV is therefore 5 L (PV/[1 – HCT]). You can indirectly determine ISF to be 9 L (ISF = ECF – PV). And because ECF is one-third of TBW, TBW is 36 L, and ICF is 24 L.

Plate 1.11   **Cell Physiology and Homeostasis**

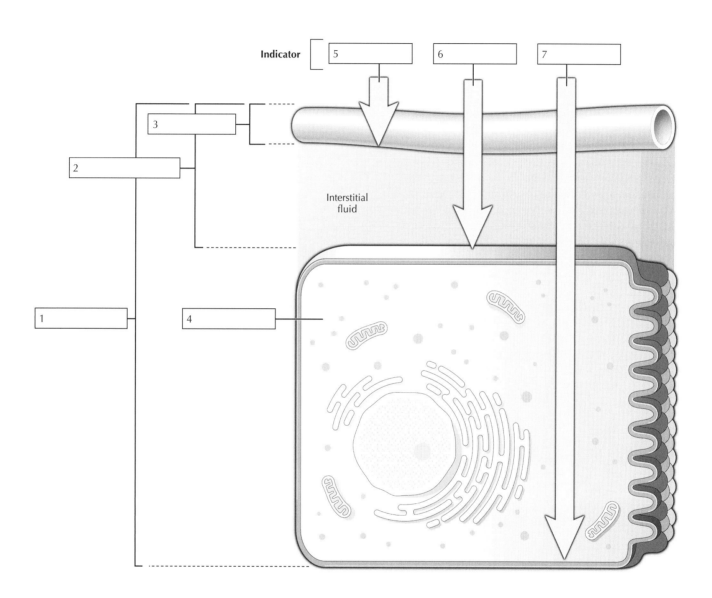

Indicator

Interstitial fluid

REVIEW QUESTIONS

A. What indicators would you infuse to determine ISF volume? ICF volume?

B. An individual with an HCT of 40 (0.40) is infused with 20 mg of inulin and 0.5 mg of Evans blue dye. After equilibrium is achieved, blood is drawn and the concentration of inulin is 1.67 mg/L and Evans blue dye is 0.17 mg/L. What compartments can be determined, and what are their volumes?

Remember that the osmolarity of our body fluid is ~290 mOsm/L (generally rounded to 300 mOsm/L for calculations). The basolateral Na^+/K^+ ATPase on cell membranes is instrumental in establishing and maintaining the intracellular and extracellular environments. The **extracellular sodium** (and the small amount of other positive ions) is balanced by **chloride** and **bicarbonate anions** and anionic proteins. For the most part, the concentrations of individual solutes are similar between plasma and ISF, with the exception of **proteins** (usually indicated as **A⁻**), which remain in the vascular space.

The primary intracellular **cation** is the **potassium ion (K^+),** which is balanced by **phosphates,** proteins, and small concentrations of other miscellaneous anions. Because of the high concentration gradients for sodium, potassium, and chloride, passive movement of these ions occurs down their gradients. The leakage of potassium out of the cell through specific K^+ channels is the key factor contributing to the resting membrane potential. The differential sodium, potassium, and chloride concentrations across the cell membrane are crucial for the generation of electrical potentials.

COLOR and **LABEL** the areas representing ions with different colors to reinforce the concentrations of the different intracellular and extracellular cations and anions:

- [ ] 1. Na^+
- [ ] 2. Cl^-
- [ ] 3. Bicarbonate ion (HCO_3^-)
- [ ] 4. K^+

REVIEW ANSWERS

A. Na^+/K^+ ATPase

B. The same

C. The sodium and potassium ion concentrations would equilibrate on either side of the cell membranes, destroying the gradients.

Plate 1.12

Cell Physiology and Homeostasis

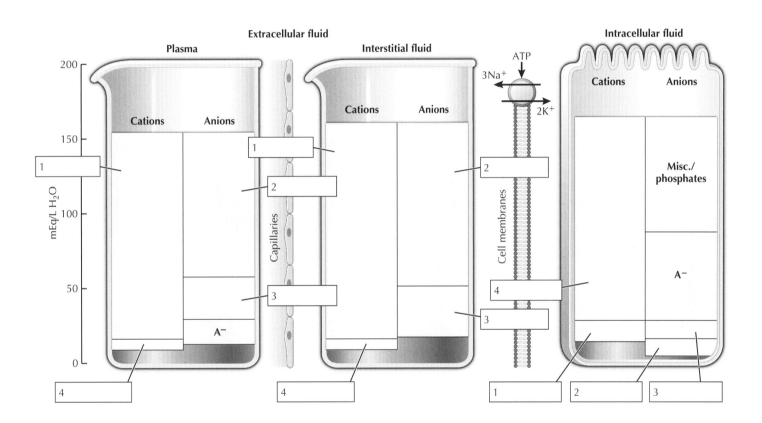

A. The intra- and extracellular ion concentrations are established and maintained by the _____ in cell membranes.

B. The osmolarity of the ECF is *lower, higher,* or *the same* as that of the ICF?

C. What would happen if the Na⁺/K⁺ ATPase stopped working?

Starling forces are the hydrostatic and oncotic pressures that produce fluid movement across the **capillary wall.** Net movement of water out of the capillaries is **filtration,** and net movement into the capillaries is **absorption.** Four forces control fluid movement:

- The **capillary hydrostatic pressure (P_c)** favors movement out of the capillaries. (P_c, like pressures in other vessels, is ultimately produced by the pumping action of the heart.)
- The **capillary oncotic pressure (π_c)** opposes filtration out of the capillaries and is dependent on the protein concentration in the blood. The only effective oncotic agent in capillaries is protein because it is ordinarily impermeable across the capillary wall.
- The **interstitial hydrostatic pressure (P_i)** opposes filtration out of capillaries, but normally this pressure is low.
- The **interstitial oncotic pressure (π_i)** favors movement out of the capillaries, but under normal conditions there is little loss of protein out of the capillaries, and therefore this value is near zero.

Movement of fluid across capillary walls can vary as a result of physical characteristics particular to capillaries in a region (e.g., pore size and fenestration) and relative permeability of these capillaries to protein, but in general the forces that describe net filtration can be expressed by the **Starling equation:**

$$\text{Net filtration} = K_f [(P_c - P_i) - \sigma (\pi_c - \pi_i)]$$

In this equation, the filtration coefficient, K_f, is a measure of the membrane's permeability to water, and σ (the reflection coefficient) describes the permeability of the membrane to proteins (where $0 < \sigma < 1$). The liver capillaries (sinusoids) are highly permeable to proteins and $\sigma = 0$. Thus, bulk movement in the liver sinusoids is controlled by hydrostatic pressure. In contrast, capillaries in most tissues have low permeability to proteins, and $\sigma = {\sim}1$, making the balance of hydrostatic and

oncotic pressures important. The Starling equation can be rearranged to express net filtration in terms of factors favoring filtration minus those favoring absorption:

$$\text{Net filtration} = K [(P_c + \pi_i) - (P_i + \pi_c)]$$

Normally, the high P_c at the **arteriolar end of the capillary** results in positive net filtration pressure, whereas the lower P_c at the **venular end of the capillary** results in net absorption (net filtration in this region has a negative value).

COLOR

☐ 1. Arterioles leading into the capillary (red)

☐ 2. Midportion of the capillary (purple), indicating the diffusion of oxygen out of the blood and replacement with CO_2

☐ 3. Last part of the capillary and into the venule (blue)

COLOR and **LABEL** outward arrows red to indicate that a force favors filtration and inward arrows blue to indicate that a force favors absorption for the following Starling forces:

☐ 4. P_c on arterial side (left) of capillary

☐ 5. P_i

☐ 6. π_c

☐ 7. π_i

☐ 8. P_c on venular side (right) of capillary

REVIEW ANSWERS

A. Net filtration = (37 + 5) − (28 + 3) = 11 mm Hg (out of the capillary)

B. Net filtration = (15 + 5) − (28 + 3) = −11 mm Hg (net absorption)

Plate 1.13

Cell Physiology and Homeostasis

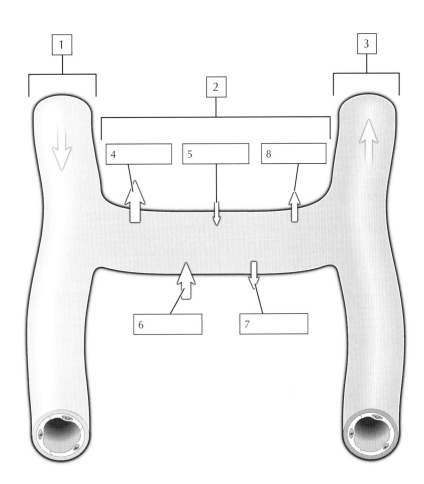

A. The pressures at the arteriolar end of the capillary above are $P_c = 37$, $P_i = 3$; $\pi_c = 28$, $\pi_i = 5$. What is the net filtration pressure at this end of the capillary?

B. The pressures at the venular end of the capillary above are $P_c = 15$, $P_i = 3$; $\pi_c = 28$, $\pi_i = 5$. What is the net filtration pressure at this end of the capillary?

Signal Transduction: G Protein–Coupled Receptors and Second Messengers

Many membrane receptors are coupled with **G proteins.** These receptors are heterotrimeric and have multiple transmembrane domains (they cross the membrane seven times), and they are linked to two main transduction systems: the **cyclic adenosine monophosphate (cAMP)** and the phosphatidylinositol (through **inositol trisphosphate [IP$_3$]**) signaling pathways. Ligand binding to the membrane-bound **G protein–coupled receptor (GPCR)** will initiate an exchange of guanosine diphosphate bound on the associated G protein for guanosine triphosphate (GTP), which causes the α **subunit of the G protein** to dissociate from the β and γ **subunits.** The α subunit then interacts with different effector proteins and, depending on the specific α subtype, initiates the intracellular signaling. The activated G proteins can also have GTPase activity, which can inactivate the complex and end the process.

There are six classes of GPCRs, and the receptors mediate or modulate physiologic processes including sensory perception (sight, smell, taste), the immune response and inflammation, autonomic nervous system transmission, and hormone action. For example, **G$_s$ protein–coupled receptors** can be activated by several hormones and peptides, including norepinephrine, epinephrine, histamine, glucagon, ACTH, and others.

The second messenger systems (cAMP and IP$_3$) signal the cellular events that produce the final effect. The cAMP signaling pathway is activated after GPCR binding initiates the translocation of the GPCR α subunit to membrane-bound **adenylyl cyclase,** which then catalyzes the formation of cAMP from ATP. The cAMP **second messenger** activates **protein kinase A (PK-A),** which phosphorylates other molecules, leading to the physiologic effect.

The IP$_3$ signal transduction pathway is activated when the α subunit of the G protein translocates to membrane-bound **phospholipase C (PLC).** The PLC cleaves phosphatidylinositol bisphosphate to form the second messengers **diacylglycerol (DAG,** which remains in the membrane and serves to insert **phosphokinase-C [PK-C]** into the membrane) and IP$_3$, which enters the cytosol. The IP$_3$ opens Ca^{2+} channels in the SER and the elevated intracellular Ca^{2+} activates the PK-C. The activated PK-C phosphorylates other molecules, resulting in altered cellular activity and leading to the physiologic effect. The important and closely related calcium-calmodulin pathway is covered in the next workbook page.

COLOR and LABEL, in Part A:

☐ 1. α-Subunit of the G protein (green) as it moves to activate the adenylyl cyclase and initiate the intracellular events

☐ 2. ATP substrate converted by adenyl cyclase to a second messenger

☐ 3. cAMP second messenger formed from ATP

☐ 4. Active PK-A, resultant kinase

COLOR and LABEL, in Part B:

☐ 5. α-Subunit of the G protein (blue) as it is stimulated to activate the PLC in the membrane and initiate intracellular events

☐ 6. IP$_3$, the intracellular second messenger directly formed by PLC action

REVIEW ANSWERS

A. The receptor may be linked to different second messenger systems or have differential effects on those second messenger systems, depending on linkage to specific G proteins (e.g., G$_s$ or G$_i$).

B. PK-C is activated by intracellular calcium (Ca^{2+}).

C. Stimulation or inhibition of the cellular message is mediated by whether the ligand-receptor complex is linked to a G$_s$ (stimulatory) or G$_i$ (inhibitory) protein.

Plate 1.14   **Cell Physiology and Homeostasis**

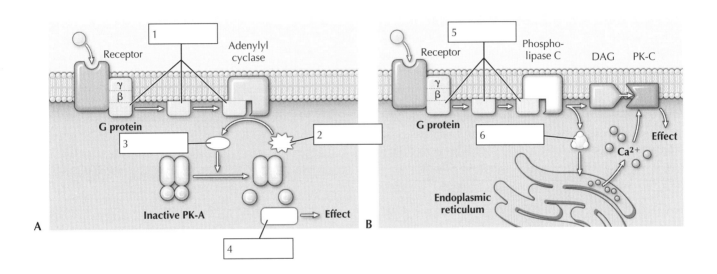

A

Receptor

1

Adenylyl cyclase

γ
β

G protein

3

2

Inactive PK-A

Effect

4

B

Receptor

5

Phospho-lipase C

DAG   PK-C

γ
β

G protein

6

Effect

Ca²⁺

Endoplasmic reticulum

REVIEW QUESTIONS

A. How can GPCRs cause different effects?

B. How is PK-C activated?

C. How can ligand binding stimulate or inhibit the cellular message?

Signal Transduction–Second Messenger Systems: Calcium-Calmodulin

Much of the basic regulation of cellular processes (e.g., secretion of substances, contraction, relaxation, activation of enzymes, cell growth) is initiated by the binding of a regulatory substance to its receptor, activation or production of a second messenger, and subsequent cellular events leading to the physiologic effect.

In a resting cell, intracellular Ca^{2+} concentration is maintained at low levels ($\sim 10^{-7}$ M) compared to ECF concentrations ($\sim 10^{-3}$ M), and increases in this cytosolic Ca^{2+} level (by various stimuli) serve to activate cellular processes. As noted earlier, IP_3 can stimulate the release of Ca^{2+} from the SER into the cytosol, and the elevation of Ca^{2+} and subsequent physiologic effects is an important part of the PLC/IP_3 pathway described in the previous workbook page.

Another important pathway for elevating cytosolic calcium is through voltage- or ligand-gated Ca^{2+} channels on the cell membrane. This mechanism plays a role in smooth muscle contraction, hormone synthesis and secretion, and neurotransmitter release. Opening of ligand- or voltage-gated calcium channels allows an influx of Ca^{2+}, which binds to calmodulin. This **Ca^{2+}-calmodulin** complex binds to other cellular proteins, including protein kinases, to alter cellular function. For example, in the gastrointestinal tract, depolarization of smooth muscle cells leads to Ca^{2+} influx and binding to calmodulin; the Ca^{2+}-calmodulin complex activates myosin light-chain kinase, initiating muscle contraction. Such kinases that are activated by a Ca^{2+}-calmodulin complex are called CaM kinases.

COLOR and LABEL

☐ 1. Open channel, to reinforce that the calcium is going down its concentration gradient into the cell

☐ 2. Ca^{2+}

☐ 3. Calmodulin, the protein that binds free calcium and becomes activated

☐ 4. Myosin light-chain kinase, the CaM kinase that is activated in gastrointestinal smooth muscle by this complex

REVIEW ANSWERS

A. Ligand, voltage

B. SER

C. 10^{-7} M

Plate 1.15

Cell Physiology and Homeostasis

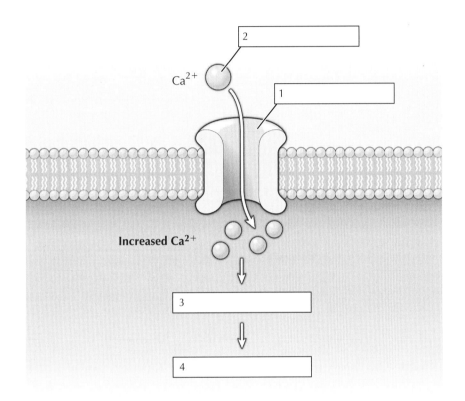

REVIEW QUESTIONS

A. Calcium can enter the cell via _____-gated or _____-gated channels.

B. Calcium can be released from what cellular organelle?

C. In a resting cell, intracellular Ca^{2+} concentration is approximately _____.

Signal Transduction: Nuclear Receptors

1

Lipophilic ligands, such as **steroid hormones, thyroid hormone, vitamin D,** and **vitamin A** (and its metabolite, **retinoic acid**) pass through the cell membrane and bind directly to their **nuclear receptors.** The receptors may also reside in the cytosol, translocating to the nucleus upon binding of the ligand. Binding of the ligand will lead to the nuclear receptor interacting with **DNA** transcription regulatory sites and increasing or decreasing the transcription of **messenger ribonucleic acid (mRNA)** from target genes.

When this pathway is stimulated, a delay occurs in presentation of the end protein because the process requires gene transcription and translation. This **delayed action** is in contrast to that of other hormones and ligands that have effects that do not require **protein synthesis.**

COLOR

☐ 1. Ligand outside the membrane and follow the arrow inside the cell

☐ 2. Ligand where it binds directly to the nuclear receptor, reinforcing that the ligand can pass through the cell membrane and initiate protein synthesis

COLOR and LABEL

☐ 3. mRNA, the result of the nuclear receptor binding to DNA

☐ 4. Protein synthesis, the final product of the cellular actions

WRITE examples of ligands that use nuclear receptors:

☐ 5. Steroid hormones

☐ 6. Thyroid hormones

☐ 7. Vitamin A

☐ 8. Vitamin D

REVIEW ANSWERS

A. Regulation of gene transcription and translation and therefore protein synthesis

B. DNA transcription and translation and protein synthesis have to occur before the effects of the synthesized protein can be observed. This is in contrast to other ligands (including peptide hormones) that have actions that often do not require transcription and translation.

C. Ligands that bind nuclear receptors are lipophilic and can pass through the cell membrane.

Plate 1.16

Cell Physiology and Homeostasis

Nuclear protein receptor

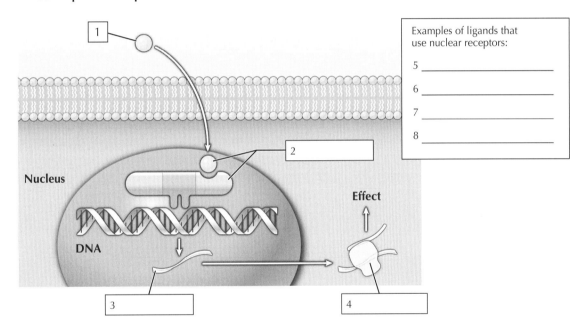

Examples of ligands that
use nuclear receptors:

5 _____

6 _____

7 _____

8 _____

Nucleus

DNA

Effect

A. What general cellular process is initiated when a ligand binds to a nuclear receptor?

B. Why are the effects of ligands that act through nuclear receptors delayed?

C. What characteristic of ligands allows them access to nuclear receptors?

Chapter 2 Nerve and Muscle Physiology

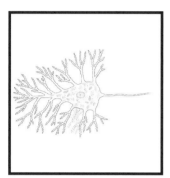
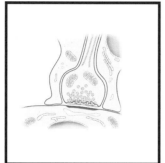
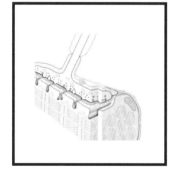
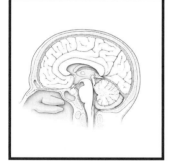

The endocrine and nervous systems are the two major regulatory systems controlling physiological activity of tissues and organs. The nervous system is particularly important in rapid physiological responses; it can also orchestrate larger, integrated responses. This section will focus on the basic principles of neuronal and muscular function.

The nervous system consists of the **central nervous system (CNS)** and the **peripheral nervous system.** The CNS includes the **brain** and **spinal cord.** The peripheral nervous system includes **nerves, ganglia** (clusters of nerve cells), and **sensory receptors** outside the CNS. The peripheral nervous system can also be divided into sensory and motor divisions. Sensory nerves transmit information from various sensory receptors to the CNS; motor nerves transmit signals from the CNS to muscles and glands, thereby controlling their activity.

The spinal cord extends from the medulla oblongata of the brain to the lumbar area through the vertebral column. It contains nerves that conduct impulses to and from areas in the brain; it also contains nerves that participate in reflex arcs. Electrical impulses *from* nerves to the brain are conducted through **sensory (afferent) nerves,** and impulses coming from the brain are conducted through **motor (efferent) nerves.**

COLOR and LABEL

☐ 1. Brain

☐ 2. Spinal cord

☐ 3. Intercostal nerves, example of peripheral nerves

☐ 4. Spinal nerves, example of peripheral nerves

REVIEW ANSWERS

A. Central

B. Nerves, ganglia, and sensory receptors

C. Afferent, or sensory nerves

D. Efferent, or motor nerves

Plate 2.1

Nerve and Muscle Physiology

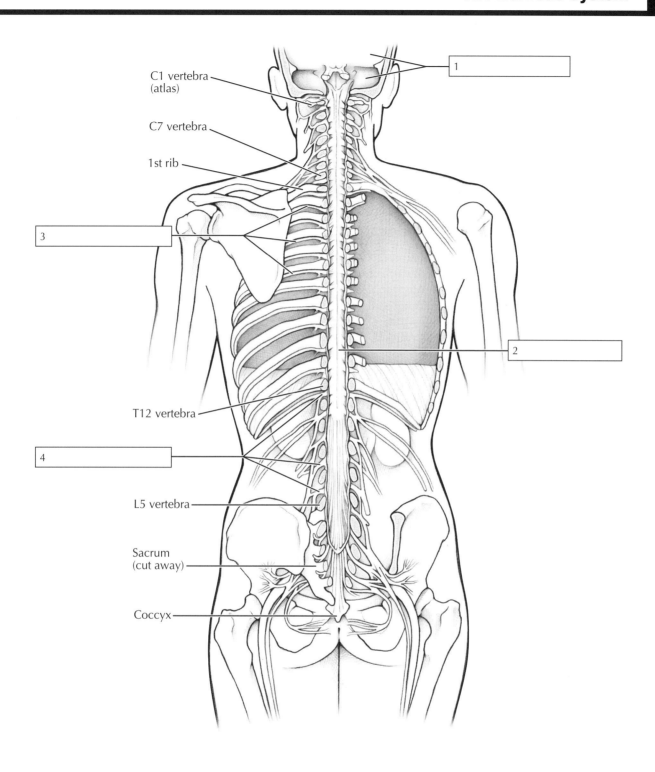

C1 vertebra (atlas)

C7 vertebra

1st rib

T12 vertebra

L5 vertebra

Sacrum (cut away)

Coccyx

1

3

2

4

REVIEW QUESTIONS

A.   The brain and spinal cord are part of the _____ nervous system.

B.   The peripheral nervous system includes _____, _____, and _____.

C.   Which nerves conduct impulses to the brain?

D.   Which nerves conduct impulses from the brain?

Neurons are electrically excitable cells in the nervous system that can receive input (electrical or chemical), process the signal, and then transmit electrical impulses through their axon to a **synapse** (the site where information is transmitted from one neuron to another) or other neuroeffector junction. The main parts of the neuron are the:

- **Soma** (or cell body)
- **Dendrites** (branches off the cell body)
- **Axon hillock** (between soma and axon)
- **Axon** (which transmits an action potential away from the neuron to other cells: the axon terminal forms a synapse with the other cells)

Axons can form synapses on the dendrites **(axodendritic synapse)** or soma **(axosomatic synapse)** of another neuron. The cellular organelles, including **nucleus,** nucleolus, mitochondria, rough endoplasmic reticulum, and **Golgi bodies,** are located in the soma. Although most neurons have the basic structures outlined above, there can be differences in type and number of dendrites and in the networks they form, characteristics that can define different neuronal systems.

Neurons rapidly communicate information between various sites in the body and to and from the brain to regulate physiological functions.

COLOR and **LABEL** the following structures:

- ☐ 1. Dendrite
- ☐ 2. Nucleus
- ☐ 3. Axon hillock; electrical impulses travel out through the axon hillock and axon
- ☐ 4. Axon; electrical impulses travel out through the axon hillock and axon
- ☐ 5. Soma
- ☐ 6. Axosomatic synapse
- ☐ 7. Axodendritic synapse

REVIEW ANSWERS

A.   Axon

B.   Axosomatic synapse

C.   Axodendritic synapse

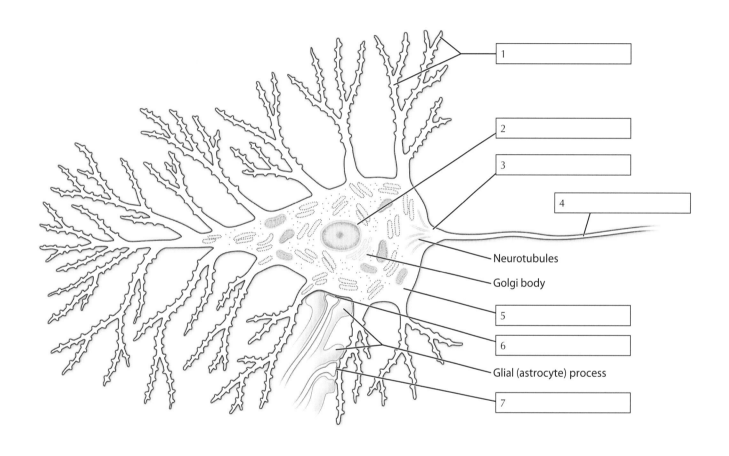

1

2

3

4

Neurotubules

Golgi body

5

6

Glial (astrocyte) process

7

A. Electrical impulses are transmitted through the _____ to synapse with cells.

B. An axon terminates on another cell body via an _____.

C. An axon terminates on another cell's dendrite via an _____.

Electrical potentials exist across cell membranes, and the inside of the cell is slightly negative compared to the charge on the extracellular side of the membrane. This membrane potential allows electrically excitable cells such as neurons and muscle to generate signals within the cell and, in the case of neurons, to other cells via axons and synapses. The next few plates describe important aspects of membrane potentials.

The term **resting membrane potential (RMP)** is synonymous with steady-state potential. An RMP is created by passive **diffusion** of ions through a selectively permeable membrane, producing **charge separation.**

In the simplest theoretical case, if a cell membrane is permeable to only one ion, and that ion is present in a higher concentration inside the cell compared with outside the cell, that ion will diffuse out of the cell **until sufficient membrane potential is established to oppose further net flux of the ion.**

For example, **if the membrane is permeable only to K⁺ and** the intracellular K⁺ concentration is higher than the extracellular concentration, then a **small outward net flux of K⁺** will occur, **resulting in a negative membrane potential,** in which the intracellular compartment is electrically negative relative to the outside of the cell.

Only a minute fraction of the ions will diffuse out of the cell, with no appreciable change in ion concentration in the compartments, before the established electrical gradient will be sufficient to oppose further outward net flux of the ion. At this point, an RMP will be established. Potassium leaking out of the cell is mainly responsible for generation of the RMP in many cells. The concentration gradients for two ions (Na^+ and K^+) are established by the Na^+/K^+ ATPase, and the RMP mainly reflects K^+ leak (K^+ is the most permeable ion across most cell membranes).

COLOR and LABEL

☐ 1. Inward Na^+ diffusion (green, to indicate passive process)

☐ 2. Outward Na^+ active transport (red, to indicate energy expenditure)

☐ 3. Outward K^+ diffusion (green)

☐ 4. Inward K^+ active transport (red)

REVIEW ANSWERS

A. Potassium

B. Potassium leak channels

C. Relatively few

D. Potassium ions are leaking out of the cell down the concentration gradient.

Plate 2.3 **Nerve and Muscle Physiology**

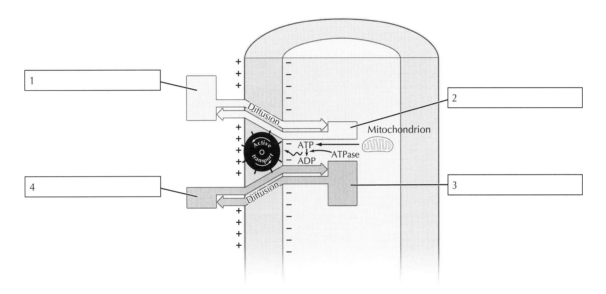

1

2

Mitochondrion

ATP

ATPase

ADP

Active Transport

Diffusion

Diffusion

4

3

Distribution of ions in an axon by charge separation and diffusion

A. The concentration of _____ ions is higher in the intracellular fluid than in the extracellular fluid.

B. Which channels (that are always open) are most important in generating the RMP of many cells?

C. Does it take relatively few ions or many ions leaking to establish an RMP?

D. In this paradigm, are ions leaking into the cell or out of the cell to establish the RMP?

The electrical potential difference between the inside and the outside of a cell (E_X) can be predicted if the membrane is permeable to only **one ion,** using the **Nernst equation:**

$$E_X = (RT/ZF) \ln ([X]_o / [X]_i)$$

where:

- E_X is the Nernst potential or **equilibrium potential**
- $\ln([X]_o/[X]_i)$ is the natural log of the ratio of the concentration of ion X outside the cell ($[X]_o$) to the concentration of the ion inside the cell ($[X]_i$)
- R is the ideal gas constant
- T is absolute temperature
- Z is the charge of the ion
- F is Faraday's number

In a simple hypothetical situation at 37°C, in which a single, monovalent cation (e.g., K^+) is permeable and its concentration inside the cell is 10-fold higher than outside (see cell in Plate 2.4), this equation becomes:

$$E_{K^+} = (61 \text{ mV}/+1) \log (0.1 \text{ mM}/1.0 \text{ mM})$$

or

$$E_{K^+} = (61 \text{ mV}) \log (0.1) = -61 \text{ mV}$$

In Plate 2.4, the **cell membrane** of the hypothetical cell on the left is impermeable to K^+, Na^+, and Cl^-, while the membrane on the cell to the right is permeable only to K^+. This selective permeability results in outward diffusion of K^+ and a membrane potential equal to the K^+ Nernst potential. The electrochemical equilibrium will be greatly changed by altering the concentration of the permeable ion inside or outside the cell. For a system in which only one ion is permeable, the Nernst potential for the permeable ion is equal to the **RMP.** In actual cells, more than one ion is permeable, and thus the RMP is a result of different permeabilities (conductances) of the ions present and the concentration differences of those ions across the cell membrane (see Plate 2.5).

COLOR in Part A:

☐ 1. Cytoplasm and membrane of the cell (the same color, indicating balance with a membrane potential [V_m] of zero)

COLOR in Part B:

☐ 1. Cytoplasm

☐ 2. Cell membrane (red) to denote potential difference between the inside and outside

LABEL

☐ 3. The RMP for the left cell; $V_m = 0$ mV

☐ 4. The RMP for the right cell; $V_m = -61$ mV

REVIEW ANSWERS

A. Membrane potential

B. $E_X = (61 \text{ mV}/Z) \log ([X]_o/[X]_i)$

C. $E_{Na^+} = (61 \text{ mV}/+1) \log (1 \text{ mM}/0.1 \text{ mM})$

which is simplified to

$E_{Na^+} = (61 \text{ mV}) \log (10) = +61 \text{ mV}$

Plate 2.4

Nerve and Muscle Physiology

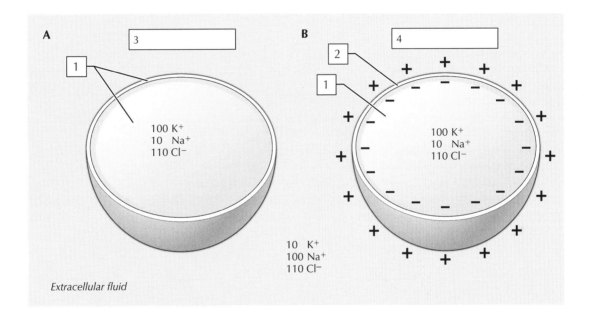

A

3

1

100 K⁺
10 Na⁺
110 Cl⁻

Extracellular fluid

B

4

2

1

100 K⁺
10 Na⁺
110 Cl⁻

10 K⁺
100 Na⁺
110 Cl⁻

REVIEW QUESTIONS

A. The Nernst potential represents the theoretical _____ if a cell is permeable to a single ion.

B. At 37°C, what is the Nernst equation for an ion X?

C. For the ion concentrations given in the right cell, if the cell is only permeable to Na⁺, the RMP will be _____.

The actual RMP (V_m) for a system involving more than one permeable ion is calculated by the **Goldman-Hodgkin-Katz equation (G-H-K equation),** which takes into account the permeabilities and concentrations of the multiple ions:

$$V_m = \left(\frac{RT}{F}\right) \ln \left(\frac{P_{K^+}[K^+_o] + P_{Na^+}[Na^+_o] + P_{Cl^-}[Cl^-_i]}{P_{K^+}[K^+_i] + P_{Na^+}[Na^+_i] + P_{Cl^-}[Cl^-_o]}\right)$$

where:

- P_X is the membrane permeability to ion X
- $[X]_i$ is the concentration of X inside the cell
- $[X]_o$ is the concentration of X outside the cell
- R is the ideal gas constant
- T is absolute temperature
- F is Faraday's number

Although cells contain many ions, this simplified G-H-K equation omits ions that are much less permeable to the cell membrane than K^+, Na^+, and Cl^- because their contribution to RMP is usually negligible. Note that the concentration of Cl^- inside appears in the top of the right-most term and the concentration of Cl^- outside appears in the bottom, whereas the situation for $[K^+]$ and $[Na^+]$ is opposite that of $[Cl^-]$ because of the difference in charge of these ions (positive vs. negative).

The RMP in many cells (including neurons) is approximately −70 millivolts (mV); in skeletal muscle it is approximately −90 mV. K^+ contributes most to the RMP because cytosolic K^+ concentration is high and extracellular K^+ concentration is low, and permeability of the plasma membrane to K^+ is high relative to other ions. Therefore, although the RMP is *similar* to the Nernst potential for K^+, other ions contribute to the RMP. Specifically, leaking of Na^+ through Na^+ channels along its electrochemical gradient contributes to the fact that the **RMP of cells is less negative (more positive) than the Nernst potential for K^+.**

REVIEW ANSWERS

A.   RMP

B.   The Nernst potential only gives the theoretical RMP if the cell was permeable to only one ion.

C. Na^+

Plate 2.5

Nerve and Muscle Physiology

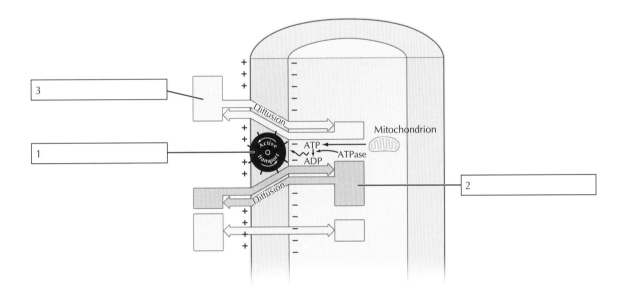

3

1

Mitochondrion

ATP

ATPase

ADP

2

REVIEW QUESTIONS

A. The G-H-K equation determines the _____ in cells.

B. The difference between the Nernst equation and the G-H-K equation is _____.

C. What ion leaking into the cells makes the RMP less negative than the Nernst potential for K+?

Electrical or chemical stimulation that increases ion permeability in the cell membrane and depolarization over a threshold potential results in an **action potential.** In neurons and skeletal muscle cells, when a stimulus produces depolarization that reaches this threshold, voltage-gated Na^+ channels open, and the inward flux of Na^+ now exceeds the ability of K^+ leakage to maintain a steady state. The further depolarization of the membrane opens more voltage-gated Na^+ channels. This positive feedback continues until all voltage-gated Na^+ channels are open, producing the rapid, **all-or-none depolarization** characteristic of an action potential. These "fast channels" are rapidly inactivated as well.

Along with these changes in **Na^+ conductance,** a delayed, slower, and smaller increase in **conductance of K^+** occurs during the action potential. This is caused by opening of voltage-gated K^+ channels; along with the fall in Na^+ conductance, it is responsible for the **repolarization** of the membrane. These K^+ channels remain open until the membrane finally returns to the equilibrium potential and are therefore responsible for the **hyperpolarization** or "**undershoot**" phase of the action potential, during which the membrane is at a more negative potential than the resting potential. This "undershoot" contributes to the **relative refractoriness** of the membrane to the generation of another action potential because a greater stimulus will be required to displace this hyperpolarized **membrane potential** to the threshold potential.

COLOR and **LABEL** the action potential and conductance changes generated in a typical neuron:

☐ 1.   Action potential

☐ 2. Na^+ conductance; Na^+ influx depolarizes the cell

☐ 3. K^+ conductance; higher K^+ conductance results in hyperpolarization and relative refractory period

---

REVIEW ANSWERS

A.   Sodium ions

B.   The threshold potential is the membrane potential at which an action potential will be initiated.

C.   The undershoot is due to voltage-gated K^+ channels, which remain open longer than necessary to restore RMP. This results in an undershoot before returning to equilibrium.

D.   Your completed graph should look like the one above it.

Plate 2.6

Nerve and Muscle Physiology

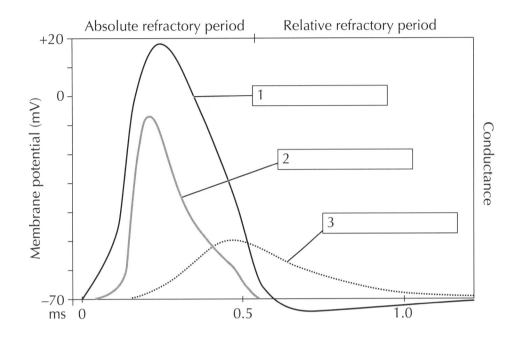

REVIEW QUESTIONS

A. In a typical action potential found in neurons or skeletal muscle cells, influx of what ion depolarizes the cell?

B. What is the threshold potential?

C. What causes the undershoot in the action potential?

D. In the graph provided below, **DRAW sodium** and **potassium conductance** to reinforce their roles in the action potential (remember the undershoot in potassium conductance!).

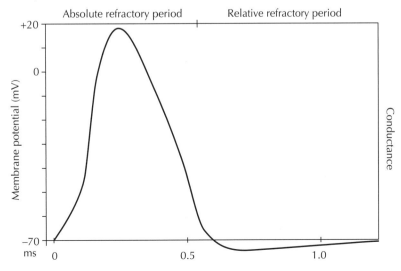

In a neuron, when threshold potential is reached, an **action potential** is generated at the axon hillock, spreads to the axon, and is conducted to the axon terminal. As depolarization occurs at a point on the membrane, Na^+ flows through the membrane from the extracellular fluid. Loss of positive charge at the point of depolarization causes **local currents,** in which positive charges flow from adjacent regions along the membrane to the area of depolarization (Part A). Local current results in depolarization of the adjacent regions; when threshold is reached, the action potential is propagated. An important characteristic of **action potential propagation** is that it occurs away from the point of initiation; it cannot travel back toward its origin. As the action potential is conducted, the area of the membrane directly behind the action potential is still in the absolute refractory state as a result of Na^+ channel inactivation, preventing retrograde conduction.

Many nerve cells in the vertebrate nervous system are **myelinated**—that is, they are covered by multiple layers of an insulating sheath of phospholipid membrane, formed by **Schwann cells** in the peripheral nervous system and **oligodendrocytes** in the CNS. This insulation decreases capacitance and increases membrane resistance, such that current travels through the interior of the axon but not across the membrane (Part B). To allow propagation of the action potential, breaks called **nodes of Ranvier** occur in the **myelin sheath.** They are present at 1- to 2-mm intervals along the axon, and the action potential thus "jumps" rapidly from node to node, bypassing the myelinated areas. The process of conduction by which the action potential "jumps" between nodes is known as **saltatory conduction** and allows very rapid propagation of the action potential despite small axon diameter.

TRACE

☐ 1. Arrows in Part A, reinforcing that in unmyelinated nerves the action potential is propagated relatively slowly by local currents

☐ 2. Arrows in Part B, indicating that the action potential jumps between nodes of Ranvier

COLOR and LABEL

☐ 3. Myelin sheaths in Part B

☐ 4. Nodes of Ranvier

REVIEW ANSWERS

A. Action potentials travel away from their point of origin because the area on the membrane behind the action potential is still in the absolute refractory state.

B. Myelin provides insulation, which increases the membrane resistance, so the charge cannot cross the membrane until there is a break in the membrane (i.e., nodes of Ranvier).

C. Oligodendrocytes form the phospholipid sheaths of myelin in the CNS; Schwann cells form the myelin sheaths in the peripheral nervous system.

D. Saltatory conduction occurs in myelinated neurons and is the process whereby the action potential "jumps" between nodes of Ranvier, resulting in rapid axonal conduction.

Plate 2.7　　　　　　　　　　　　　　　　**Nerve and Muscle Physiology**

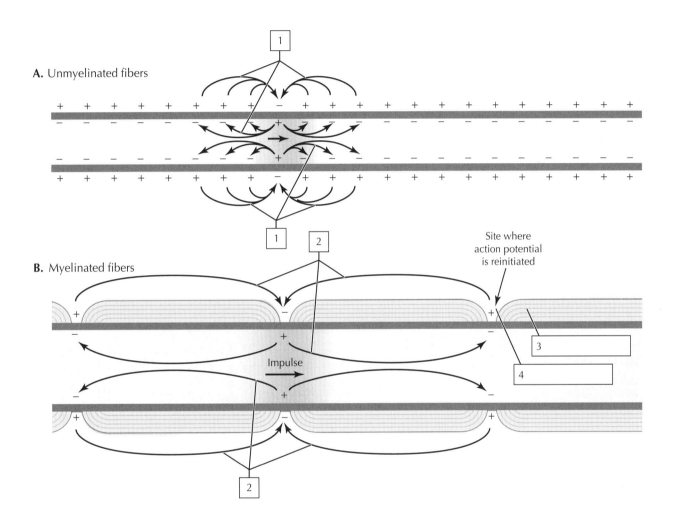

A. Unmyelinated fibers

B. Myelinated fibers

Site where action potential is reinitiated

Impulse

REVIEW QUESTIONS

A. Why do action potentials travel away from their point of origin?

B. What is the function of myelin on axons?

C. What cells form myelin in the CNS? The peripheral nervous system?

D. Explain saltatory conduction.

The terminal fibers of **axons** branch and form synaptic **boutons** (terminals), the sites at which an electrical response in one cell is transmitted to another cell. This transmission can occur through electrical or chemical synapses. Some neurons can use both types of synapses.

- **Electrical synapses** allow passage of electrical current directly from one cell to another through **gap junctions** (regulated connections between the cytoplasm of two cells). In addition to neurons, cardiac myocytes and some types of smooth muscle use electrical synapses. These synapses allow rapid transmission of impulses between cells as electrical current flows freely through the gap junction.
- **Chemical synapses** conduct signals between neurons using neurotransmitters. When an electrical signal reaches the axonal terminal, neurotransmitter is released into the **synaptic cleft** and binds to its receptor on the **postsynaptic cell** to propagate the electrical signal. Transmission via chemical synapses is slower than transmission through electrical synapses. Many neurons in the CNS and peripheral nervous system use chemical synapses; we will focus on chemical transmission.

Depending on the **presynaptic** neuron (and thus transmitter released), the chemical transmission may result in either an **excitatory postsynaptic potential** (depolarization) or an **inhibitory postsynaptic potential** (hyperpolarization) as a result of Na^+ or Cl^- influx at the **postsynaptic membrane,** respectively.

Chemical transmission in these synapses is unidirectional, from the presynaptic fiber to the postsynaptic cell.

A given neuron will have input from multiple excitatory and inhibitory neurons, and generation of an action potential depends on summation of these inputs.

- **Temporal summation** occurs when a series of impulses is generated by an excitatory presynaptic fiber.
- **Spatial summation** occurs when local potentials are generated by multiple excitatory fibers on the postsynaptic cell.

Inhibitory fibers can synapse on an excitatory axon **(presynaptic inhibition)** or directly on the target soma **(postsynaptic inhibition).**

COLOR and LABEL

- ☐ 1. Axon
- ☐ 2. Synaptic vesicles
- ☐ 3. Synaptic cleft
- ☐ 4. Presynaptic membrane
- ☐ 5. Postsynaptic membrane

REVIEW ANSWERS

A. Electrical and chemical synapses

B. Synaptic boutons (also known as axonal terminals)

C. The neurotransmitter that is released from the presynaptic bouton

D. Temporal summation

E. Spatial summation, resulting from local potentials generated by multiple excitatory fibers on the postsynaptic cell.

Plate 2.8   **Nerve and Muscle Physiology**

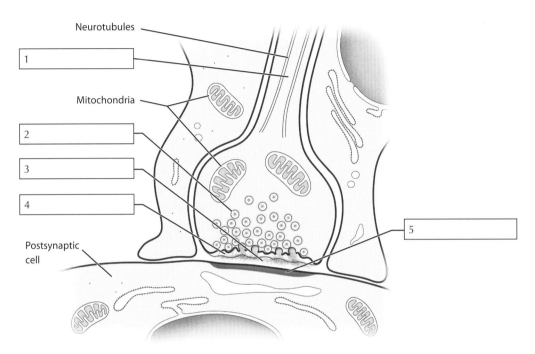

Neurotubules

1

Mitochondria

2

3

4

Postsynaptic cell

5

Enlarged section of bouton

A. What are the two types of synapses found in the nervous system?

B. Axon fibers branch and terminate in _____.

C. In a chemical synapse, what determines whether the postsynaptic potential is excitatory or inhibitory?

D. What type of summation is produced by rapid, repeated firing of a presynaptic fiber?

E. What type of summation results when multiple fibers release sufficient neurotransmitter to produce firing of a target neuron?

Motor neurons are efferent nerves that originate in the CNS and communicate with skeletal muscle fibers at specialized synapses known as **motor endplates** or **neuromuscular junctions.** Among the several types of motor neurons, the most common is the α-**motor neuron.** Branches of an α-motor neuron may form multiple neuromuscular junctions in depressions in the **sarcolemmae** (muscle cell membranes) of muscle fibers. Each α-motor neuron may thus innervate multiple muscle fibers, although each fiber is innervated by only one α-motor neuron. An α-motor neuron and the fibers it innervates are called a **motor unit.** All of the motor neurons innervating a muscle are collectively known as a **motor neuron pool.**

Stimulation of a motor nerve results in the release of **acetylcholine (ACh)** from vesicles at the **presynaptic membrane** in the motor endplate; ACh diffuses and binds to postsynaptic receptors, producing depolarization of the sarcolemma and leading to an action potential and, ultimately, contraction of the muscle fiber.

COLOR and **LABEL** the following parts of the motor endplate:

☐ 1.   Presynaptic membrane

☐ 2.   Synaptic vesicles; containing ACh

☐ 3.   Sarcolemma

☐ 4.   Postsynaptic membrane

☐ 5.   Synaptic cleft

☐ 6.   ACh receptor sites on the postsynaptic membrane

Clinical Note

Myasthenia gravis (MG) is an autoimmune disease affecting skeletal muscle function. In MG, antibodies are formed that block or damage the ACh receptor of the motor endplate, thus blocking the action of ACh. The most commonly affected muscles are those of the eyes and face and muscles involved in swallowing, talking, and chewing, although other muscles can be affected. A myasthenic crisis may be associated with an infectious disease or adverse drug reaction and can affect the muscles of breathing. Hospitalization and artificial respiration may be required. MG is usually an episodic disease, often occurring after high physical activity. It may be treated with rest and, if necessary, corticosteroids and cholinesterase inhibitors. The latter drugs inhibit acetylcholinesterase, prolonging ACh action.

REVIEW ANSWERS

A.   Motor endplates

B.   α-Motor neuron

C.   The muscle cell membrane

D.   The α-motor neuron and the fibers it innervates comprise the motor unit.

E.   ACh

Plate 2.9

Nerve and Muscle Physiology

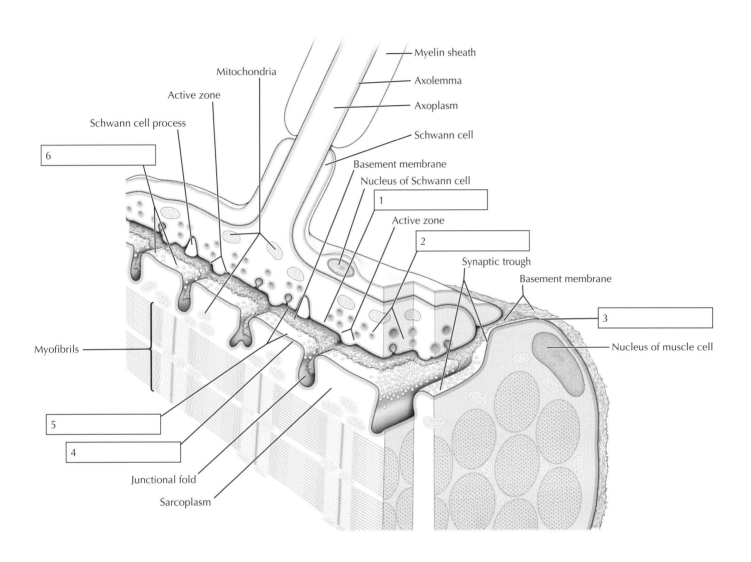

Myelin sheath

Axolemma

Axoplasm

Schwann cell

Basement membrane

Nucleus of Schwann cell

Mitochondria

Active zone

Schwann cell process

6

Active zone

1

2

Synaptic trough

Basement membrane

3

Nucleus of muscle cell

Myofibrils

5

4

Junctional fold

Sarcoplasm

REVIEW QUESTIONS

A. Neuromuscular junctions are also called _____.

B. What is the most common motor neuron?

C. What is the sarcolemma?

D. What makes up a motor unit?

E. What neurotransmitter is released from the presynaptic membrane?

When ACh is released into the synaptic cleft of the neuromuscular junction at the presynaptic membrane, it diffuses to nicotinic ACh receptors on the postsynaptic membrane, causing the opening of ligand-gated cation channels permeable to Na^+ and K^+. As a result, an excitatory postsynaptic potential (endplate potential) is produced. When the threshold is reached, an action potential is produced; ultimately, this action potential is responsible for contraction of the muscle fiber, although several more steps must take place.

The **sarcoplasmic reticulum (SR)** is a complex network surrounding the myofibrils (left figure), containing high concentration of Ca^{2+} sequestered from the sarcoplasm by the action of Ca^{2+}-ATPase. An action potential is conducted to the SR from the sarcolemma by **transverse (T) tubules.** The T tubules form triads with two **terminal cisternae of the SR,** providing for close communication between the interior of the muscle cell and extracellular fluid. When depolarization spreads into the T tubules, it reaches voltage-gated Ca^{2+} channels known as **dihydropyridine (DHP) receptors.** Although DHP receptors are voltage-gated Ca^{2+} channels, ion flux through these channels is not a requisite for muscle contraction. Rather, a conformational change in the DHP receptor, caused by T tubule depolarization, is required. These receptors are in close apposition to calcium channel proteins known as **ryanodine receptors**, which are large proteins of the SR that extend into the gap between the cisternae of the SR and the T tubules. The conformational change in the DHP receptors causes a conformational change in the ryanodine receptors and release of

stored Ca^{2+} from the SR, initiating the contraction process. The term **excitation-contraction coupling** refers to this linking of depolarization to Ca^{2+} release. This release of Ca^{2+} results in the sliding of filaments and the contraction of skeletal muscle (see Plate 2.11).

COLOR and LABEL

- ☐ 1. T tubule
- ☐ 2. SR
- ☐ 3. Terminal cisternae of the SR
- ☐ 4. Thin actin filaments
- ☐ 5. Thick myosin filaments

Clinical Note

The action of ACh at nicotinic receptors can be blocked by **curare** and **α-bungarotoxin.** Curare was first known as the alkaloid plant toxin used in arrow poison in Central and South America. It competitively blocks the binding of ACh to its nicotinic receptors. Medical applications were eventually developed for curare and related compounds. α-Bungarotoxin, a toxin in venom of the Southeast Asian banded krait snake, is a noncompetitive nicotinic antagonist that binds the receptor irreversibly. At sufficient doses, curare and α-bungarotoxin cause muscle paralysis, asphyxiation resulting from paralysis of the diaphragm, and death.

REVIEW ANSWERS

A. DHP

B. Ryanodine receptor

C. Ca^{2+}

Plate 2.10 | **Nerve and Muscle Physiology**

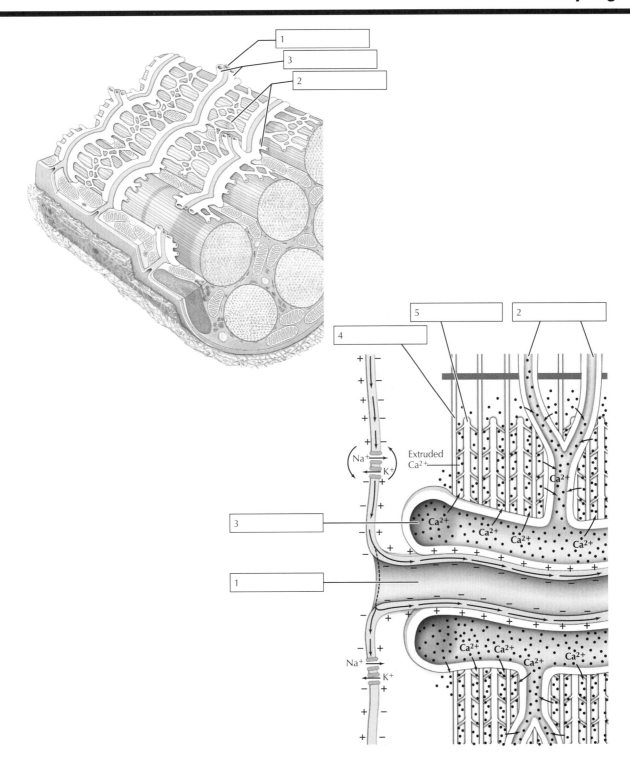

A. Spread of the wave of depolarization into the T tubules results in a conformational change in the _____ of the T tubules.

B. That conformational change results in a subsequent change in conformation of _____ in the SR.

C. Release of _____ from the SR results in sliding of actin and myosin filaments.

Contraction of skeletal muscle is the basis for voluntary movement. It occurs upon stimulation of the muscle at the neuromuscular junction, followed by a sequence of events leading to shortening of **sarcomeres.** In Part B, note that skeletal muscle consists of **fascicles** that are in turn composed of **multinucleated muscle fibers.** These fibers are composed of smaller **myofibrils,** which contain the sarcomeres, the site at which sliding of **actin** and **myosin** produces muscle contraction. The organization of sarcomeres within the skeletal muscle produces its **striated appearance.** The **Z line** marks the boundary between two sarcomeres. The **I band** consists of only actin filaments, which extend from the Z line toward the center of the sarcomere. Thick myosin filaments are found in the dark **A band.** The **H zone** is the area in which there is no actin-myosin overlap. The **M line** at the center of the sarcomere is the site at which myosin filaments are anchored. Note the **crossbridges** between thin actin filaments and thick myosin filaments.

The **sliding filament theory** explains how events at the sarcomere produce skeletal muscle contraction (Part C). The thick filaments contain myosin, anchored at the M line; the thin filaments are actin and associated **tropomyosin** and **troponin,** anchored at the Z line. Actin has binding sites for myosin, covered by the protein tropomyosin. When muscle is relaxed (low cytosolic Ca^{2+} concentration), binding of myosin to actin is blocked by the tropomyosin, and adenosine diphosphate (ADP) is bound to the myosin head groups. When depolarization occurs, Ca^{2+} is released from the SR. Binding of Ca^{2+} to troponin results in exposure of the myosin binding sites and formation of crossbridges between the myosin head group and actin. This is followed by a ratcheting motion of the myosin head group, shortening the sarcomere as actin and myosin slide past each other. ADP and inorganic phosphate are released. Subsequently, binding of adenosine triphosphate (ATP) to the myosin head group causes detachment from actin, after which ATP is partially hydrolyzed by ATPase to ADP, causing "recocking" of the headgroup. If Ca^{2+} is still elevated, myosin and actin rapidly bind, and crossbridge cycling in this manner causes contraction to continue. Muscle relaxation takes place as free Ca^{2+} falls when it is resequestered into the SR.

COLOR and **LABEL** the following, noting the relaxed vs. contracted state:

- [ ] 1. Actin
- [ ] 2. Myosin
- [ ] 3. Crossbridges

REVIEW ANSWERS

A. ATP

B. H zone

C. M line

D. Tropomyosin

Plate 2.11

Nerve and Muscle Physiology

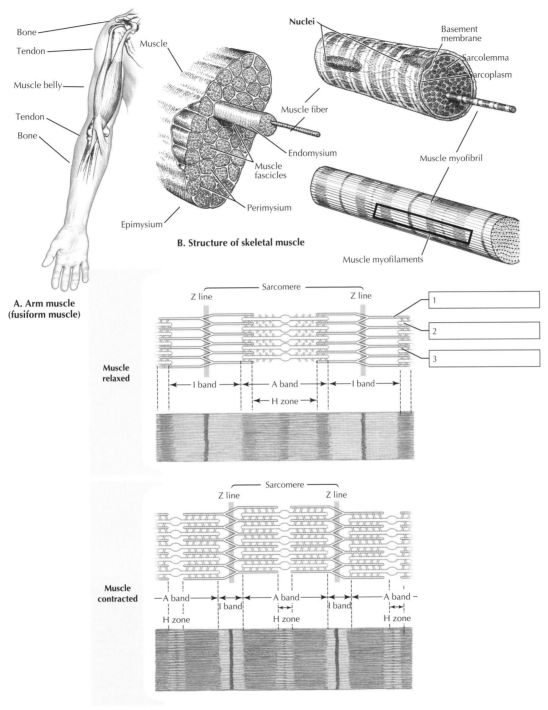

Bone
Tendon
Muscle belly
Tendon
Bone

**A. Arm muscle
(fusiform muscle)**

Muscle
Muscle fiber
Endomysium
Muscle
fascicles
Perimysium
Epimysium

B. Structure of skeletal muscle

Nuclei
Basement
membrane
Sarcolemma
Sarcoplasm
Muscle myofibril
Muscle myofilaments

Sarcomere
Z line   Z line

1
2
3

Muscle
relaxed

I band — A band — I band
H zone

Sarcomere
Z line   Z line

Muscle
contracted

A band — I band — A band — I band — A band
H zone   H zone   H zone

C. Sliding filament theory

A. The energy for actin and myosin sliding and thus shortening of the sarcomere is derived from _____.

B. Within the sarcomere, actin is not found in the _____.

C. Myosin is anchored within the sarcomere to the _____.

D. The binding site for myosin on actin is blocked in relaxed muscle by _____.

Smooth muscle is a type of nonstriated muscle found in organs. Its contractile proteins are not organized as sarcomeres and thus smooth muscle is not striated in appearance. The contractile elements are anchored to the cell membrane and dense bodies within the cell, and **actin**-myosin interaction is the basis of contraction. In contrast to skeletal muscle, which is controlled by motor neurons, smooth muscle is controlled by the autonomic nervous system (ANS) (see Plate 2.18) and various neurotransmitters and other chemical ligands that affect cytosolic free Ca^{2+} concentration. Smooth muscle is classified as either unitary smooth muscle or multiunit smooth muscle. **Unitary smooth muscle cells** have gap junctions between them, allowing direct and rapid spread of action potentials and synchronous contraction of cells. On the other hand, **multiunit smooth muscle** has no gap junctions, and cells function independently, allowing fine motor control, for example, in the ciliary body of the eye and the piloerector muscles in the skin.

Excitation-contraction coupling is illustrated in the figure. Binding of a ligand to the cell membrane produces either depolarization and opening of calcium channels or activation of the enzyme **phospholipase C,** which results in IP_3 formation. IP_3 binds to **receptors** on the SR within the smooth muscle cells, releasing stored Ca^{2+}. Once Ca^{2+} is elevated through one of these mechanisms, it binds to **calmodulin,** which activates **myosin kinase,** initiating the actin-myosin interaction and contraction. The **contraction cycle** continues as long as Ca^{2+} is elevated. The **latch state** occurs when myosin is dephosphorylated by **myosin phosphatase.** In this state, contraction is maintained without further **ATP** utilization and thus without further energy consumption.

COLOR and LABEL

- ☐ 1. Ca^{2+} ions
- ☐ 2. Myosin head groups
- ☐ 3. Inorganic phosphates
- ☐ 4. Actin

TRACE

- ☐ 5. The movement of Ca^{2+} into the cytosol through the calcium channel and from the SR. Note the binding of myosin and actin, ratcheting of the headgroup to produce contraction, and the role of ATP and ADP in the contraction cycle.

REVIEW ANSWERS

A. Latch state

B. Calcium channels, SR

C. Calmodulin

Plate 2.12   **Nerve and Muscle Physiology**

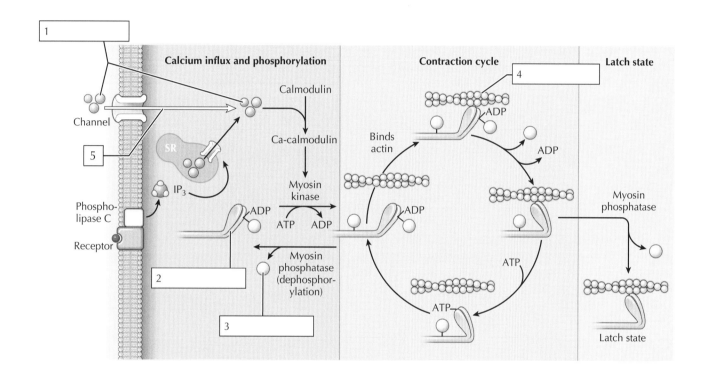

Calcium influx and phosphorylation

Contraction cycle

Latch state

Calmodulin

Channel

Ca-calmodulin

Phospho-
lipase C

Myosin
kinase

Receptor

ATP ADP

Myosin
phosphatase
(dephosphor-
ylation)

IP₃

SR

Binds
actin

ADP

ADP

ADP

ATP

ATP

ATP

Myosin
phosphatase

Latch state

REVIEW QUESTIONS

A. Prolonged contraction of smooth muscle is maintained without further expenditure of energy when myosin and actin are in the

_____

B. In smooth muscle contraction, the elevation of intracellular Ca^{2+} is achieved by influx of Ca^{2+} into the cytosol through
_____ or release of Ca^{2+} stored in the _____.

C. Intracellular free Ca^{2+} binds to the calcium binding protein _____, producing the complex that activates myosin kinase.

Cardiac muscle shares some characteristics with skeletal muscle and smooth muscle but is dissimilar in other respects. Contraction of skeletal muscle is under voluntary control by the CNS, whereas cardiac and smooth muscle contraction are involuntary. Like unitary smooth muscle, cardiac muscle is capable of spontaneous electrical activity, with contraction of the latter normally under control of cardiac pacemaker cells in the sinoatrial node. Gap junctions allow synchronous contraction of cardiac muscle, similar to unitary smooth muscle. Gap junctions are found in the **intercalated disks** between cardiac muscle cells. The high degree of organization of actin and myosin fibers into sarcomeres in cardiac and skeletal muscle produces the striated appearance of these muscle types (see illustration). Cardiac muscle, like smooth muscle, uses both extracellular and intracellular sources of Ca^{2+} (from the **SR**) for contraction, whereas skeletal muscle relies solely on Ca^{2+} from the SR.

In contrast to the **triads** of one T tubule and two terminal cisternae of the SR found in skeletal muscle, **dyads** of one T tubule and one terminal cisterna of SR are observed in cardiac muscle.

COLOR and LABEL each of the following:

- ☐ 1. Actin filaments in a section of the illustration
- ☐ 2. Myosin filaments in that section
- ☐ 3. Intercalated disk
- ☐ 4. SR
- ☐ 5. Basement membrane
- ☐ 6. Capillary

REVIEW ANSWERS

A. Cardiac muscle and skeletal muscle are striated; smooth muscle is not.

B. T tubules, terminal cisternae of the SR

C. Extracellular source, SR

D. Intercalated disks

Plate 2.13   **Nerve and Muscle Physiology**

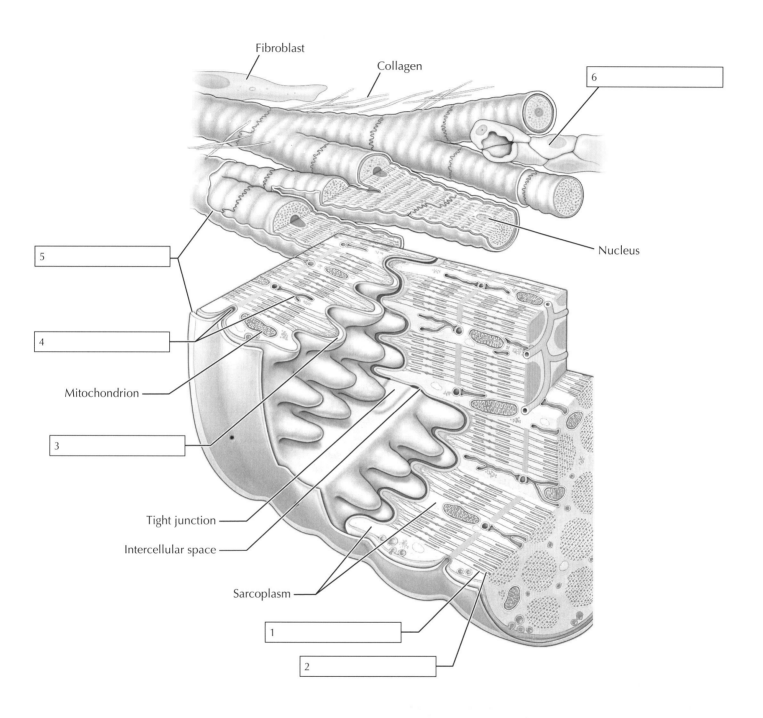

Fibroblast

Collagen

6

Nucleus

5

4

Mitochondrion

3

Tight junction

Intercellular space

Sarcoplasm

1

2

REVIEW QUESTIONS

A. Among the three types of muscle, which are striated and which lack striations?

B. Dyads are formed in cardiac muscle between _____ and _____.

C. Ca²⁺ for cardiac muscle contraction is derived from _____ and _____.

D. Gap junctions between cardiac muscle cells are located in the _____.

The nervous system consists of the CNS and the peripheral nervous system. The CNS includes the brain and spinal cord, whereas the peripheral nervous system includes nerves, ganglia, and sensory receptors outside the CNS. The peripheral nervous system is further subdivided into sensory and motor divisions. Sensory nerves transmit information from sensory receptors throughout the body to the CNS; motor nerves send signals from the CNS to muscles and glands to control their activity.

The brain consists of the **telencephalon** (also known as the **cerebrum** or cerebral hemispheres), diencephalon (thalamus and hypothalamus), cerebellum, and brainstem (midbrain, pons, and medulla). The general structure of the CNS and the vertebral column is shown in the illustration. Some key points are:

- The **right and left cerebral hemispheres** (telencephalon) consist of an outer **cerebral cortex** (gray matter) and inner white matter. Gray matter contains unmyelinated axons, and white matter contains myelinated axons. Areas of the cerebral cortex receive and integrate sensory information, integrate motor function, and perform other high-level functions such as learning and reasoning. Much of the sensory information (except olfactory signals) is received indirectly through the thalamus. For the most part, the right and left hemispheres receive input from the contralateral (opposite) side of the body. The large **corpus callosum** and smaller anterior, posterior, and hippocampal commissures functionally and anatomically connect the two hemispheres. The **basal ganglia** are nuclei deep within the cerebral hemispheres that are involved in movement regulation and other functions. The **hippocampus** and **amygdala** are deep formations that are part of the **limbic system,** involved in emotion and long-term memory, and affect endocrine and ANS function, among other functions.

- The **diencephalon** is located between the cerebral hemispheres and the brainstem and is part of the limbic system. The **thalamus** processes sensory input before passing it to the cerebral cortex as well as motor signals leaving the cerebral cortex. The hypothalamus (not labeled), separated from the thalamus by the **hypothalamic sulcus,** has an important role in regulation of body temperature, the reproductive system, hunger and thirst, salt and water balance, circadian rhythms, the endocrine system, and the ANS.

- The **cerebellum,** located between the cerebral cortex and spinal cord and in close proximity to the brainstem, integrates sensory and motor information, as well as information regarding proprioception received from muscles, joints, tendons, and the inner ear.

- The **brainstem** is the lowest portion of the brain, consisting of the midbrain (mesencephalon), pons, and medulla oblongata (medulla). The medulla, continuous with the spinal cord, regulates autonomic functions as well as swallowing, vomiting, and coughing reflexes. The pons is involved in regulation of breathing and relays sensory information from cerebrum to cerebellum. The midbrain is involved in eye movement and transmission of visual and auditory information; it has a role in regulation of motor activity. Cranial nerves III to XII originate from the brainstem.

COLOR and **LABEL** these major parts of the brain:

- ☐ 1. Left cerebral hemisphere
- ☐ 2. Corpus callosum
- ☐ 3. Diencephalon (thalamus and hypothalamic sulcus as illustrated)
- ☐ 4. Brainstem
- ☐ 5. Cerebellum

REVIEW ANSWERS

A. Corpus callosum

B. Diencephalon (function of the thalamus)

C. Cerebral hemispheres

D. Brainstem

E. Cerebellum

Plate 2.14

Nerve and Muscle Physiology

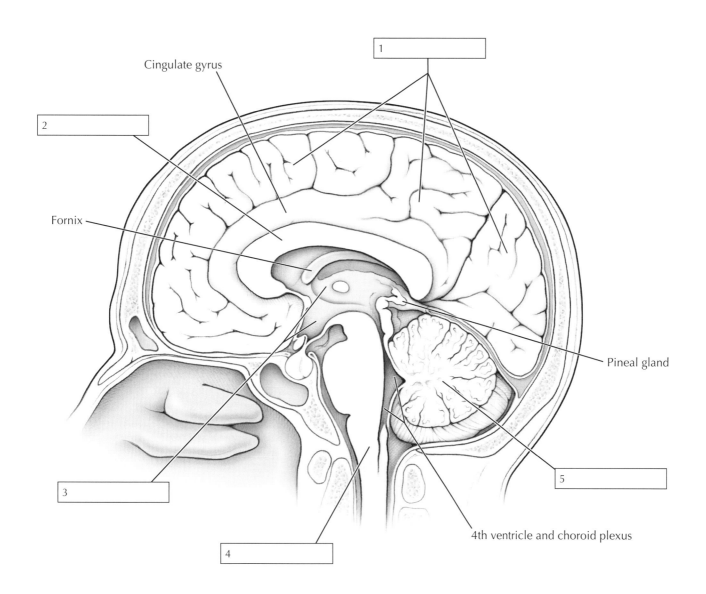

Cingulate gyrus

1

2

Fornix

3

4

Pineal gland

5

4th ventricle and choroid plexus

REVIEW QUESTIONS

A. _____ functionally connects the right and left cerebral hemispheres.

B. _____ processes sensory input and passes it to the cerebral cortex; it processes motor signals leaving the cerebral cortex.

C. _____ receive and integrate sensory information and integrate motor function, learning, and reasoning.

D. _____ regulates autonomic functions and vomiting and coughing reflexes.

E. _____ integrates sensory and motor information and information regarding proprioception.

The environment of neurons within the CNS is maintained in part by the **blood-brain barrier.** Endothelial cells of capillaries within the CNS are joined by tight junctions, preventing movement of water-soluble substances, highly charged molecules, and cells between blood and brain. Astrocytes (nonneuronal cells in the CNS) are also involved in maintaining integrity of the blood-brain barrier.

Cerebrospinal fluid (CSF) formation, circulation, and regulation are also a key aspect in maintaining homeostasis within the CNS. Its composition is somewhat different than that of **blood plasma;** it is secreted by the **choroid plexus** and circulates through the two **lateral ventricles** and the **third** and **fourth ventricles** of the brain. It leaves the fourth ventricle through the lateral and medial apertures and enters the **subarachnoid space** of the spinal cord. Much of the fluid is reabsorbed at the arachnoid granulations into the venous system and into the capillaries of the CNS and **pia mater,** one of the three **meninges** (membranes) covering the neural tissue of the spinal cord.

The spinal cord originates at the medulla at the base of the skull and extends into and down the cervical and thoracic regions of the vertebral column to its lumbar region. The three meninges include the inner pia mater adhering to the surface of the spinal cord, the middle **arachnoid membrane,** and outer **dura mater.** These membranes are continuous with the membranes covering the brain.

COLOR and LABEL the following structures of the CNS:

- [ ] 1. Right lateral ventricle
- [ ] 2. Left lateral ventricle
- [ ] 3. Central aqueduct
- [ ] 4. Fourth ventricle
- [ ] 5. Central canal of the spinal cord
- [ ] 6. Third ventricle
- [ ] 7. Subarachnoid space
- [ ] 8. Superior sagittal sinus

TRACE

- [ ] 9. Arrows indicating the flow of CSF

Clinical Note

In a healthy person, the dura mater and arachnoid membrane are in close contact. In pathophysiological situations, the "potential space" between these meninges, the subdural space, may be an actual space. This can occur with a subdural hematoma (bleeding into the potential space between the inner leaflet of the dura mater and the arachnoid membrane, usually associated with injury). Compression of neural tissue may occur, with damaging results. Similarly, trauma may also produce subarachnoid bleeding into the CSF-containing space between the arachnoid membrane and the pia mater.

REVIEW ANSWERS

A. Choroid plexus

B. Tight junctions

C. Pia mater, arachnoid membrane, and dura mater

Plate 2.15   **Nerve and Muscle Physiology**

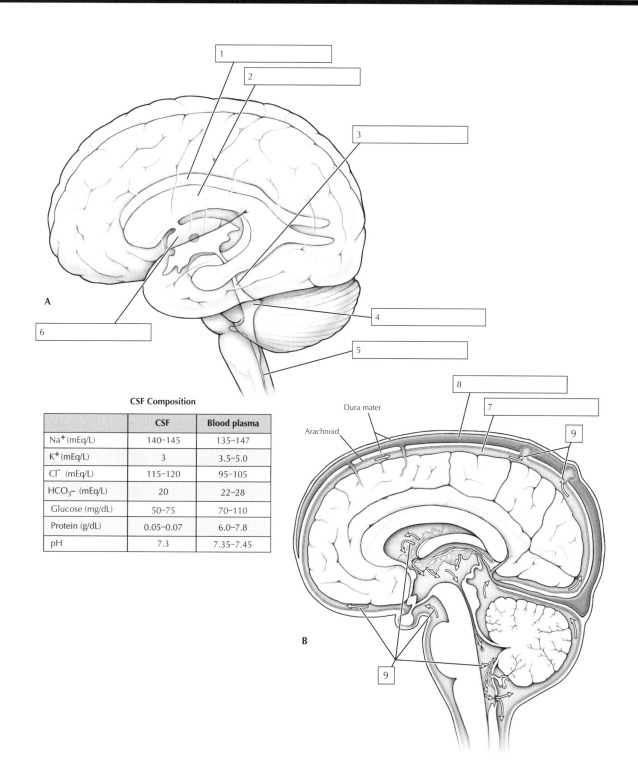

A

CSF Composition

	CSF	Blood plasma
Na$^+$ (mEq/L)	140–145	135–147
K$^+$ (mEq/L)	3	3.5–5.0
Cl$^-$ (mEq/L)	115–120	95–105
HCO$_3^-$ (mEq/L)	20	22–28
Glucose (mg/dL)	50–75	70–110
Protein (g/dL)	0.05–0.07	6.0–7.8
pH	7.3	7.35–7.45

Dura mater

Arachnoid

B

REVIEW QUESTIONS

A. CSF is secreted by the _____.

B. The blood-brain barrier is maintained by _____ between endothelial cells.

C. From innermost to outermost, the three meninges are _____, _____ and _____.

2 The Sensory System

As part of the peripheral nervous system, sensory receptors detect various kinds of stimuli, including visual, auditory, gustatory (taste), and somatosensory stimuli. Stimulation of these receptors produces opening or closing of ion channels, which results in a membrane potential change in the receptor. When the threshold is reached, information is transmitted via **afferent pathways** to the CNS, which receives and integrates such information and transmits efferent signals to effector systems. The **somatosensory system** includes **mechanoreceptors, thermal receptors,** and **nociceptive (pain) receptors,** which respond to stimuli in the skin and visceral organs, muscles, and joints (thus the term *somatovisceral sensory system* is also used). Although the specifics of somatosensory receptors are beyond the scope of this volume, briefly, somatosensory signals (pain, **touch, pressure, temperature**) originating below the head are transmitted to the primary somatosensory area, located in the **postcentral gyrus** of the **parietal lobe** of the **cerebral cortex.** They are conveyed to the dorsal root ganglia and then through the **spinothalamic** and spinoreticular **tracts** of the anterolateral system, eventually reaching the primary somatosensory cortex (see illustration). Signals involved in **proprioception** and signals generated by **vibration** and tactile stimuli are carried through the **fasciculus gracilis** and **fasciculus cuneatus** to the ventral posterolateral nucleus of the thalamus. The lateral cervical system also carries some proprioceptive, vibratory, and tactile information. These various pathways reach synapses in the thalamus before projecting to the cerebral cortex.

Somatosensory and **proprioceptive signals** originating in the head produce afferent signals to nerve cell bodies in specific ganglia through the **trigeminal nerve (cranial nerve V).** Projections in this system are mainly to contralateral nuclei in the thalamus, with signals eventually reaching the primary somatosensory cortex.

The **special senses** are those senses that have specific sensory organs associated with them. These are vision (eyes), taste (tongue), hearing and balance (ears with their auditory and vestibular apparatuses), and smell (nose). Sensory information from these organs is carried by special visceral afferents and special somatic afferents associated with cranial nerves (see Plate 2.20). The specifics of sensory perception by these organs and ultimately by the brain are complex and beyond the scope of this workbook.

COLOR and **LABEL** the pathways for transmission of the following types of stimuli, starting outside the spinal cord and proceeding to the brain:

☐ 1. Proprioception, position

☐ 2. Touch, pressure, vibration

☐ 3. Pain, temperature

REVIEW ANSWERS

A. Trigeminal nerve (cranial nerve V)

B. Pain

C. Thalamus

D. Special senses

E. Parietal, cerebral cortex

Plate 2.16

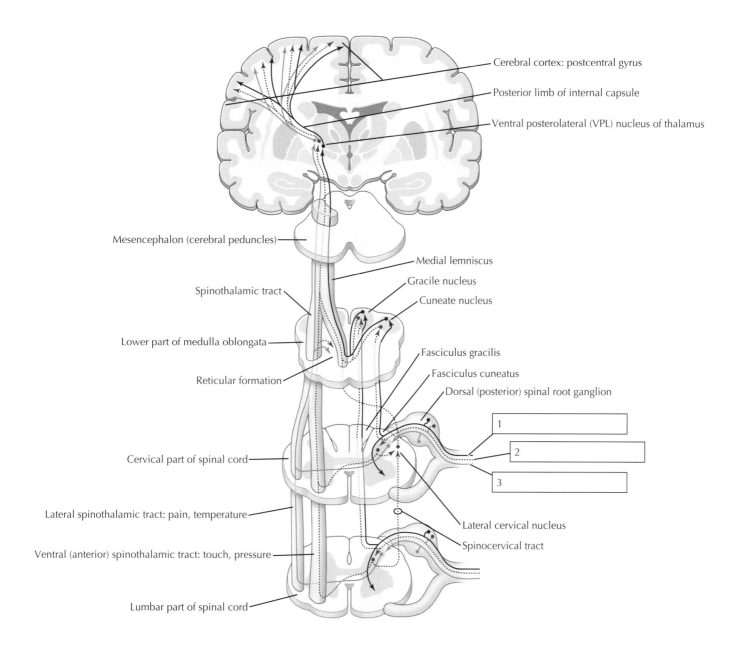

Cerebral cortex: postcentral gyrus

Posterior limb of internal capsule

Ventral posterolateral (VPL) nucleus of thalamus

Mesencephalon (cerebral peduncles)

Medial lemniscus

Gracile nucleus

Cuneate nucleus

Spinothalamic tract

Lower part of medulla oblongata

Reticular formation

Fasciculus gracilis

Fasciculus cuneatus

Dorsal (posterior) spinal root ganglion

Cervical part of spinal cord

1

2

3

Lateral spinothalamic tract: pain, temperature

Lateral cervical nucleus

Spinocervical tract

Ventral (anterior) spinothalamic tract: touch, pressure

Lumbar part of spinal cord

REVIEW QUESTIONS

A. Somatosensory and proprioceptive signals originating in the head travel through the _____ to nerve cell bodies in ganglia.

B. Nociception refers to perception of _____.

C. Various afferent neural pathways of the somatosensory systems reach synapses in the _____ before projecting to the cerebral cortex.

D. Senses that are associated with specific sensory organs are called _____.

E. The primary somatosensory area is located in the _____ lobe of the _____.

The motor system consists of two subdivisions, the **somatic motor system** and the ANS, controlling **voluntary muscle activity** and **involuntary muscle activity,** respectively. The somatic motor system is responsible for controlling movement and posture, a task accomplished through involuntary spinal reflexes and voluntary, coordinated muscle action involving contraction and relaxation. Most skeletal muscle fibers are the **extrafusal fibers** that are innervated by α-**motor neurons** and contract to generate movement and postural adjustments. **Intrafusal** skeletal muscle fibers act as specialized sensors and have important roles in coordinating fine muscle movement and proprioception; they are innervated by γ-**motor neurons.**

The simplest motor responses are **spinal reflexes**, in which a sensory signal is integrated completely within the spinal cord to produce a stereotypic motor response. An example is the **knee jerk reflex.** More complex motor responses require control involving the **spinal cord,** brainstem, cerebellum, basal ganglia, and **cerebral motor cortex.** Voluntary movement often involves patterns of skeletal muscle activity regulated by lower centers after activation by the **motor cortex.** Fine motor movement, particularly by the muscles of the fingers and hands, is controlled more directly by the cerebral cortex.

The most important descending pathway for control of fine motor activity originating in the cerebral cortex is the **corticospinal** tract, also known as the **pyramidal tract.** Nerve fibers in this tract originate in the **primary motor cortex** and the adjacent **premotor** and **supplemental motor areas,** as well as somatosensory areas posterior to the motor cortex. The descending pathway is illustrated in Plate 2.17, as sections through the brain and spinal cord. Most of the fibers cross (decussate) in the lower medulla to form the **lateral corticospinal tract;** others descend through the **anterior corticospinal tract.** At various levels of the spinal cord, some fibers from these tracts synapse directly with second-order motor neurons (anterior horn cells). Secondary motor neurons innervated by axons of the lateral corticospinal tract are mainly those controlling distal limb muscles, whereas those innervated by the anterior tract are mainly those controlling axial muscles.

TRACE and **LABEL** the nerve bundles illustrated in the corticospinal tract, starting at their origin in or near the motor cortex and extending to the synapses with second-order motor neurons (anterior horn cells); continue tracing to the synapses with the motor endplates.

☐ 1. Anterior corticospinal tract

☐ 2. Lateral corticospinal tract

REVIEW ANSWERS

A. Extrafusal, α-motor neurons

B. Intrafusal, γ-motor neurons

C. Fine motor activity, particularly of the hands and fingers

D. Distal limb, axial

Plate 2.17　　　　　　　**Nerve and Muscle Physiology**

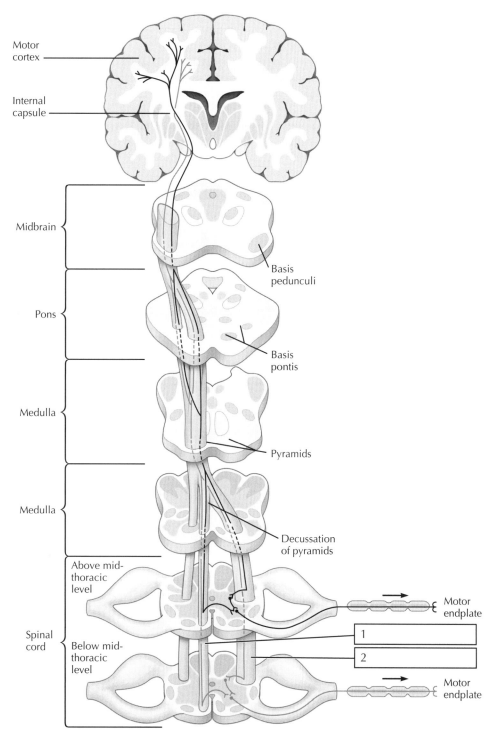

Motor cortex

Internal capsule

Midbrain

Pons

Medulla

Medulla

Spinal cord

Above mid-thoracic level

Below mid-thoracic level

Basis pedunculi

Basis pontis

Pyramids

Decussation of pyramids

Motor endplate

1

2

Motor endplate

REVIEW QUESTIONS

A. The majority of skeletal muscle fibers are _____ fibers innervated by _____.

B. Fibers that act as specialized sensors involved in coordinating fine muscle movement and proprioception are _____ fibers; they are innervated by _____.

C. What type of motor activity is most directly controlled by the cerebral cortex?

D. Secondary motor neurons innervated by the axons of the lateral corticospinal tract are mainly those controlling _____ muscles, whereas those innervated by the anterior tract are mainly those controlling _____ muscles.

As part of the peripheral nervous system, the **ANS** is the primary effector for **involuntary control** and coordinated activity of smooth muscle of visceral organs, cardiac muscle, and glands. It is essential for most homeostatic processes. Within the brain, sensory information is integrated and the activity of the ANS is modulated to orchestrate this involuntary control of physiological processes.

The two divisions of the ANS are the **sympathetic nervous system (SNS)** and the **parasympathetic nervous system (PNS).** In many cases the SNS and PNS have opposing actions, and regulation of bodily function often involves reciprocal actions of the two systems. For example, heart rate is elevated by SNS activity and decreased by PNS activity.

The SNS has an important role in the response to **stress** through the classic *fight-or-flight* response, whereas the PNS is important in **"vegetative"** resting state activities such as digestion. The SNS response is often a generalized reaction to fear, stress, or physical activity and results in a patterned response in many organs, including elevated heart rate, cardiac output, and blood pressure, as well as bronchial dilation, mydriasis (dilation of the pupils), and sweating. The PNS can produce selective effects such as on the digestive tract during feeding or during the sexual response *(feed and breed).*

The **central components** regulating the ANS are the **hypothalamus,** brainstem **(midbrain, pons, medulla),** and spinal cord; the **peripheral components** are the cranial nerves (III, VII, IX, X, see Plate 2.21) and the **sympathetic and parasympathetic nerves** and ganglia. Areas within the hypothalamus and brainstem regulate and coordinate various processes through the ANS, including temperature regulation, responses to thirst and hunger, micturition (urination), respiration, and cardiovascular function.

COLOR and **LABEL** the CNS sites regulating the ANS:

- ☐ 1. Hypothalamus
- ☐ 2. Midbrain
- ☐ 3. Pons
- ☐ 4. Medulla
- ☐ 5. Spinal cord

REVIEW ANSWERS

A. SNS

B. PNS

C. Hypothalamus, brainstem (midbrain, pons, medulla), and spinal cord.

Plate 2.18   **Nerve and Muscle Physiology**

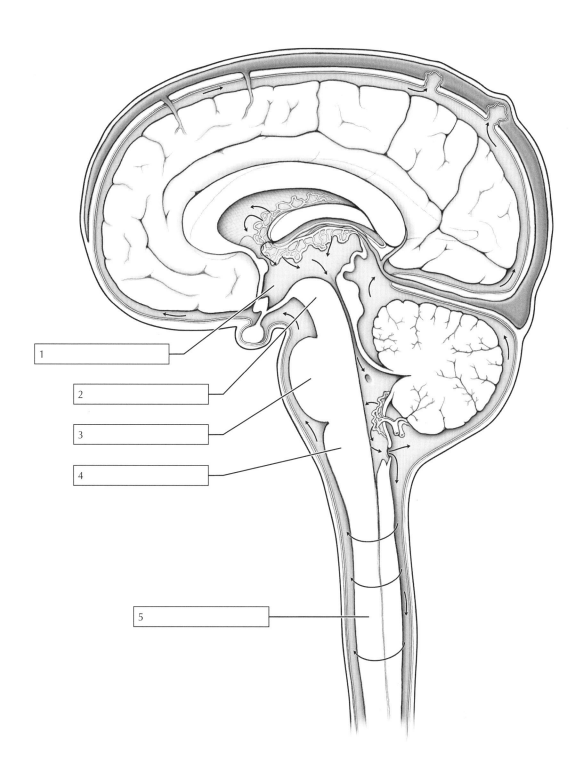

1

2

3

4

5

REVIEW QUESTIONS

A. Stress *(fight or flight)* responses are mediated by what division of the ANS?

B. Vegetative *(feed or breed)* responses are mediated by what division of the ANS?

C. What central structures are key regulators of the ANS?

Netter's Physiology Coloring Book

Plate 2.18

One physical difference between peripheral sympathetic and parasympathetic nerves is that although both the SNS and PNS have **preganglionic fibers** that synapse on autonomic ganglia, the sympathetic nerves have relatively short preganglionic fibers arising from the spinal cord that synapse with long **postganglionic fibers** in the **sympathetic chain ganglia.**

For both parasympathetic and sympathetic **preganglionic neurons, ACh** is the ganglionic neurotransmitter. Sympathetic postganglionic fibers release mainly **norepinephrine (NE),** although ACh is released at the sweat glands.

TRACE the following fibers in the SNS using different colors. Note the long postganglionic fibers in the SNS, in contrast to the very short postganglionic fibers in the PNS (see Plate 2.20).

☐ 1. Preganglionic fibers

☐ 2. Postganglionic fibers

REVIEW ANSWERS

A. The pre- and postganglionic fibers of the SNS synapse within the paravertebral sympathetic chain ganglia.

B. ACh is the preganglionic neurotransmitter for both the SNS and PNS.

C. NE is the typical postganglionic neurotransmitter in the SNS.

D. ACh

Plate 2.19   **Nerve and Muscle Physiology**

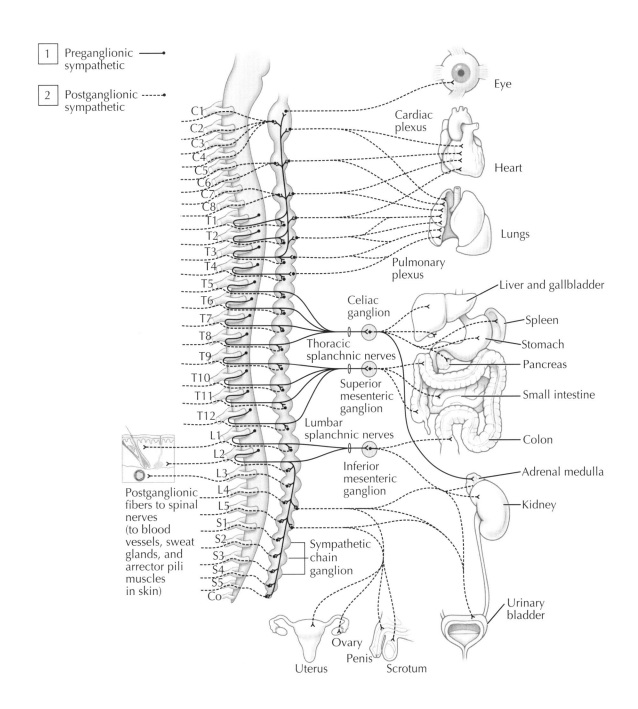

1 Preganglionic ——•
  sympathetic

2 Postganglionic -----•
  sympathetic

C1
C2
C3
C4
C5
C6
C7
C8
T1
T2
T3
T4
T5
T6
T7
T8
T9
T10
T11
T12
L1
L2
L3
L4
L5
S1
S2
S3
S4
S5
Co

Eye

Cardiac plexus

Heart

Lungs

Pulmonary plexus

Celiac ganglion

Thoracic splanchnic nerves

Superior mesenteric ganglion

Lumbar splanchnic nerves

Inferior mesenteric ganglion

Postganglionic fibers to spinal nerves (to blood vessels, sweat glands, and arrector pili muscles in skin)

Sympathetic chain ganglion

Liver and gallbladder

Spleen

Stomach

Pancreas

Small intestine

Colon

Adrenal medulla

Kidney

Urinary bladder

Uterus
Ovary
Penis
Scrotum

REVIEW QUESTIONS

A. Where are the ganglia of the SNS located?

B. What is the preganglionic neurotransmitter in the SNS?

C. What is the usual postganglionic neurotransmitter(s) in the SNS?

D. In contrast to the usual postganglionic neurotransmitter in the SNS, at sweat glands, the SNS postganglionic transmitter is

_____.

Plate 2.20, note the role of **cranial nerves III, VII, IX, and X** in most of the PNS effects throughout the body. Note also that the **pelvic splanchnic nerves** that emerge from the sacral spinal cord at levels S2–S4, not cranial nerves, are responsible for PNS regulation of the lower gastrointestinal tract (colon) and urogenital system. In contrast to the long postganglionic nerves in the SNS, the **postganglionic nerves of the PNS** are short and originate from ganglia on or near the end organ. These PNS postganglionic nerves release ACh, which acts at muscarinic receptors at the end organs. The role of the ANS can be considered mainly one of maintaining homeostasis. This is accomplished usually through reciprocal changes in the two limbs: when SNS activity is stimulated, PNS activity is reduced, and vice versa. As an example, when blood pressure acutely falls below the normal level, the SNS is activated and the long postganglionic sympathetic nerves carry signals from the sympathetic chain ganglion to the heart to elevate heart rate and contractility (see Plate 2.19). Concomitantly, PNS activity is diminished, resulting in reduced signals through CN X (vagus nerve) to the **parasympathetic** ganglia associated with the heart and subsequently through the postganglionic nerves to the heart (see Plate 2.19). Thus it is the elevated SNS activity and reduced PNS activity that raise heart rate in this example.

TRACE the following fibers in the PNS using different colors. Note the very short postganglionic fibers in the PNS, in contrast to the long postganglionic fibers seen in the SNS.

☐ 1.   Preganglionic fibers

☐ 2.   Postganglionic fibers

REVIEW ANSWERS

A.   CN III, VII, IX, X

B.   The pre- and postganglionic fibers of the PNS synapse within ganglia close to or on the end organs

C.   ACh is the preganglionic neurotransmitter for both the PNS and SNS.

D.   ACh is the postganglionic neurotransmitter in the PNS; it acts at muscarinic receptors.

Plate 2.20   **Nerve and Muscle Physiology**

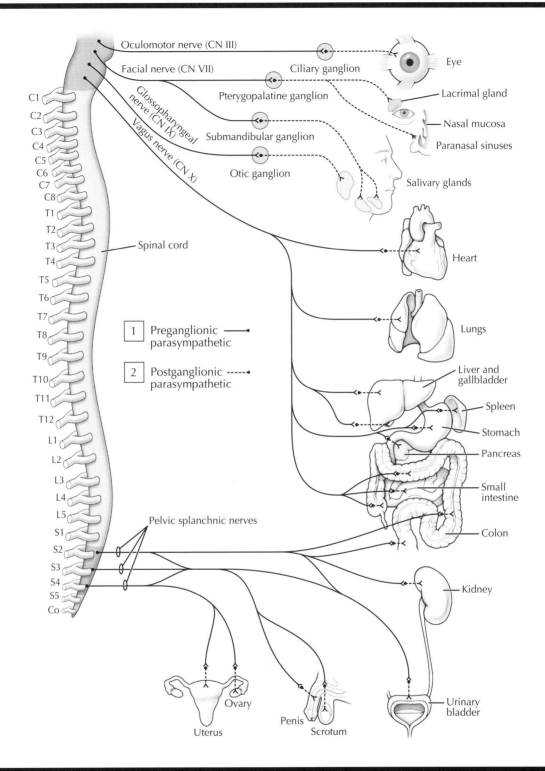

Oculomotor nerve (CN III)

Facial nerve (CN VII)

Glossopharyngeal nerve (CN IX)

Vagus nerve (CN X)

Ciliary ganglion

Pterygopalatine ganglion

Submandibular ganglion

Otic ganglion

C1
C2
C3
C4
C5
C6
C7
C8
T1
T2
T3
T4
T5
T6
T7
T8
T9
T10
T11
T12
L1
L2
L3
L4
L5
S1
S2
S3
S4
S5
Co

Spinal cord

| 1 | Preganglionic parasympathetic |
| 2 | Postganglionic parasympathetic |

Pelvic splanchnic nerves

Eye

Lacrimal gland

Nasal mucosa

Paranasal sinuses

Salivary glands

Heart

Lungs

Liver and gallbladder

Spleen

Stomach

Pancreas

Small intestine

Colon

Kidney

Urinary bladder

Ovary

Uterus

Penis

Scrotum

REVIEW QUESTIONS

A. Which cranial nerves function as part of the peripheral PNS?

B. Where are the ganglia of the PNS located?

C. What is the preganglionic neurotransmitter in the PNS?

D. What is the postganglionic neurotransmitter in the PNS and what type of receptors does it act at?

The **cranial nerves,** part of the peripheral nervous system, originate in the brain, with 10 of the 12 nerves originating in the brainstem, one of the key central components affecting the ANS (see Plate 2.18). The cranial nerves carry information between the brain and other parts of the body, including the head and neck, salivary glands, heart, lungs, digestive tract and associated organs, kidneys and bladder, and reproductive organs. Thus information can be relayed to the brain and back for proper physiological function.

The cranial nerves are **paired** (to serve both sides of the body), and are designated by Roman numerals (I–XII), with the numbering starting at the front of the head. They can be further assigned to either a sensory or motor function.

CRANIAL NERVE	FUNCTION	NOTES
CN I, olfactory nerve	Sensory	Transmits information about inhaled aromatic molecules
CN II, optic nerve	Sensory	Transmits information from the rods and cones in eye to the optic chiasm
CN III, oculomotor nerve	Motor	Controls movement of four of the six muscles of the eye, allowing movement and focus; also controls pupil size
CN IV, trochlear nerve	Motor	Controls the superior oblique muscle of the eye, which allows downward, outward, and inward movement
CN V, trigeminal nerve	Sensory and motor	3 divisions, the ophthalmic (transmits sensory information from upper face including scalp, forehead, and upper eyelid), maxillary (transmits sensory information from the middle face including cheeks, upper lip, and nasal cavity), and mandibular (transmits sensory information from the lower face including ear, lower lip, and chin and carries motor signals back to the region)
CN VI, abducens nerve	Motor	Controls the lateral rectus muscle of the eye (used when looking to the side)
CN VII, facial nerve	Sensory and motor	Controls movement of facial muscles and stimulates salivary and tear gland activity; transmits afferent sensory information from the tongue (taste), and outer ear tactile sensation
CN VIII, vestibulocochlear nerve	Sensory	Provides information on hearing (through the cochlear portion) and balance (through the vestibular portion)

CRANIAL NERVE	FUNCTION	NOTES
CN IX, glossopharyngeal nerve	Sensory and motor	The sensory root provides information from the tongue, inner ear, and back of the throat, and the motor portion stimulates voluntary movement of the stylopharyngeus muscle at the back of the throat
CN X, vagus nerve	Sensory and motor	Conducts afferent sensory signals from the back of the throat and ear canal and taste information from the tongue; the motor portion controls areas of the throat, heart, and digestive tract (this is the longest cranial nerve, with the most diverse functions)
CN XI, accessory nerve	Motor	Controls neck muscles that allow rotation, flexion, and extension of neck and shoulders
CN XII, hypoglossal nerve	Motor	Controls most of the muscles of the tongue

COLOR the sensory nerves the same color:

☐ 1. CN I, olfactory nerve
☐ 2. CN II, optic nerve
☐ 3. CN VIII, vestibulocochlear nerve

COLOR the motor nerves the same color:

☐ 4. CN III, oculomotor nerve
☐ 5. CN IV, trochlear nerve
☐ 6. CN VI, abducens nerve
☐ 7. CN XI, accessory nerve
☐ 8. CN XII, hypoglossal nerve

COLOR the nerves that have sensory and motor functions the same color:

☐ 9. CN V, trigeminal nerve
☐ 10. CN VII, facial nerve
☐ 11. CN IX, glossopharyngeal nerve
☐ 12. CN X, vagus nerve

Clinical Note

Helpful mnemonic: On Old Olympic Towering Tops A Finn And German Vinned Some Hops

REVIEW ANSWERS

A. Brainstem

B. CN X, the vagus

C. CN V, VII, IX, X

Plate 2.21

Nerve and Muscle Physiology

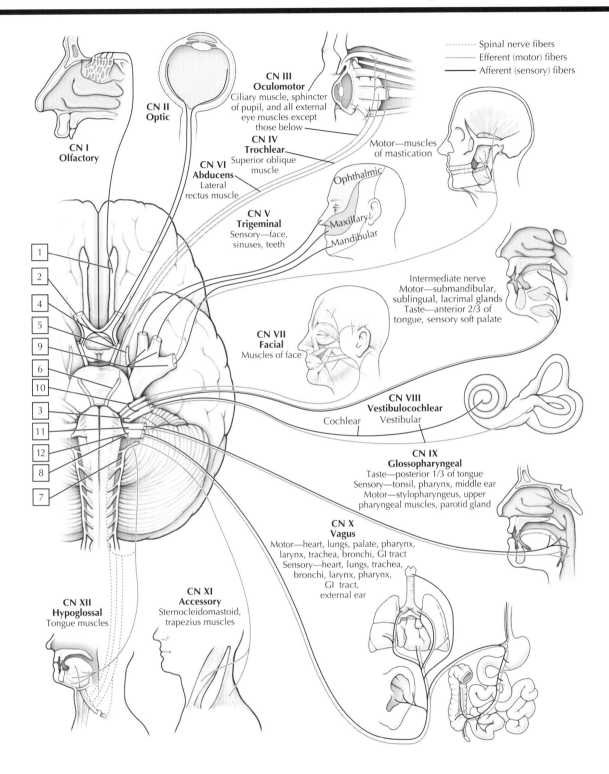

Spinal nerve fibers
Efferent (motor) fibers
Afferent (sensory) fibers

CN I
Olfactory

CN II
Optic

CN III
Oculomotor
Ciliary muscle, sphincter of pupil, and all external eye muscles except those below

CN IV
Trochlear
Superior oblique muscle

CN VI
Abducens
Lateral rectus muscle

CN V
Trigeminal
Sensory—face, sinuses, teeth

Motor—muscles of mastication

Ophthalmic
Maxillary
Mandibular

Intermediate nerve
Motor—submandibular, sublingual, lacrimal glands
Taste—anterior 2/3 of tongue, sensory soft palate

CN VII
Facial
Muscles of face

CN VIII
Vestibulocochlear
Cochlear   Vestibular

CN IX
Glossopharyngeal
Taste—posterior 1/3 of tongue
Sensory—tonsil, pharynx, middle ear
Motor—stylopharyngeus, upper pharyngeal muscles, parotid gland

CN X
Vagus
Motor—heart, lungs, palate, pharynx, larynx, trachea, bronchi, GI tract
Sensory—heart, lungs, trachea, bronchi, larynx, pharynx, GI tract, external ear

CN XII
Hypoglossal
Tongue muscles

CN XI
Accessory
Sternocleidomastoid, trapezius muscles

1
2
4
5
9
6
10
3
11
12
8
7

REVIEW QUESTIONS

A. Ten of the 12 cranial nerves arise from the _____.

B. Which is the longest cranial nerve?

C. Which nerves have both sensory and motor functions?

Chapter 3 Cardiovascular Physiology

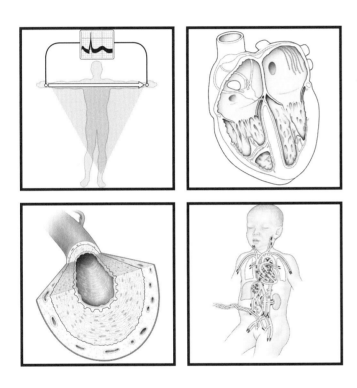

The **four-chambered human heart,** with its one-way valves, pumps blood through a **series circulation** in which there is no mixing of oxygenated and deoxygenated blood. Freshly oxygenated blood from the lungs is collected into the **left atrium (LA)** and pumped by the **left ventricle (LV)** into the aorta, which distributes blood into the rest of the **systemic circulation.** The arteries of the systemic circulation perfuse the organs and tissues throughout the body, resulting in exchange of gases, nutrients, and wastes between blood and tissues at the capillaries. Deoxygenated blood from the tissue capillaries then collects into the veins and flows down its pressure gradient toward the heart, back to the **right atrium (RA)** and then the **right ventricle (RV).** The RV pumps the blood back through the pulmonary artery (PA) to the lungs, where it is reoxygenated. Thus, because all flow follows the same course (left heart to systemic circulation, to the right heart and then lungs, back to the left heart), oxygenated and deoxygenated blood do not mix, and a series circulation is maintained.

The systemic circulation is a high-pressure, high-resistance circulation, whereas the pulmonary circulation is a low-pressure, low-resistance circulation. Pressures in some areas of the circulation are expressed as **systolic/diastolic pressure,** representing pressure during ventricular contraction and ejection of blood into the arterial system **(systole)** and pressure during relaxation and filling of the ventricle and runoff of blood from the arteries **(diastole).** In veins and the atria, it is more meaningful to express pressure as a range. Typical resting pressures in regions of the circulation are listed below, in millimeters of mercury (mm Hg). Note that left atrial pressure (LAP) is typically measured as **pulmonary capillary wedge pressure (PCWP).** Pressures through the system are shown in the table.

SITE	PRESSURES (mm Hg) (SYSTOLIC/DIASTOLIC)
Left atrium (LA)	4–12
Left ventricle (LV)	120/0
Aorta	120/80
Right atrium (RA)	2–8
Right ventricle (RV)	25/0
Pulmonary artery (PA)	25/10

COLOR

☐ 1. Areas of the circulation where fully oxygenated blood is found (red)

☐ 2. Areas containing deoxygenated blood (blue)

☐ 3. Areas where diffusion between blood and tissues or blood and air occur (purple)

Clinical Note

Hypertension, or high blood pressure, is usually used to describe chronically elevated arterial pressure. The American College of Cardiology/American Heart Association High Blood Pressure Guidelines are as follows:

- **Normal:** Less than 120/80 mm Hg
- **Elevated:** Systolic between 120 and 129 and diastolic less than 80
- **Stage 1:** Systolic between 130 and 139 or diastolic between 80 and 89
- **Stage 2:** Systolic at least 140 or diastolic at least 90 mm Hg
- **Hypertensive crisis:** Systolic over 180 and/or diastolic over 120, with patients needing prompt changes in medication if there are no other indications of problems or immediate hospitalization if there are signs of organ damage.

Hypotension is low arterial blood pressure, although in general lower arterial pressure is a sign of good health. Thus hypotension is not typically diagnosed unless it is symptomatic (dizziness and fainting are two symptoms). **Orthostatic hypotension** is transient low arterial blood pressure (and thus lightheadedness or even fainting) associated with postural change, for example, from a lying to standing position. It is usually associated with dehydration or side effects of medication.

REVIEW ANSWERS

A. Pulmonary

B. 120/80

C. 25/10

D. 120/0

E. 25/0

F. Dehydration, side effects of medications

Plate 3.1

Cardiovascular Physiology

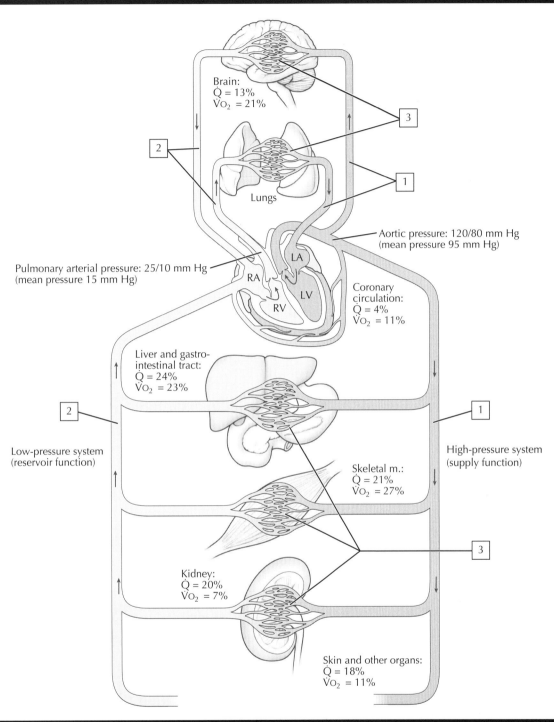

Brain:
$\dot{Q}$ = 13%
$\dot{V}O_2$ = 21%

Lungs

Pulmonary arterial pressure: 25/10 mm Hg
(mean pressure 15 mm Hg)

Aortic pressure: 120/80 mm Hg
(mean pressure 95 mm Hg)

LA

RA

LV

RV

Coronary
circulation:
$\dot{Q}$ = 4%
$\dot{V}O_2$ = 11%

Liver and gastro-
intestinal tract:
$\dot{Q}$ = 24%
$\dot{V}O_2$ = 23%

Low-pressure system
(reservoir function)

High-pressure system
(supply function)

Skeletal m.:
$\dot{Q}$ = 21%
$\dot{V}O_2$ = 27%

Kidney:
$\dot{Q}$ = 20%
$\dot{V}O_2$ = 7%

Skin and other organs:
$\dot{Q}$ = 18%
$\dot{V}O_2$ = 11%

REVIEW QUESTIONS

A. The _____ circulation is a low-pressure, low-resistance circulation.

B. Normal, resting, arterial blood pressure is approximately _____ mm Hg (systolic/diastolic).

C. Normal, resting, pulmonary arterial blood pressure is approximately _____ mm Hg (systolic/diastolic).

D. Normal, resting, LV pressure is approximately _____ mm Hg (systolic/diastolic).

E. Normal, resting, RV pressure is approximately _____ mm Hg (systolic/diastolic).

F. Two common causes of orthostatic hypotension are _____ and _____.

The total volume of blood in a 70-kg person is approximately 5 L. At rest, most of that volume (approximately 64%) is in the systemic veins. **Veins** are able to accommodate this large volume at a low pressure as a result of their **capacitance** and can act as a **reservoir** of blood when blood volume is reduced (by hemorrhage or dehydration). The entire **pulmonary circulation** contains about 9% of blood volume. Note that capillaries contain the smallest fraction of blood volume, only about 5%.

Flow of blood is governed by the equation

$$Q = \Delta P/R$$

where Q is flow, ΔP is the pressure gradient in a tube or system, and R is resistance. The overall flow rate in the circulation can be defined as **cardiac output (CO),** or the flow rate from one ventricle; for a resting 70 kg person, it is approximately 5 L/min. Note that because the circulation is in series, on average, the CO of the two ventricles will be the same. Because blood is pumped by the heart each time it beats, CO can be defined in terms of **heart rate (HR)** and the volume pumped with each beat **(stroke volume [SV]):**

$$CO = HR \times SV$$

Resting HR is normally about 70 beats/min, and resting SV is about 70 mL, yielding the resting CO of approximately 5 L/min. In Plate 3.2, the percentage of this CO flowing through various organs is given as $\dot{Q}$; similarly, the proportion of total **oxygen consumption** rate by organs is given as $\dot{V}O_2$. During exercise, CO increases, reaching values of up to 25 L/min or more in a healthy, well-trained athlete.

Considering the resistance to flow through the systemic circulation, the **greatest resistance** is in the **small arteries** and **arterioles** (the vessels that feed the capillaries). Contraction and relaxation of the systemic arterioles and small arteries play an important part in regulation of blood pressure and control of blood flow. Normally, at rest, these vessels account for about 47% of **systemic vascular resistance** but, more importantly, that resistance can be regulated widely, and it responds as well to local conditions.

COLOR and **LABEL** in Part A the pie chart showing the volume distribution of blood to:

☐ 1. Veins
☐ 2. Lungs
☐ 3. Small arteries and arterioles
☐ 4. Large arteries
☐ 5. Heart in diastole
☐ 6. Capillaries

COLOR and **LABEL** in Part B the pie chart showing the distribution of vascular resistance through:

☐ 7. Small arteries and arterioles
☐ 8. Capillaries
☐ 9. Large arteries
☐ 10. Veins

Clinical Note

During low volume states (**hemorrhage** or **dehydration**), veins constrict in response to the sympathetic nervous system (SNS). This results in a redistribution of blood from veins to other parts of the circulation, allowing for better perfusion of tissues and helping to maintain arterial blood pressure in the face of the reduced volume.

REVIEW ANSWERS

A.	5, 5
B.	Small arteries and arterioles
C.	9
D.	64

Plate 3.2   **Cardiovascular Physiology**

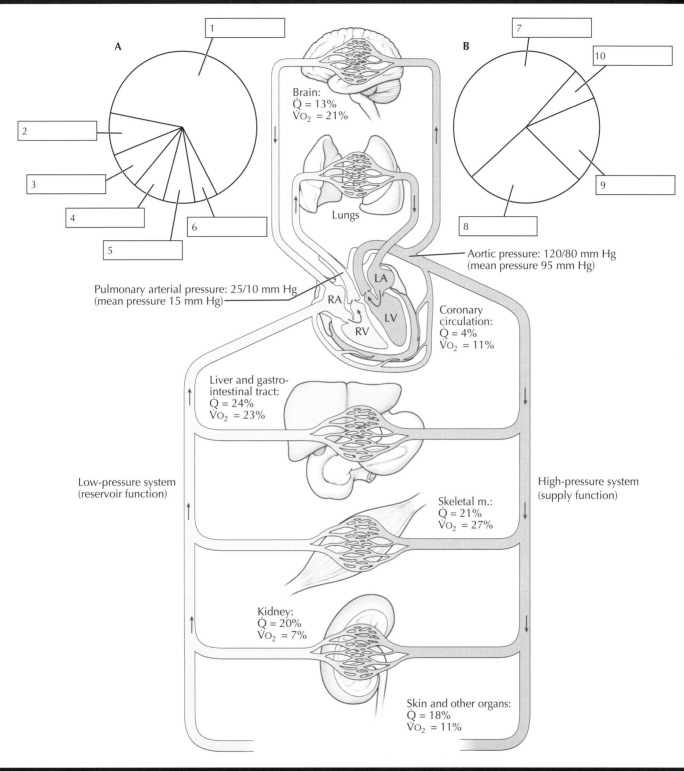

A

1

2

3

4

6

5

Brain:
$\dot{Q}$ = 13%
$\dot{V}O_2$ = 21%

Lungs

B

7

10

9

8

Aortic pressure: 120/80 mm Hg
(mean pressure 95 mm Hg)

Pulmonary arterial pressure: 25/10 mm Hg
(mean pressure 15 mm Hg)

LA

RA

LV

RV

Coronary
circulation:
$\dot{Q}$ = 4%
$\dot{V}O_2$ = 11%

Liver and gastro-
intestinal tract:
$\dot{Q}$ = 24%
$\dot{V}O_2$ = 23%

Low-pressure system
(reservoir function)

High-pressure system
(supply function)

Skeletal m.:
$\dot{Q}$ = 21%
$\dot{V}O_2$ = 27%

Kidney:
$\dot{Q}$ = 20%
$\dot{V}O_2$ = 7%

Skin and other organs:
$\dot{Q}$ = 18%
$\dot{V}O_2$ = 11%

REVIEW QUESTIONS

A. Average blood volume is _____ L, and average CO is _____ L/min.

B. The greatest resistance in the circulation occurs in the _____.

C. The pulmonary circulation contains approximately _____% of blood volume.

D. The systemic veins contain approximately _____% of blood volume.

Plate 3.3 shows a human heart, sectioned and laid open to reveal the chambers and valves. Note that the ventricular **myocardium** (muscle layer) is much thicker than the atrial myocardium. The **interventricular septum,** which separates the ventricles, is a thick muscular structure that functionally behaves as part of the **LV.** The difference in thickness in left and right ventricular walls is consistent with the higher pressures generated in the LV. Blood enters the left heart from the **pulmonary veins,** flowing freely into the **LA.** During diastole, blood passes from LA to LV through the open **mitral valve.** During systole, the period of ventricular contraction, the mitral valve is closed, and contraction of the ventricles pumps blood into the **aorta** through the now-open aortic valve.

Turning to the right side, blood returns from the systemic circulation to the **RA.** During diastole, blood passes from the RA to the **RV** through the open **tricuspid valve.** During systole, the tricuspid valve is closed, and blood is pumped from the RV through the now open **pulmonic valve** into the PA. Over the course of systole and diastole, the valves open and close as a result of pressure gradients. The **papillary muscles** and **chordae tendineae** have the function of holding the tricuspid valve and mitral valve in place during ventricular contraction, preventing inversion or prolapse of the valves (see Clinical Note).

COLOR and LABEL

☐   1.   Pulmonary trunk
☐   2.   LA
☐   3.   Pulmonary veins
☐   4.   Aorta
☐   5.   Mitral valve
☐   6.   RA
☐   7.   Tricuspid valve
☐   8.   Chordae tendineae
☐   9.   RV
☐ 10.   Papillary muscles
☐ 11.   Interventricular septum
☐ 12.   LV
☐ 13.   Myocardium

Clinical Note

Mitral valve prolapse is a condition in which the mitral valve balloons back into the LA during ventricular contraction, sometimes accompanied by regurgitation (leaking) of blood backward into the LA. Mitral valve prolapse can be asymptomatic but may result in lightheadedness, arrhythmias, fatigue, and chest pain not associated with coronary artery disease. The condition may go undetected for years without serious consequences but can also lead to **endocarditis** (infection and inflammation of the inner lining of the heart, in this case, of the valves).

REVIEW ANSWERS

A.   Tricuspid valve

B.   Aortic

C.   LV

D.   Papillary muscles, chordae tendineae

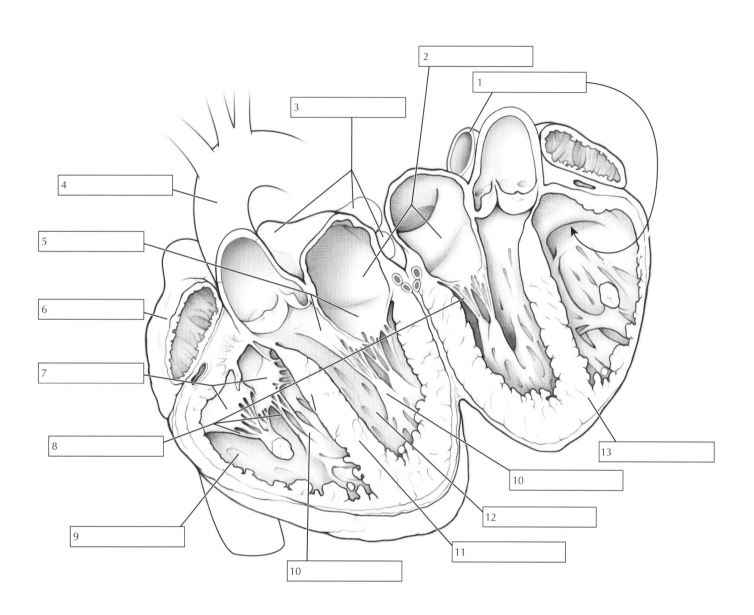

2

1

3

4

5

6

7

8

9

10

13

10

12

11

REVIEW QUESTIONS

A. The valve between the RA and RV is the _____.

B. The LV pumps blood out to the systemic circulation through the _____ valve.

C. The most muscular chamber of the heart is the _____

D. During ventricular contraction, the atrioventricular valves are held in place, preventing prolapse, by the _____ and _____.

Like other excitable cells, cells in the heart have the ability to generate action potentials. These action potentials result in the rhythmic cycle of contraction and relaxation of the heart muscle that allows the heart to pump blood. In a healthy heart, the **pacemaker** for this electrical activity is the **sinoatrial (SA) node,** and the resting HR is approximately **70 beats/min.**

The SA nodal cells have a resting membrane potential of around −60 mV but undergo spontaneous, gradual depolarization as a result of an inward current of Na^+ and Ca^{2+} and reduced outward K^+ current. When this **diastolic depolarization** reaches a threshold, **T-type and L-type Ca^{2+} channels** open, producing upstroke of the action potential. **Repolarization** occurs because of **increased K^+ conduction and closure of Ca^{2+} channels.**

Action potentials generated in the **SA node** cause a depolarization that passes along the **internodal tracts** in the upper part of the wall of the RA, spreading across the atria and initiating atrial contraction. They eventually reach the **atrioventricular (AV) node,** the only site for normal propagation of the depolarization between the atria and ventricles. Conduction velocity is slow through the AV node, allowing time for final filling of the ventricles by atrial contraction. From the AV node, depolarization reaches the **bundle of His** and is rapidly conducted through the **left and right bundle branches** to **Purkinje fibers** and, ultimately, the ventricular muscle, producing a powerful and coordinated contraction of the ventricles.

COLOR and **LABEL** these structures that are part of the conduction system of the heart and note their placement in the right and left sides of the heart:

- [ ] 1.   SA node
- [ ] 2.   Internodal tracts
- [ ] 3.   Purkinje fibers
- [ ] 4.   Right bundle branch of His
- [ ] 5.   Common AV bundle of His
- [ ] 6.   AV node
- [ ] 7.   Left bundle branch of His
- [ ] 8.   Interventricular septum

REVIEW ANSWERS

A.   Internodal tracts

B.   SA node

C.   70 beats/min

D.   SA node; Na^+ and Ca^{2+}; K^+

E. Ca^{2+} channels

Plate 3.4   **Cardiovascular Physiology**

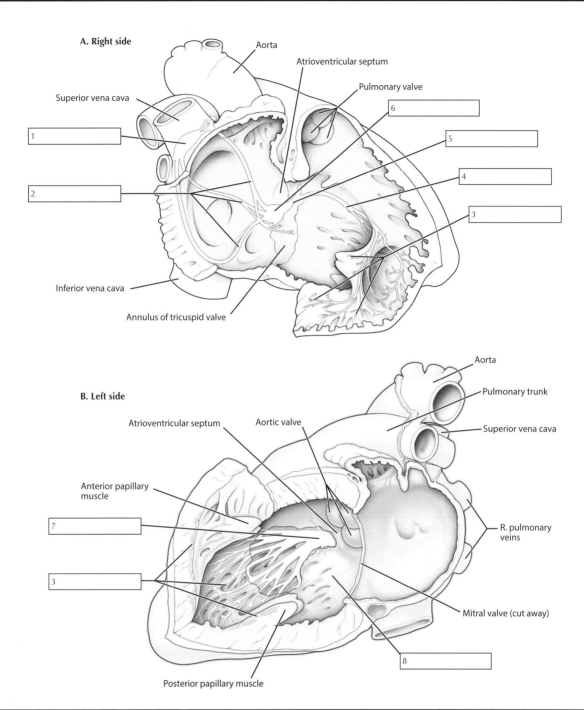

A. Right side

Aorta

Atrioventricular septum

Superior vena cava

Pulmonary valve

6

1

5

2

4

3

Inferior vena cava

Annulus of tricuspid valve

Aorta

B. Left side

Pulmonary trunk

Atrioventricular septum

Aortic valve

Superior vena cava

Anterior papillary muscle

7

R. pulmonary veins

3

Mitral valve (cut away)

8

Posterior papillary muscle

REVIEW QUESTIONS

A. The wave of depolarization is transmitted between the SA node and the AV node through the _____.

B. The normal cardiac pacemaker is the _____.

C. The normal resting HR is _____.

D. The pacemaker rate of the heart is linked to diastolic depolarization of the _____, caused by inward current of _____ and reduced outward current of _____.

E. When threshold is reached, an action potential is initiated in the cardiac pacemaker cells. This action potential is associated with the opening of _____.

In Part A, **action potentials** are illustrated for various parts of the cardiac conduction system. The last tracing in the top panel represents the normal **electrocardiogram (ECG),** which is the recording of changes in electrical potential at the surface of the body produced by the cardiac electrical events. The **P wave** of the ECG is produced by **atrial depolarization; the QRS** complex results from **ventricular muscle depolarization,** and the **T wave** is associated with **ventricular repolarization.** As depolarization spreads sequentially through the conducting system, the wave is propagated as the action potential in a cell results in adjacent cells depolarizing to their threshold, initiating an action potential in those cells.

Note the sharp upstroke during depolarization of all but the nodal action potentials, consistent with the rapid conduction of the wave of depolarization in most parts of the heart (**atrial muscle,** His-Purkinje system, **ventricular muscle**). In Part C, the action potential of ventricular muscle and the underlying changes in ion currents are illustrated. The phases of the ventricular action potential and associated changes in ion conduction are:

- **Phase 4** resting membrane potential, mainly a function of K^+ efflux and close to the Nernst potential for K^+;
- **Phase 0** upstroke;
- **Phase 1** rapid repolarization to the plateau;
- **Phase 2** plateau; and
- **Phase 3** repolarization leading back to the resting membrane potential.

Note the large role of Na^+ conductance in the upstroke. Inactivation of those channels and opening of voltage-sensitive K^+ channels causes phase 1. In contrast, the upstrokes of the action potentials of the **SA** and **AV nodes** are less steep, which is important in the delayed conduction of the wave of depolarization through the AV node. In Part B, the changes in ion conductance associated with the action potential in the SA node are illustrated (the AV node is similar).

The areas labeled **ERP** and **RRP** in the ventricular action potential represent the **effective refractory period,** when another action potential cannot be elicited, and the **relative refractory period,** during which it is more difficult to elicit an action potential than during phase 4. The presence of refractory periods is important in maintaining normal cardiac rhythm and avoiding arrhythmias.

COLOR and **LABEL** the seven action potentials in the heart (on right) and the associated structure in the heart in Part A:

- ☐ 1. SA node
- ☐ 2. Atrial muscle
- ☐ 3. AV node
- ☐ 4. Common bundle of His
- ☐ 5. Bundle branches
- ☐ 6. Purkinje fibers
- ☐ 7. Ventricular muscle

Clinical Note
The normal resting HR, set by the pacemaker rate of the AV node, is approximately 70 beats/min and has a regular rhythm. When the heart beats too quickly or slowly or with an irregular rhythm, this is an arrhythmia. Resting HRs above 100 or below 60 beats/min are referred to as **tachycardia** and **bradycardia,** respectively, although resting HRs below 60 beats/min are often seen in runners and endurance-trained athletes.

REVIEW ANSWERS

A. Ventricular repolarization

B. Na^+ influx

C. Arrhythmias

D. 60 beats/min; 100 beats/min

Plate 3.5　　　　　　　　　　　　　　　**Cardiovascular Physiology**

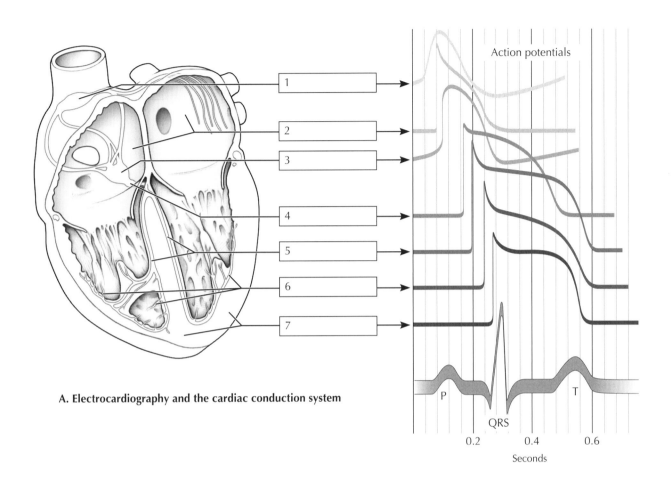

A. Electrocardiography and the cardiac conduction system

Action potentials

P   T

QRS

0.2   0.4   0.6

Seconds

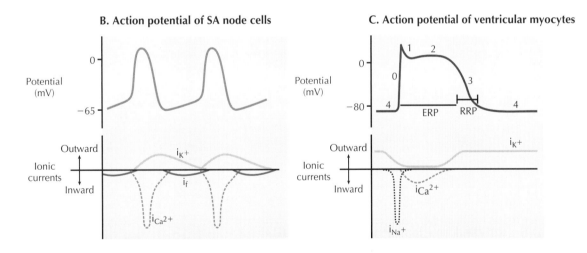

B. Action potential of SA node cells

Potential (mV)
0
−65

Outward
Ionic currents
Inward

i_{K^+}
i_f
$i_{Ca^{2+}}$

C. Action potential of ventricular myocytes

Potential (mV)
0
−80

1   2
0
3
4   ERP   RRP   4

Outward
Ionic currents
Inward

i_{K^+}
$i_{Ca^{2+}}$
i_{Na^+}

REVIEW QUESTIONS

A. The T wave of the ECG corresponds to _____ in the heart.

B. The ion flux mainly responsible for the sharp phase 0 upstroke in the ventricular action potential is _____.

C. The presence of the refractory periods is important in preventing cardiac _____.

D. Bradycardia is defined as resting HR below _____; tachycardia is resting HR above _____.

Electrocardiography

The **ECG** is a recording made at the surface of the body, of the rhythmic electrical potential changes occurring there as a result of the cycle of depolarization and repolarization of the heart. Various lead configurations are useful in evaluation of heart function.

The **standard limb leads I, II, and III** are used to record voltage differences between (I) right and left arm, (II) right arm and left leg, and (III) left arm and left leg (with the first in each pair of electrodes being negative and the second being positive). In the three **augmented leads (aVR, aVL, aVF),** two of the limb electrodes are combined as the negative electrode and the third limb lead is positive. For the six **precordial leads** (leads placed on the precordium, the area above the heart and lower chest), all three limb electrodes are combined to form the negative electrode, and the positive electrode is placed in the designated locations for the **unipolar leads** (V_1, V_2, V_3, V_4, V_5, and V_6).

At any point during the sequential electrical events in a cardiac cycle, if current flows toward the arrowheads in the diagram, upward deflection occurs in the ECG. When current flows away from the arrowheads, downward deflection occurs, and no deflection (or biphasic deflection) occurs when current flow is perpendicular to the arrow. Evaluation of specific cardiovascular disease types is aided by simultaneous evaluation of tracings made using multiple leads.

COLOR the arrows in each of the diagrams (red), indicating the direction of current that will result in an upward ECG deflection in the given lead configuration.

- ☐ 1. Limb leads
- ☐ 2. Augmented limb leads
- ☐ 3. Precordial leads

Clinical Note

Electrocardiography is useful in revealing:

- Cardiac arrhythmias and conduction defects
- Presence, location, and extent of ischemia or infarction
- Orientation of the heart in the thoracic cavity and the size of its chambers
- Effects of some drugs and effects of abnormal electrolyte levels.

The orientation of the heart and size of its chambers can be altered in some acute and chronic disease states.

REVIEW ANSWERS

A. True

B. False

C. True

D. False

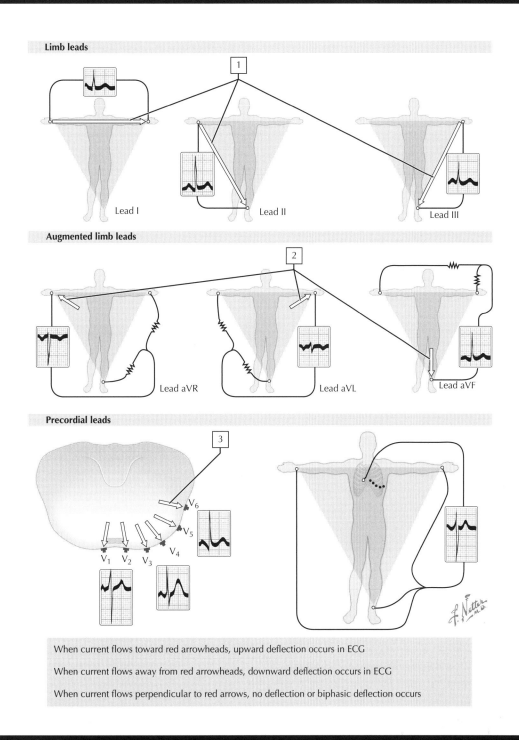

Limb leads

Lead I

Lead II

Lead III

Augmented limb leads

Lead aVR

Lead aVL

Lead aVF

Precordial leads

V₁ V₂ V₃ V₄ V₅ V₆

When current flows toward red arrowheads, upward deflection occurs in ECG

When current flows away from red arrowheads, downward deflection occurs in ECG

When current flows perpendicular to red arrows, no deflection or biphasic deflection occurs

REVIEW QUESTIONS

Answer the following True or False questions:

A. Enlargement of the heart may be inferred from an ECG recording.

B. Poor contractile function of the heart can be inferred from an ECG recording.

C. The simultaneous recording of multiple leads in an ECG is useful in assessing some pathophysiological changes in the heart.

D. The QRS complex of the ECG is always an upward deflection on the tracing.

As discussed in Plate 3.2, flow (Q) through the circulation is a function of the pressure gradient (ΔP) from arteries to the central veins, and the resistance (R) of the circulation to flow:

$$Q = \Delta P/R$$

As the heart ejects its SV during systole, arterial pressure, rises; it falls during diastole as blood flows downstream. **Systolic arterial pressure** is the peak pressure in the artery during ventricular ejection, whereas **diastolic pressure** is the lowest pressure, just before the next systole. Thus arterial pressure is often expressed as systolic/diastolic pressures, and **normal resting arterial pressure** is approximately **120/80 mm Hg.** The **pulse pressure** is the difference between the extremes in pressure in a region of the circulation, and thus the pulse pressure in the arteries is approximately 40 mm Hg (120 to 80 mm Hg).

Part A illustrates pressure curves in different regions of the circulation at rest. Part B depicts the rhythmic changes in pressures as may be measured starting at the **LA** and proceeding downstream through the entire circulation. Note the **left ventricular pressure (LVP) of 120/0** is the largest pulse pressure (120 mm Hg). The high systolic pressure of 120 mm Hg creates the gradient for flow of blood through the systemic circuit, whereas the low diastolic pressure (near zero) allows filling of the LV during diastole. On the "right side" of the circulation, the resting **right ventricular pressure** is approximately 25/0, and the **pulmonary artery pressure** is approximately 25/10 mm Hg.

In Part C, note the **mean arterial pressure (MAP)** is not simply the mean of systolic and diastolic pressures but is best approximated as diastolic arterial pressure plus one-third the pulse pressure. This MAP is a function of **CO** and **peripheral resistance.** Pulse pressure is a function of several factors, including, as illustrated, **SV** and **arterial compliance** (the distensibility of the arterial vessels). An increase in SV produces larger pulse pressure, as will a *decrease* in arterial compliance. HR and peripheral resistance also affect pulse pressure. Rapid HR is usually associated with low pulse pressure, and low peripheral resistance is associated with greater pulse pressure. Also note the **dicrotic notch** in the arterial pressure curve, which is associated with closure of the aortic valve**.**

COLOR the segments of the pressure wave continuum associated with each region of circulation in Part B:

- [ ] 1. LA
- [ ] 2. LV
- [ ] 3. Aorta
- [ ] 4. Large arteries
- [ ] 5. Small arteries
- [ ] 6. Arterioles
- [ ] 7. Capillaries
- [ ] 8. Veins
- [ ] 9. RA
- [ ] 10. RV
- [ ] 11. Pulmonary arteries

COLOR the individual pressure panels in Part A using the same colors from Part B to designate the part of the circulation being illustrated. Note the changes in pulse pressures in the different regions of the circulation.

- [ ] 12. LAP (use same color as 1 in Part B)
- [ ] 13. LVP (use same color as 2 in Part B)
- [ ] 14. Aortic pressure (use same color as 3 in Part B)
- [ ] 15. RAP (use same color as 9 in Part B)
- [ ] 16. Right ventricular pressure (use same color as 10 in Part B)

Clinical Note

Arteriosclerosis is the loss of compliance, thickening and hardening of arteries. With arteriosclerosis, arterial pulse pressure is large as a result of the diminished compliance. In dehydration or hemorrhage, the loss of blood volume translates to a small SV and therefore a small pulse pressure. A **"weak pulse"** is felt upon palpitation during physical exam.

REVIEW ANSWERS

A. LV

B. 93 mm Hg (DP + ⅓ PP = 80 + 13)

C. SV, arterial compliance, peripheral resistance, HR

D. It will lower MAP.

E. 67 mL/stroke

Plate 3.7   **Cardiovascular Physiology**

A. Pulse Pressures Through the Circulation

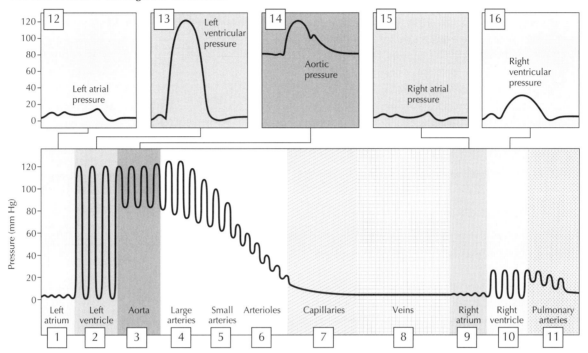

B. Pressure Wave Continuum

C. The Arterial Pressure Wave

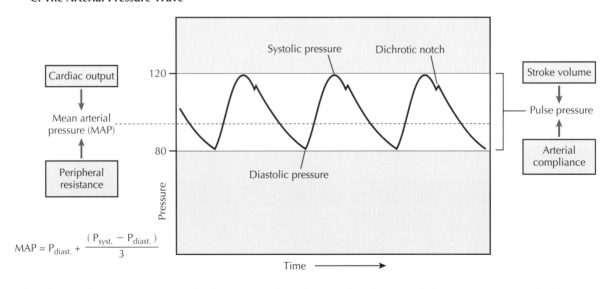

$$MAP = P_{diast.} + \frac{(P_{syst.} - P_{diast.})}{3}$$

REVIEW QUESTIONS

A. Which part of the circulation has the largest pulse pressure?

B. If systolic arterial pressure is 120 and diastolic pressure is 80, what is the MAP?

C. The magnitude of pulse pressure in the arterial system is a function of what factors?

D. Reducing peripheral resistance will have what effect on MAP?

E. If measured CO is 6 L/min and HR is 90 beats/min, what is SV?

3 Biophysics of the Circulation I: Poiseuille's Law

In the basic flow equation presented in Plate 3.7, **Q = ΔP/R,** we can also view the pressure gradient, ΔP, as the **MAP** minus the **pressure in central veins (central venous pressure [CVP])**, and R is the total peripheral resistance (TPR). For flow through a single tube or vessel, **Poiseuille's law** states this relationship specifying the components of R:

$$Q = \Delta P \Pi r^4/\eta 8L$$

where *r* is the radius of the tube, η is the viscosity of the fluid, and *L* is the length of the tube.

Because Q = ΔP/R, the following relationship results:

$$R = \eta 8L/\Pi r^4$$

These relationships are illustrated in the vessels shown in Parts A and B.

Part C illustrates the resistance (per unit tube length) of vessels along the circulation. As vessels branch, they become smaller, leading to the smallest radius at the level of the arterioles (the smallest arteries) and into the capillaries; it is at the arterioles that resistance is the highest. Note that it is also in the smaller arteries and arterioles where adjustments to resistance, through contraction and relaxation of the vessels and changes in radius, lead to changes in local blood flow as physiological needs vary. Along the path of blood from capillaries to venules, small veins, and larger veins toward the heart, vessel radius increases, reducing resistance of individual vessels.

COLOR the arrows illustrating upstream vs. downstream pressures (left vessel), net pressure, and flow direction (right vessel).

- ☐ 1. P_1
- ☐ 2. ΔP
- ☐ 3. P_2
- ☐ 4. Blood flow (Q)
- ☐ 5. Resistance to flow

TRACE in Part C:

- ☐ 6. Graph line, noting the relationship between resistance per unit length and vessel radius

REVIEW ANSWERS

A. 5

B. 5

C. 160

D. 15

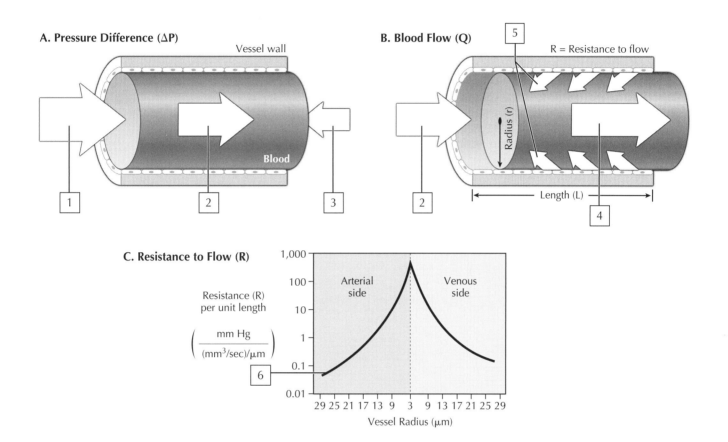

A. Pressure Difference (ΔP)

Vessel wall

Blood

1

2

3

B. Blood Flow (Q)

5

R = Resistance to flow

Radius (r)

2

Length (L)

4

C. Resistance to Flow (R)

Resistance (R)
per unit length

$$\left(\frac{mm\ Hg}{(mm^3/sec)/\mu m} \right)$$

6

1,000

100

10

1

0.1

0.01

Arterial
side

Venous
side

29 25 21 17 13 9   3   9 13 17 21 25 29

Vessel Radius (μm)

REVIEW QUESTIONS

Assume that flow through a tube is 10 mL/min. For each of the changes below, assume that other parameters are controlled (unchanged) and predict the change in flow using Poiseuille's law:

A. If the length of the tube is doubled, flow will be _____ mL/min.

B. If viscosity of the fluid is doubled, flow will be _____ mL/min.

C. If the radius of the tube is doubled, flow will be _____ mL/min.

D. If the pressure gradient is increased by 50%, flow will be _____ mL/min.

Flow (Q) through a tube (or set of parallel tubes) will be a function of the **cross-sectional area (A)** of the tube (or the sum of the cross-sectional area of parallel tubes) and the **linear velocity of the flow (V):**

$$Q = VA$$

Within a single, non-branching tube, because Q will be the same along the entire length of the tube, in segments where the tube narrows, the velocity will be higher, and in segments where the tube is wider, the velocity will be lower.

To apply this principle to the cardiovascular system, the overall blood flow is the same at each level of the system, but as the total cross-sectional area of the system varies, the velocity will vary inversely. Referring to the right illustration, as the arterial system branches, eventually leading to the **capillaries,** because the total cross-sectional area increases *(dotted line)* the velocity falls *(solid line),* reaching a minimum velocity at the capillaries where all exchange of gases, nutrients, and wastes with the interstitial fluid takes place.

As blood travels back toward the heart and veins converge, the total cross-sectional area of the circulation again falls (right figure, *dotted line*) and velocity rises *(solid line).* Of course, pressure falls along the entire course of the systemic circulation from the aorta to the venae cavae, with the greatest fall in pressure taking place in the **arterioles.**

COLOR the type of vessels:

- [ ] 1. Arteries
- [ ] 2. Arterioles
- [ ] 3. Capillaries

TRACE

- [ ] 4. Velocity arrows, noting the large velocity in the large vessels (V_1), where total cross-sectional area is low, compared to the smaller velocity arrow (V_2) in the capillaries, where total cross-sectional area is high.
- [ ] 5. Velocity (V) curves through the circulatory system
- [ ] 6. Area (A) curves through the circulatory system

REVIEW ANSWERS

A. 20 (flow will be the same along the entire length of the tube)

B. Higher

C. Aorta

D. Capillaries

Plate 3.9

Cardiovascular Physiology

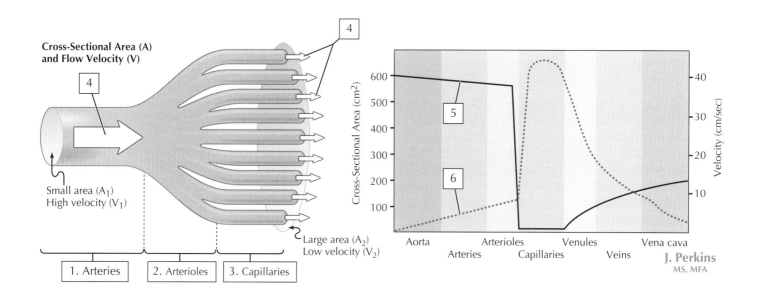

Cross-Sectional Area (A) and Flow Velocity (V)

4

4

Small area (A_1)
High velocity (V_1)

Large area (A_2)
Low velocity (V_2)

1. Arteries   2. Arterioles   3. Capillaries

Cross-Sectional Area (cm^2)

600
500
400
300
200
100

5

6

Velocity (cm/sec)

40
30
20
10

Aorta   Arterioles   Venules   Vena cava
  Arteries   Capillaries   Veins

J. Perkins
MS, MFA

REVIEW QUESTIONS

A. Flow measurements are made along a vessel that has a uniform cross-sectional area of 1 cm^2, except in one narrower segment where the cross-sectional area is reduced to 0.5 cm^2. If flow in most of the vessel is 20 mL/min, the flow in the narrow segment is _____ mL/min.

B. Compared to the rest of the vessel, velocity in the narrow segment will be lower/the same/higher (circle one).

C. In the human circulation, the velocity is highest in which vessel?

D. In the human circulation, the velocity is lowest in which vessels?

Netter's Physiology Coloring Book

Plate 3.9

Blood flow through vessels is, for the most part, **laminar flow,** meaning that flow occurs linearly, in a **streamlined** manner (left vessel), with flow in the center of the stream occurring at a higher velocity than flow toward the vascular wall, resulting from shear stress associated with flow of fluid across the face of the vascular wall. In fact, the rate of flow approaches zero near the wall.

In **turbulent flow,** by contrast, flow is irregular, with vortices, whorls, and eddies (right vessel). Vascular disease often begins in areas of turbulence because irregularities in the flow pattern present sites for adherence and infiltration into the wall of formed elements, lipoproteins, and other material.

Reynold's number (R$_e$) relates the factors associated with turbulence:

$$R_e = VD\rho/\eta$$

where *V* is velocity of flow, *D* is diameter of the tube, *ρ* is density of the fluid, and *η* is fluid viscosity. When R$_e$ is below 2000, flow is usually laminar. Thus turbulence is promoted by high velocity, large vessel diameter, high fluid density (not usually a factor in blood), or low fluid viscosity. Turbulence also is associated with branch points, abrupt changes in vessel diameter (see Clinical Note), and flow obstructions.

The third important biophysical relationship is **Laplace's law,** which defines **wall tension (T)** in terms of **transmural pressure (P$_t$)** and **vessel radius (r):**

$$T = P_t r$$

Wall tension can be conceptualized as the force that would rend a vessel wall apart if the wall is slit (or as the force necessary to hold together a theoretical slit in a vessel wall). Thus high wall tension would favor bursting of a vessel and is associated with high P$_t$ (transmural pressure is the difference between pressure within the vessel and pressure in the interstitium) and large vessel radius (r).

COLOR and **LABEL** the arrows in the vessels illustrating:

☐ 1. Laminar flow

☐ 2. Turbulent flow

Clinical Note

Anemia is the condition of **reduced red blood cell count (low hematocrit)** or **low hemoglobin** in blood. **Blood viscosity** is greatly reduced with serious anemia, resulting in turbulent blood flow and flow murmurs, and other potentially serious pathophysiology. An **aneurysm** is a bulging in a segment of blood vessel, caused by weakening of the vessel wall. An **aortic aneurysm** is susceptible to continued expansion and eventual rupture, resulting from progression of the underlying disease and further increase in wall tension as the radius increases. Vascular wall disease and aneurysm are most common in areas where flow is turbulent.

REVIEW ANSWERS

A. ↑

B. ↑

C. ↑

D. ↓

E. ↑

Plate 3.10   **Cardiovascular Physiology**

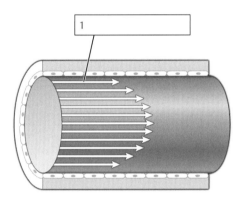

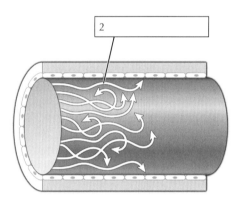

REVIEW QUESTIONS

In each of the blanks below, draw an up or down arrow to illustrate the direction of change (assume a well-controlled experiment).

A. Tendency toward turbulence if vessel diameter is increased _____

B. Tendency toward turbulence when velocity of flow increases _____

C. Tendency toward turbulence when viscosity falls _____

D. Wall tension in smaller vessels, compared to larger vessels _____

E. Wall tension when pressure within a vessel rises _____

3 Measurement of Blood Pressure

Indirect measurement of **arterial blood pressure** by **sphygmomanometry** using a blood pressure cuff is ubiquitous in clinical settings, arterial blood pressure being one of the four "vital signs" (along with body temperature, HR, and respiratory rate). However, measurement of blood pressure in other parts of the circulation can be clinically important in diagnosing disease and monitoring patients. Arterial pressure can be measured directly through an arterial catheter, which can be passed back to the heart in the retrograde direction (against the flow), back to the aorta and LV to determine **LVP.**

Measurement and monitoring of pressures in the central veins, right heart, and pulmonary system can also be important in diagnosis and in critical care settings. Pulmonary capillary wedge pressure, or "wedge pressure," is one such measurement. A flexible **Swan-Ganz catheter** can be passed in the **antegrade** direction (with the flow) from a large vein (such as femoral) back to the **RA** and **RV,** into the pulmonary arterial system, with the aid of a partially inflated balloon (see Plate 3.11). Once advanced as far as possible into a branch of the pulmonary arterial system, the balloon is fully inflated temporarily to measure PCWP through the lumen at the end of the catheter. That pressure, beyond the vascular occlusion caused by the balloon, will have fallen to equilibrate with the downstream pressure and is an indicator of pulmonary venous pressure and LAP (which also give an approximation of the left ventricular end-diastolic pressure, the loading pressure of the LV). Wedge pressure is useful in hemodynamic assessment in heart failure and for differential diagnosis when pulmonary edema is present.

COLOR

☐ 1. Swan-Ganz catheter, using different colors for the individual tubes at its proximal end

COLOR and **LABEL** the structures signifying the path of the catheter (starting from either the superior or inferior vena cava):

☐ 2. Superior vena cava
☐ 3. Inferior vena cava
☐ 4. RA
☐ 5. Tricuspid valve
☐ 6. RV
☐ 7. Pulmonic valve
☐ 8. Pulmonary artery trunk
☐ 9. Pulmonary artery branch

REVIEW ANSWERS

A. Sphygmomanometer

B. Pulmonary venous pressure, LAP

C. Arterial catheterization (with retrograde advancement of the catheter to the LV)

D. Pulmonary edema (also, potentially, heart failure)

Plate 3.11   **Cardiovascular Physiology**

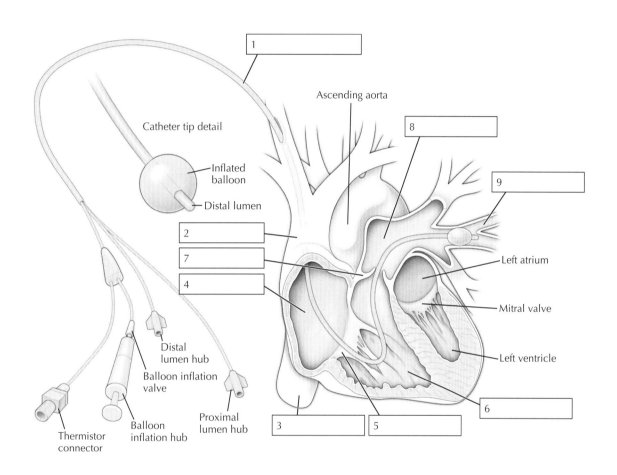

Catheter tip detail

Ascending aorta

Inflated balloon

Distal lumen

Distal lumen hub

Balloon inflation valve

Balloon inflation hub

Thermistor connector

Proximal lumen hub

Left atrium

Mitral valve

Left ventricle

1

8

9

2

7

4

3

5

6

A. The instrument typically used for indirect measurement of arterial blood pressure is known as a _____.

B. PCWP is measured as an approximation of _____ and _____.

C. LVP can be measured through _____.

D. Wedge pressure is useful in differential diagnosis of causes of _____.

---

3 Cardiac Cycle

The **cardiac cycle diagram,** also known as a **Wiggers diagram,** is a graphic representation of one cardiac cycle of systole and diastole, illustrating changes in various parameters over the course of time (less than 1 second at an HR of 70 beats/min). In Plate 3.12, the cardiac cycle is illustrated for the "left side" of the circulation (LA and LV and systemic circuit), showing the progression of changes in **LVP, aortic pressure, LAP, LV volume,** heart sounds, and **electrocardiogram (ECG).** The tracings begin at the point corresponding to the P wave of the ECG (bottom tracing). The phases of the cycle labeled at the top of Plate 3.12, beginning from the left, are as follows:

- **Atrial systole:** Period during ventricular diastole when the atrium contracts to achieve the final filling of the ventricle
- **Isovolumetric contraction:** Short interval between the closing of the mitral valve initiated by the beginning of ventricular contraction and opening of the aortic valve. During this phase, LVP rises rapidly to the aortic pressure; isovolumetric contraction ends with opening of the aortic valve when LVP rises above aortic pressure.
- **Ejection phase:** Ventricular systole continues, but now blood is ejected from the ventricle into the aorta, raising aortic pressure to its peak of approximately 120 mm Hg at rest.
- **Isovolumetric relaxation:** Toward the end of ejection, the T wave of the ECG signals the repolarization and beginning of relaxation of the ventricle. Closure of the aortic valve marks the end of systole and the beginning of diastole with the short isovolumetric relaxation phase. Pressure in the ventricle plummets; when it falls below atrial pressure, the mitral valve opens, ending isovolumetric relaxation.
- **Ventricular filling:** Opening of the mitral valve results first in rapid, then reduced, ventricular filling followed by atrial systole and the start of a new cycle.

The **atrial pressure curve** has three upward waves, **a, c,** and **v.** The a wave is caused by atrial contraction. The c wave is associated with isovolumetric contraction; when the ventricles contract isometrically, the mitral valve bulges into the atrium. The v wave is produced by gradual return of blood to the atrium during ventricular systole while the atrioventricular valve (mitral, in this case) is closed.

The **phonocardiogram** tracing consists of four possible **heart sounds.** S_1, the first heart sound, is generated by the closure of the mitral (and tricuspid) valve; S_2 is associated with the closure of the aortic (and pulmonic) valve; S_3 is associated with passive filling of the ventricle; S_4 is associated with active filling of the ventricle. These heart sounds can vary in intensity, and S_1 and S_2 can be "split," consisting of two distinct sounds resulting from asynchrony between valve closure on the left and right sides of the heart, depending on various physiological and pathophysiological considerations. In a healthy adult, often only S_1 and S_2 are audible.

COLOR the various regions of the Wiggers diagram:

- ☐ 1. Atrial systole
- ☐ 2. Isovolumetric contraction
- ☐ 3. Rapid ejection
- ☐ 4. Reduced ejection
- ☐ 5. Isovolumetric relaxation
- ☐ 6. Rapid ventricular filling
- ☐ 7. Reduced ventricular filling (diastasis)

TRACE each of the curves in the diagram, while considering the physiological basis of the shapes of the curves:

- ☐ 8. Electrocardiogram
- ☐ 9. Heart sounds
- ☐ 10. LV volume (mL)
- ☐ 11. LVP (mm Hg)

REVIEW ANSWERS

A. S_1, closure of AV valves (mitral and tricuspid); S_2 closure of the aortic and pulmonic valves; S_3, passive filling for the ventricle; S_4 active filling of the ventricle.

B. Beginning of isovolumetric contraction

C. Reduced ejection (late systole)

D. Venous return of blood to the atrium while the mitral valve is closed

Plate 3.12   **Cardiovascular Physiology**

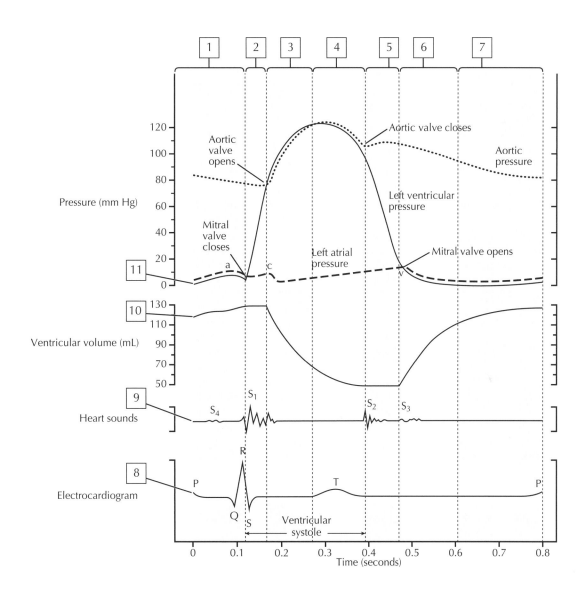

A. Name the physiological basis for the generation of the four heart sounds, S_1, S_2, S_3, and S_4.

B. Ventricular pressure rises above atrial pressure at what point in the cardiac cycle?

C. The T wave of the ECG occurs during the _____ phase of the cardiac cycle?

D. The v wave of the LAP curve is caused by _____.

Normal blood pressure is maintained in the face of challenges to homeostasis through the **autonomic nervous system** and **arterial baroreceptor reflex** (Plate 3.13, Parts A and B). Arterial baroreceptors are specialized cells in the wall of the **aortic arch** and **carotid artery sinus.** They respond to stretch (when arterial pressure rises) by adjusting their rate of firing and therefore the afferent neural signals to the cardiovascular centers in the ventral medulla. The medullary center, in response, adjusts **SNS** activity and **parasympathetic nervous system (PNS)** activity to maintain pressure homeostasis.

The **PNS,** through the **vagus nerve,** innervates the **SA node** and **AV node;** increased PNS activity produces a *decrease* in the pacemaker rate of the SA node and thus a fall in HR, through release and action of acetylcholine (Part A). The PNS also innervates specific vascular beds in the lower gastrointestinal tract and sexual organs through sacral PNS tracts, where it produces vasodilation under certain physiologic conditions.

The **SNS** innervates the SA and AV nodes, *increasing* HR and conduction velocity. The SNS also innervates ventricular myocardium, increasing its **contractility,** with all actions through the release of norepinephrine (upper right illustration). The **adrenal** medulla acts as part of the SNS, releasing epinephrine into the bloodstream.

In Part C, the response to a rise in arterial pressure is illustrated. When a person goes from a standing to a lying position, CO and arterial blood pressure rise as venous return from the lower part of the body increases. Higher arterial pressure results in a higher firing rate of the baroreceptors, which is detected by the medullary center. PNS activity is increased while SNS outflow decreases; HR falls, arterioles and veins relax, and SV is reduced, all contributing to a return to normal blood pressure. SV falls as part of this response because of reduced ventricular filling pressure associated with lower venous tone (relaxation), as well as reduced cardiac contractility. When blood pressure falls, for example, upon standing, the effects are reversed.

Note that HR is also affected by various other factors, including the following:

- Hormones (e.g., thyroid hormone increases HR)
- **Bainbridge reflex:** right atrial stretch increases HR
- Respiration (HR may be increased by the Bainbridge reflex during inspiration as blood return to the heart is increased as the thorax expands)
- Chemoreceptor reflexes

COLOR and LABEL

- ☐ 1. Midbrain
- ☐ 2. Sacral spinal cord
- ☐ 3. Thoracic region

TRACE

- ☐ 4. In Part A, the PNS (vagus) path to the endpoints at the SA and AV nodes and the small arteries and arterioles where ACh is released.
- ☐ 5. In Part B, the SNS path to the endpoints on the SA and AV nodes, left ventricular muscle, and small arteries and arterioles, where norepinephrine is released.

COLOR in Part C:

- ☐ 6. Open arrows illustrating how a change in posture from standing to lying results in a rise in MAP and a signal from the baroreceptors to the central nervous system (CNS)/medulla.

TRACE in Part C:

- ☐ 7. Path noting the upward and downward open arrows indicating the responses generated by the increase in PNS.
- ☐ 8. Path noting the upward and downward open arrows indicating the responses generated by the decrease in SNS. Note that all responses contribute to a decrease in MAP.

REVIEW ANSWERS

PARAMETER	EFFECT OF SNS	EFFECT OF PNS
Heart rate	↑	↓
Stroke volume	↑	—
Cardiac contractility	↑	—
Peripheral vascular resistance	↑	—
Venous tone	↑	—
Cardiac output	↑	↓
Mean arterial pressure	↑	↓

Plate 3.13   **Cardiovascular Physiology**

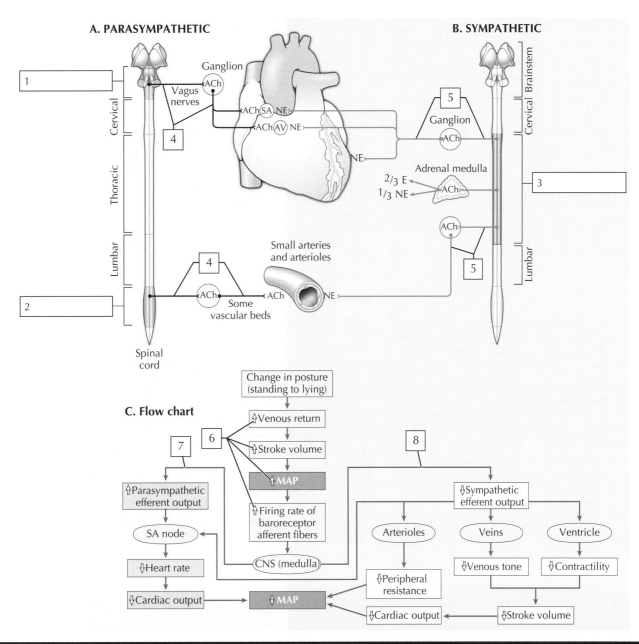

A. PARASYMPATHETIC

B. SYMPATHETIC

C. Flow chart

REVIEW QUESTIONS

In this table, refer to the flowchart and draw an upward arrow or a downward arrow to signify an increase or a decrease in a parameter expected when the SNS or PNS is activated (assume there is no effect on the other branch of the autonomic nervous system). For no effect, draw a dash (—).

PARAMETER	EFFECT OF SNS	EFFECT OF PNS
Heart rate		
Stroke volume		
Cardiac contractility		
Peripheral vascular resistance		
Venous tone		
Cardiac output		
Mean arterial pressure		

The **Frank-Starling mechanism** is an important property of cardiac muscle and ventricular function: it describes that the **force of contraction,** and therefore **SV,** is dependent on the degree of stretch or filling of the ventricle during diastole. The degree of stretch before contraction is called the **preload** on the heart. With more ventricular filling (preload), SV increases, up to an optimal degree of stretch. In Part A, this Frank-Starling effect is illustrated by the **cardiac function curve.**

It is important to note that when preload is higher, the increase in SV is due to a greater force of contraction, **_without_** a change in the underlying contractility or **inotropic state** of the cardiac muscle. Contractility or **inotropism** is defined as the intrinsic ability of the heart muscle to generate force (the strength or the "fitness" of the muscle). The degree of force attained during heart contraction is a function of three factors: the preload and the contractility, as well as the afterload, where afterload is the arterial pressure against which the heart contracts.

In Part B, the effects of sympathetic stimulation and heart failure on the cardiac function curve are illustrated. With **sympathetic stimulation** or with administration of **inotropic drugs** (e.g., dopamine, dobutamine, epinephrine), the cardiac function curve shifts upward (i.e., has a steeper slope), whereas **heart failure** or **myocardial ischemia** or **infarction** will cause the curve to shift downward (lower slope). A steeper slope of the cardiac function curve is an indication of greater contractility: with the same preload, the heart is able to achieve greater force of contraction. Because the PNS does not significantly innervate ventricular muscle (see Plate 3.13), activation of the PNS does not directly have an effect on contractility of the human ventricles.

TRACE and **LABEL** the slopes for the Frank-Starling curves:

- ☐ 1.   Normal, resting state
- ☐ 2.   Sympathetic stimulation
- ☐ 3.   Heart failure

In Part B, note the slope of the top line (sympathetic stimulation) is the steepest, and the slope of the bottom line (heart failure) is the shallowest.

REVIEW ANSWERS

A.   Frank-Starling mechanism

B.   Higher preload ↑

     Higher afterload ↓

     Sympathetic stimulation ↑

     Heart failure ↓

     Inotropic drug administration ↑

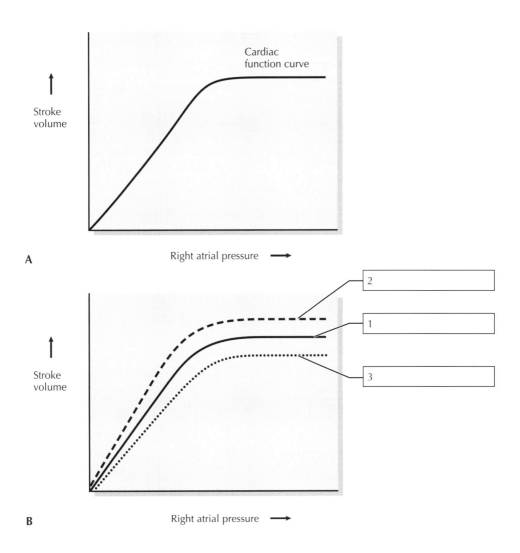

A

B

REVIEW QUESTIONS

A. Increasing the end diastolic volume of the LV will result in greater SV through increased contractility or the Frank-Starling mechanism?

B. For each of the following, draw an arrow (↑ or ↓) showing the effect on SV.

Higher preload _____

Higher afterload _____

Sympathetic stimulation _____

Heart failure _____

Inotropic drug administration _____

Assessment of cardiac function can be accomplished by several methods experimentally and clinically. In addition to analysis of the cardiac function curve and its slope (Plate 3.14), analysis of the **force-velocity relationship** illustrates the effects of preload and contractility changes on heart function. The **velocity of shortening** of a segment of cardiac muscle is inversely related to the **afterload** against which the muscle is contracting (Part A). Thus cardiac muscle has the highest velocity of shortening at zero afterload; in other words, when there is no opposing force. That highest velocity of shortening is known as the V_{max} (at the Y intercept of the graph, as noted).

At the other end of the spectrum, when the opposing force (afterload) is too great, muscle generates force but cannot actively contract, making the velocity of shortening zero. At that point, on the X intercept of the graph, the contraction can be described as **isometric.** In Parts A and B, compare the effects on this relationship of (A) **increased preload** and (B) **increased contractility.** In the first case, with increased preload, velocity of shortening is increased. This is a result of the **Frank-Starling relationship,** whereby increased preload produces more forceful (and therefore higher velocity) contraction. However, with alteration of preload, there is no change in V_{max} because there has been no change in the underlying contractility of the muscle. Changes in contractility, however, shift the entire curve, either upward (increased contractility) or downward (decreased contractility), with concomitant change in V_{max}.

Clinical Note

Heart failure refers to reduced ability of the heart to pump blood to supply the tissues of the body. It is most often caused by coronary heart disease, chronic hypertension, or diabetes. Poor cardiac function can cause **peripheral edema** (swelling of ankles and legs resulting from retention of fluid), **pulmonary edema** (fluid in the alveoli of the lungs caused by high pulmonary vascular pressures), and **tiredness, shortness of breath,** and **limited exercise capacity.** It is treated through lifestyle changes, diet, and medications and is potentially a lethal disease. A variety of medical approaches are used to treat this complicated condition; these can include the use of inotropic drugs such as dopamine and dobutamine to increase contractility of the heart and diuretics to reduce excess fluid volume in the body.

REVIEW ANSWERS

A.   Zero

B.   Zero

C.   Contractility

D.   Preload

E.   In Part A, the third line should meet the other two at V_{max}, whereas in Part B, the third curve should illustrate a parallel shift downward with lower V_{max} as shown below.

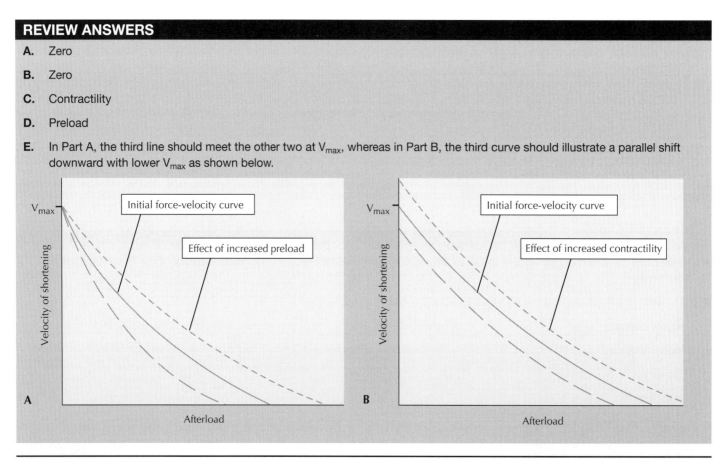

Plate 3.15

Cardiovascular Physiology

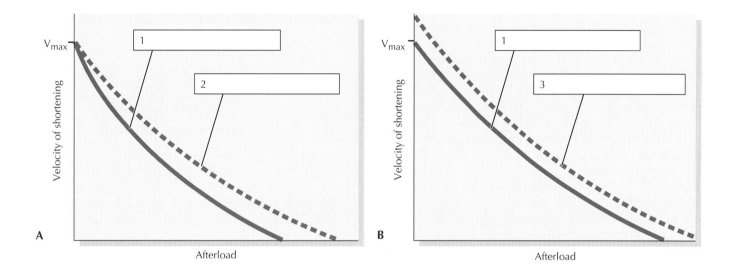

A

B

Afterload

Afterload

REVIEW QUESTIONS

A. The velocity of shortening is highest when afterload is _____.

B. With isometric contraction of cardiac muscle, velocity of shortening is, by definition, _____.

C. V_{max} is increased when _____ is elevated.

D. An increase in _____ will result in higher velocity of shortening except when the afterload is zero.

E. On each graph below, draw a third line, showing the effect of *reducing preload* (Part A) and *reducing contractility* (Part B).

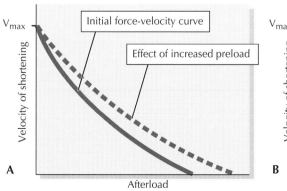

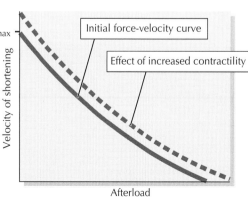

Initial force-velocity curve

Effect of increased preload

Initial force-velocity curve

Effect of increased contractility

A

B

Afterload

Afterload

A continuous plot of LVP against **left ventricular volume** during the cardiac cycle yields a closed loop. In Part A, the normal, resting loop is illustrated. When the loop is recorded starting at opening of the mitral valve (bottom left corner of the loop), the line segment traced until closing of that valve (bottom right corner of the loop) demonstrates the large increase in volume that occurs during diastole with only a modest rise in pressure. When the LV begins to contract, the closing of the mitral valve (bottom right corner of the loop) signals the start of **isometric contraction.** Pressure rises quickly while volume remains constant. When LVP reaches the aortic pressure (at the top right of the loop), the **aortic valve** opens, and ventricular **ejection** of blood into the aorta commences. At the end of ejection, the aortic valve closes (top left corner of the loop); the now relaxing ventricle enters into **isometric relaxation,** during which pressure falls rapidly while volume remains constant (at the **end-systolic volume [EDV]).**

Parts B through D of Plate 3.16 illustrate the effects of various manipulations on this loop. In Part B, an increase in preload (end-diastolic volume) results in an expansion of the loop to the right, and thus a greater **SV** is achieved through the Frank-Starling mechanism. An increase in **afterload** (arterial pressure) causes the loop to be taller because higher pressure must be achieved within the LV to open the aortic valve and eject blood (Part C). The loop is also narrower because the SV that can be ejected against the higher arterial pressure is diminished. In Part D, the effect of increased contractility of the LV (increasing **CO**) on the loop is illustrated. For example, with better **inotropic status** (also known as an increase in **cardiac contractility**) caused by administration of an inotropic drug, despite preload and initial afterload being unchanged, the SV is greater (thus the lower end-systolic volume).

LABEL the heart in Part A depicting:

- ☐ 1. Isometric period
- ☐ 2. Diastolic period

COLOR

- ☐ 3. Blood in RV (blue) to indicate the isometric state of the ventricles with valves closed
- ☐ 4. Blood in LV (red) to indicate the isometric state of the ventricles with valves closed
- ☐ 5. Arrow from the lumen of the RA into the RV, indicating the filling process taking place (blue)
- ☐ 6. Arrow from the LA into the LV (red)
- ☐ 7. Flow from the RV into the PA (blue)
- ☐ 8. Flow from the LV into the aorta, illustrating the flow during systole (red)

Clinical Note
Ejection fraction (EF) is defined as the proportion of EDV of a ventricle that is ejected:

$$EF = SV/EDV$$

This is a useful parameter in describing the pumping effectiveness of the ventricles. In a healthy heart (one with normal contractility), EF will be greater than 0.5 (50%).

EF is a more valid indicator of contractility of the heart than **dP/dt$_{max}$,** the maximum instantaneous rate of rise of the ventricular pressure during isometric contraction. The latter measurement requires catheterization of the heart and is load dependent, whereas EF can be measured with **echocardiographic techniques.**

REVIEW ANSWERS

- **A.** Isometric contraction
- **B.** Isometric relaxation
- **C.** SV
- **D.** Systolic pressure
- **E.** Preload (end-diastolic volume), contractility
- **F.** Afterload (arterial pressure)

Plate 3.16   **Cardiovascular Physiology**

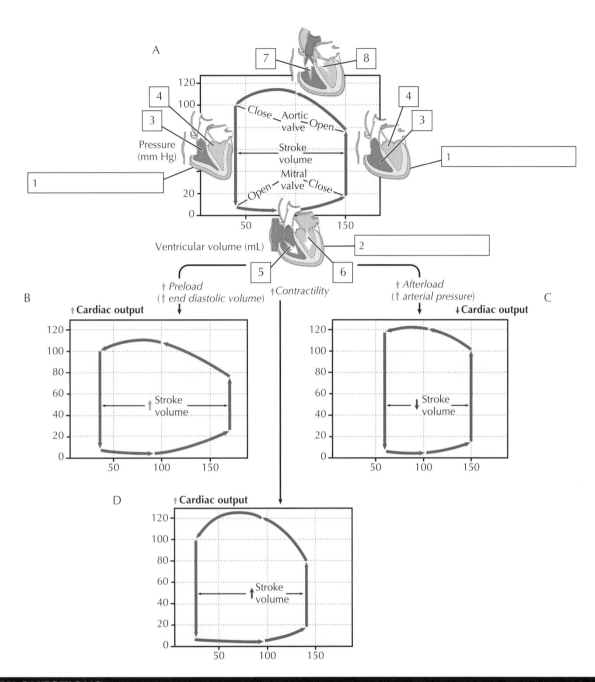

REVIEW QUESTIONS

A. The vertical line segment on the right side of the pressure-volume loop represents what phase of the cardiac cycle?

B. The vertical line segment on the left side of the pressure-volume loop represents what phase of the cardiac cycle?

C. The horizontal distance between the two vertical line segments represents _____.

D. The highest point reached in the loop is the left ventricular _____.

E. In this graphical paradigm, SV is increased by an increase in _____ or _____.

F. In this graphical paradigm, SV is diminished by an increase in _____.

The primary function of veins is to carry blood back to the heart, and thus the **systemic veins** carry **deoxygenated blood** toward the RA. At rest, systemic veins contain nearly two-thirds of our total blood volume, but **central venous pressure** (**CVP**, the pressure in the **venae cavae** near the RA) is only a few mm Hg. This CVP is the basis for preload on the heart and, under normal conditions, is approximately the same as RA pressure. Because of the great **compliance** of veins, they are able to accommodate the large volume at low pressure. Part A illustrates compliance of arteries and veins. Note that small changes in volume of the arterial system result in large changes in pressure, in contrast to the small changes in venous pressure. This **venous reservoir** of blood can be mobilized through **venoconstriction** to provide for adequate filling of the heart when blood volume is low or when additional preload is required to maintain high **CO,** for example, during aerobic exercise. The venous reservoir is mobilized through venoconstriction by the **SNS.** Constriction of veins raises the venous pressure and thus the CVP and preload on the heart.

Part B is a **vascular function curve,** which depicts the effect of CO on CVP or RA pressure. Under controlled, experimental conditions, alterations in CO have an opposite effect on CVP. A rise in CO produces a fall in CVP as the heart pumps blood more rapidly from the venous space toward the arterial side of the circulation. Conversely, when CO falls, CVP rises. If the heart were to stop beating suddenly (CO = 0 L/min), vascular pressures would equilibrate throughout the circulation at the mean circulatory pressure (MCP) of approximately 7 mm Hg.

Clinical Note

In a standing position, hydrostatic pressure in veins is significantly affected by gravity. Pressure in the veins of the lower part of the body is high as a result of the hydrostatic pressure exerted by the column of blood above, up to the RA. Because the veins are compliant, blood pools in the lower part of the body upon standing, causing a fall in CO and arterial blood pressure until the arterial baroreceptor reflex mechanism results in higher SNS activity. Higher HR, increased contractility, increased peripheral resistance, and, importantly, venoconstriction, all caused by the SNS, act to correct the fall in arterial blood pressure. **Orthostatic hypotension** is a clinical term referring to low blood pressure associated with a sudden change in posture from sitting or lying position to standing upright. **Lightheadedness** commonly occurs; **vertigo** (dizziness) and **syncope** (fainting) and other symptoms also may occur until physiological adjustments take place to correct arterial blood pressure. This condition can result from various causes of hypovolemia (dehydration, diarrhea, bleeding), anemia, various medications, and prolonged bed rest.

Plate 3.17

Cardiovascular Physiology

A. Compliance of arteries and veins

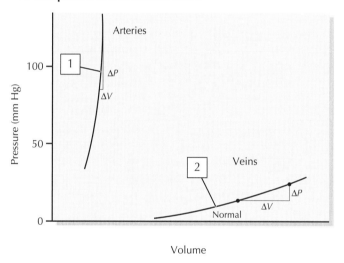

B. Vascular function curve

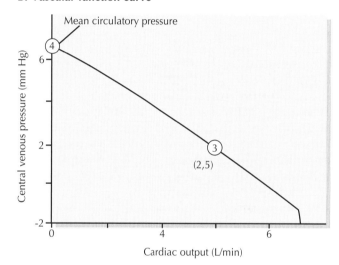

A. When CVP is measured while experimentally manipulating CO, CVP is highest when CO is _____.

B. Physiologically, venous compliance can be reduced through _____.

C. Orthostatic hypotension is more likely to occur when blood volume is _____.

D. The vascular function curve illustrates the effect of _____ on _____.

The interactions between vascular function and cardiac function can be illustrated by the simultaneous consideration of two relationships: the **cardiac function curve** (previously considered in Plate 3.14) and the **vascular function curve** (shown in Plate 3.17). The cardiac function curve results from the Frank-Starling relationship, in which **RAP** (preload) is the independent variable and **CO** is the dependent variable. Thus a rise in RAP (preload) results in a rise in CO. The vascular function curve is illustrated in an unconventional graph, in which the independent variable (CO) is plotted on the y-axis and the dependent variable (RAP) is on the x-axis (note that either RAP or CVP may be used to represent preload). This is an inverse relationship: a rise in CO produces a fall in RAP (or preload). Thus greater CO will result in redistribution of blood volume, with reduction of preload. Note that the x-intercept of the vascular function curve is **MCP,** which is the pressure in the system when CO is zero. It is dependent on blood volume and the compliance of the vascular system as a whole. Thus if the heart is stopped, pressure equilibrates across the entire system. Note that a positive MCP is necessary for the heart to pump blood effectively.

In Part A, the normal, resting relationship between the two curves is illustrated. The two lines intersect at the point where CO = 5 L/min and RAP = 2 mm Hg, the approximate values for these variables at rest. Conceptually, then, we can think about this intersection as the point of equilibrium between two opposing relationships (the effect of RAP on CO and the effect of CO on RAP); this is where the system achieves balance at rest. When one of the curves is displaced—for example, by a change in blood volume (Part B) or contractility (Part C)—the intersections will change. Note that changes in blood volume produce different intersections on the cardiac function curve (Part B), a result of the Frank-Starling mechanism; a change in contractility (Part C) produces altered intersection on the vascular function curve. With such manipulations, a new equilibrium point is established.

Clinical Note

In **heart failure,** the inotropic state (contractility) of the heart is weakened, most often as a result of coronary artery disease. This results in a shifting downward and to the right of the cardiac function curve (Part C), resulting in lowered CO and higher venous pressures. Over time, the body will respond, mainly through renal mechanisms, by retaining fluid, shifting the vascular function up and to the right. Although this has the effect of increasing CO to a point closer to normal, it is at the cost of even higher venous pressures, causing the "congestion" of congestive heart failure (peripheral and pulmonary edema) and greater work for an already failing heart.

REVIEW ANSWERS

A.   5 L/min, 2 mm Hg

B.   Depressed, depressed

C.   Increase, decrease

D.   Elevated

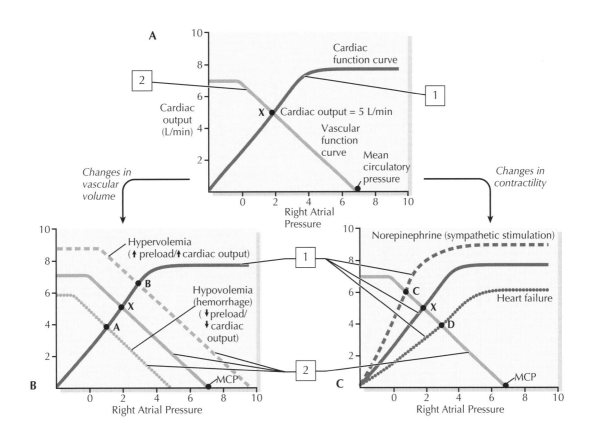

REVIEW QUESTIONS

A. At rest, the normal value for CO is _____ and the normal value for RAP is approximately _____.

B. With a fall in blood volume (e.g., due to hemorrhage) CO will tend to be _____ (depressed or elevated) and preload (RAP) will tend to be _____.

C. Administration of an inotropic drug will tend to _____ (increase or decrease) CO and _____ (increase or decrease) RAP or preload.

D. With heart failure, MCP will be _____ (depressed or elevated).

To fully appreciate the physiology of the peripheral circulation, it is important to understand the anatomy and histology of the vessels and the microcirculation. The vascular walls of arteries and veins have three tissue layers:

- **Tunica intima.** This innermost layer consists of a single layer of **endothelial cells,** which form the inner lining of the vessel and rest on a **basement membrane** that separates them from the second layer, the media.
- **Tunica media.** This second layer consists mainly of vascular smooth muscle cells, making it the contractile portion of the vessel wall.
- **Tunica adventitia.** This third layer consists mainly of connective tissue.

The vessel illustrated (Part A) is a large artery with prominent medial smooth muscle. Veins and arteries differ in absolute and relative thickness of media and adventitia, as do vessels of different sizes. Vessels also differ in types of connective tissue and cellular constituents in these layers. For example, large arteries are rich in elastic tissue and have relatively thick adventitia compared to smaller arteries. Smaller arteries have, on the other hand, a relatively more prominent, muscular medial layer. The walls of large arteries and veins have their own vascular supply within the adventitial layer, the **vaso vasora.** The tunica media of arteries is bounded by an **internal elastic membrane** and an **external elastic membrane. Capillaries,** unlike other vessel types, have only a tunica intima, consisting of a single layer of endothelial cells (endothelium) and basement membrane.

In Part B, the components of the microcirculation are illustrated. These include the **arterioles,** capillaries, and **venules. Metarterioles** are much like arterioles but have discontinuous smooth muscle in their medial layer. **Precapillary sphincters** are cuffs of smooth muscle found at the point where blood enters a capillary from an arteriole or metarteriole. It is the constriction of the smallest arteries, arterioles, and precapillary sphincters that regulates blood flow into capillary beds.

COLOR and LABEL

- [ ] 1. Tunica intima
- [ ] 2. Tunica media
- [ ] 3. Tunica adventitia
- [ ] 4. Arterioles
- [ ] 5. Metarterioles
- [ ] 6. Venules
- [ ] 7. Precapillary sphincter

REVIEW ANSWERS

A. Vaso vasora

B. Arteries

C. Tunica media

D. Endothelial cell layer, basement membrane (tunica intima)

Plate 3.19

Cardiovascular Physiology

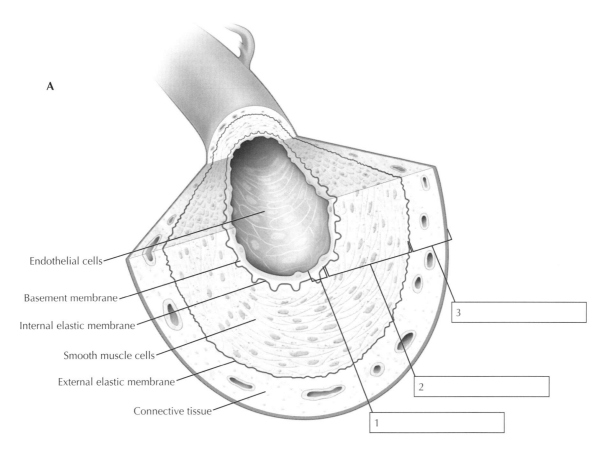

A

Endothelial cells
Basement membrane
Internal elastic membrane
Smooth muscle cells
External elastic membrane
Connective tissue

3

2

1

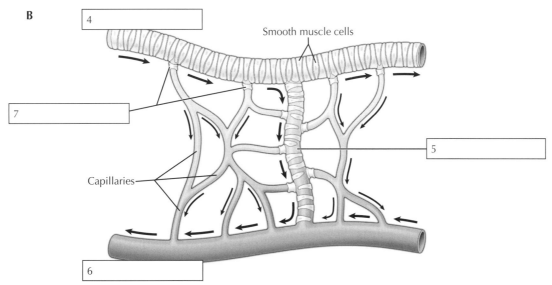

B

4

Smooth muscle cells

7

5

Capillaries

6

REVIEW QUESTIONS

A. In large arteries and veins, the vessel wall receives its own blood supply through the _____.

B. Internal and external elastic membranes are found in what type of vessel?

C. In arteries, the _____ is bounded by internal and external elastic membranes.

D. The capillary wall consists only of _____ and _____.

As blood flows through the circulation, it encounters the greatest resistance at the level of the small arteries and arterioles. The state of contraction or relaxation of these vessels is regulated by various **factors that act directly on vascular smooth muscle to cause contraction** (e.g., **norepinephrine acting at α-adrenergic receptors, vasopressin [ADH]), angiotensin II,** or relaxation (e.g., **epinephrine acting at β-adrenergic receptors, atrial natriuretic peptide [ANP]**). However, the endothelium can also play a role in determining the tone of underlying vascular smooth muscle through the production of vasoactive substances. Thus **shear stress, histamine, acetylcholine, bradykinin,** and other **"endothelium-dependent vasodilators"** activate the enzyme **nitric oxide synthase,** which converts the amino acid **arginine** to **nitric oxide (NO)** and the byproduct citrulline. This endothelium cell product NO, a short-lived free radical, readily diffuses to smooth muscle, where it stimulates vasodilation by elevating production of the second messenger cyclic guanosine monophosphate. Ultimately, free intracellular Ca^{2+} is sequestered, resulting in the smooth muscle relaxation. **Prostacyclin (PGI$_2$)** is also produced by endothelial cells in circumstances that stimulate NO production (i.e., elevated free intracellular Ca^{2+} in the endothelial cells). It is a product of the polyunsaturated membrane fatty acid **arachidonic acid** and is related to the **prostaglandins;** it, too, causes relaxation of smooth muscle cells and thus vasodilation.

In addition to the endothelium-derived vasodilators NO and PGI$_2$, endothelium can also be a source of **endothelin,** a vasoconstrictor peptide that is released during **pulmonary hypertension** and **vessel injury.** It acts directly on smooth muscle cells to elevate the level of free intracellular Ca^{2+} and thereby causes **vasoconstriction.** Thus vasodilation or vasoconstriction can be the direct result of a mediator acting on smooth muscle or may occur when endothelium, in response to a stimulus, releases a mediator that subsequently acts on underlying smooth muscle in the vascular wall. In Plate 3.20, endothelium-dependent and -independent pathways for vasoconstriction and vasodilation are illustrated.

TRACE the arrows showing:

☐ 1. Shear stress, histamine, acetylcholine, and bradykinin stimulate NO and PGI$_2$ synthesis by endothelial cells

☐ 2. NO and PGI$_2$ diffuse from the endothelium to the smooth muscle and cause vasodilation

☐ 3. Pulmonary hypertension and vessel injury stimulate endothelin release by endothelial cells

☐ 4. Endothelin produced by endothelium acts on smooth muscle to cause vasoconstriction

☐ 5. ANP acts directly on smooth muscle to cause vasodilation

☐ 6. Vasopressin (ADH) acts directly on smooth muscle to cause vasoconstriction

REVIEW ANSWERS

A. Peptide, vasoconstrictor (contraction)

B. Independent, vasodilator

C. Arachidonic acid, vasodilation (relaxation)

D. 6 seconds, endothelial cells

Plate 3.20

Cardiovascular Physiology

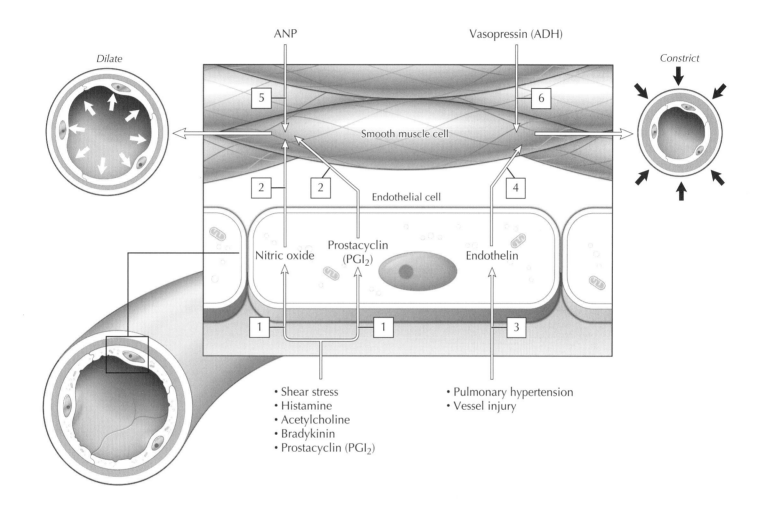

ANP

Vasopressin (ADH)

Dilate

Constrict

5

6

Smooth muscle cell

2

2

4

Endothelial cell

Nitric oxide

Prostacyclin (PGI₂)

Endothelin

1

1

3

• Shear stress
• Histamine
• Acetylcholine
• Bradykinin
• Prostacyclin (PGI₂)

• Pulmonary hypertension
• Vessel injury

REVIEW QUESTIONS

A. Chemically, endothelin is a _____; when released by endothelial cells, it causes _____.

B. Atrial natriuretic peptide is an endothelium- _____ (dependent or independent) _____ (vasoconstrictor or vasodilator).

C. Prostacyclin (PGI₂) is a product of _____ in endothelial cells and stimulates _____ in vascular smooth muscle.

D. NO has a biological half-life of _____; it is a vasodilator produced by _____.

Three mechanisms in regulation of local blood flow are metabolic regulation, autoregulation (also called *myogenic regulation*), and shear stress–induced vasodilation.

Metabolic regulation refers to the coupling of blood flow to a tissue to the rate of metabolism in that tissue. When metabolism in a tissue rises, the rate of production of metabolic products by that tissue is increased, and those metabolic products produce vasodilation. As an example, exercising skeletal muscle produces local accumulation of CO_2, H^+, K^+, lactic acid, adenosine, prostaglandins, and other products of metabolic activity. These accumulating substances produce vasodilation, which increases blood flow to the region and matches tissue perfusion to the level of metabolism. This relationship is illustrated in Part B. A period of increased metabolism produces increased blood flow. This phenomenon is also referred to as **active hyperemia** because the **increased blood flow** (hyperemia) is an active response to altered metabolism. **Reactive hyperemia** is a closely related phenomenon in which occlusion of blood flow to a tissue produces a large increase in blood flow (relative to the original flow rate) upon release of the occlusion. This reactive hyperemia is caused by buildup of substances mentioned previously (CO_2, H^+, lactic acid, K^+, adenosine) during the period of occlusion.

Myogenic regulation, or **autoregulation,** in contrast, is a mechanism for keeping flow relatively constant in the face of fluctuating perfusion pressure when tissue metabolism is relatively constant. Part C illustrates this effect. When perfusion pressure to a vascular bed rises, the flow rate rises as a result. However, within a short period, flow in vascular beds (where this mechanism is operant) returns to a level closer to the baseline. This happens because smooth muscle of the arteries and arterioles of the microcirculation constricts in response to stretch caused by the rise in transmural pressure, thus autoregulating blood flow. Note that myogenic regulation is a function of smooth muscle response to stretch and is not mediated by the endothelium of the vessels. In other words, it is an **endothelium-independent** phenomenon.

Shear stress–induced vasodilation is a third mechanism for local regulation. When blood flow velocity through an arterial vessel rises, the increased shear stress associated with the flow of blood along the endothelial surface stimulates the endothelium to produce the short-lived free radical vasodilator NO, which in turn stimulates relaxation of the underlying smooth muscle, thus further augmenting flow (see Plate 3.20). Obviously, this is an **endothelium-dependent** effect of shear stress.

To put these three mechanisms in context, they are not effective mechanisms for control of blood pressure or CO but are important in blood flow regulation within a local area, to maintain local blood flow at the appropriate level for local needs.

COLOR the area, if present, between the actual blood flow and the original blood flow representing:

☐ 1.   Increased blood flow
☐ 2.   Reduced blood flow

LABEL the period of:

☐ 3.   Basal blood flow
☐ 4.   Vascular occlusion
☐ 5.   Reactive hyperemia

REVIEW ANSWERS

A. Active, reactive hyperemia

B. Increased blood flow velocity across the endothelial cell surface

C. Endothelium independent

D. Shear stress–induced vasodilation

Plate 3.21   **Cardiovascular Physiology**

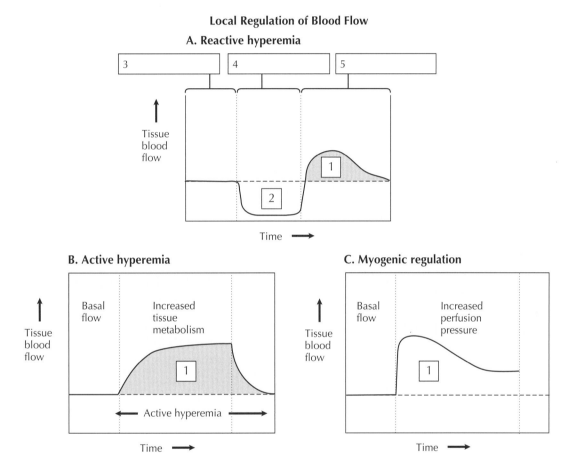

Local Regulation of Blood Flow

A. Reactive hyperemia

B. Active hyperemia

C. Myogenic regulation

REVIEW QUESTIONS

A. Two types of metabolic regulation are _____ and _____.

B. The physiological change that initiates shear stress induced vasodilation is _____.

C. Is myogenic regulation endothelium dependent or endothelium independent?

D. A drug that inhibits NO synthesis would be expected to block which of the mechanisms for local regulation of blood flow?

In contrast to mechanisms that regulate local blood flow (see Plate 3.21), neural and humoral mechanisms should be conceptualized mainly as systems for regulating broader parameters such as arterial blood pressure, blood volume, and blood osmolarity, as well as, in the case of the SNS, *distribution pattern* of blood flow.

The SNS, along with the arterial baroreceptor system, is the primary mechanism for **short-term regulation of arterial blood pressure** under normal conditions. Smooth muscle cells and the heart have several types of adrenergic receptors, including α- and β-receptors:

- **α-Receptors** mediate constrictor responses to catecholamines. **α_1-Receptors** are the primary vasoconstrictor receptor; these activate the IP_3 second messenger system, elevating free intracellular Ca^{2+} and thus causing contraction.
- **β_2-Receptors** mediate vasodilator responses to catecholamines; binding of these receptors activates the cyclic adenosine monophosphate second messenger system.
- **β_1-Receptors** mediate adrenergic effects on the SA node and AV node (increasing HR and conduction velocity) as well as cardiac muscle (increasing contractility). These receptors are also linked to the **cyclic adenosine monophosphate** second messenger system.

Responses of vessels to stimulation of sympathetic nerves depend on the type of adrenergic receptors present. In the arterial system, the major response is constriction, elevating peripheral resistance and thus raising arterial blood pressure. SNS activation also causes widespread constriction of veins, increasing venous pressure and enhancing preload on the heart. Note that sympathetic activation can also cause release of epinephrine from the adrenal medulla, with the circulating epinephrine acting as a hormone at many sites. In the vasculature, epinephrine is a much better agonist for β_1-receptors than norepinephrine, but both have strong affinity for α- and β_1-receptors.

Plate 3.22 illustrates several of the mechanisms regulating arterial blood pressure. This regulation is critical for maintaining adequate and relatively stable pressure necessary for perfusion of tissues throughout the body. Based on the biophysical relationship between pressure, flow, and resistance (see Plate 3.8) and the effects of blood volume and venous function on CO (see Plates 3.8 and 3.9), short-term regulation of arterial pressure involves regulation of CO and peripheral resistance, whereas long-term regulation of blood pressure requires control of blood volume. Monitoring of blood pressure occurs at these key points:

- Aortic arch and carotid sinus baroreceptors
- Renal juxtaglomerular apparatus
- Low-pressure (cardiopulmonary) baroreceptors

The extreme importance of the **arterial baroreceptors** in moment-to-moment regulation of arterial pressure has been discussed (see Plate 3.13). Afferent arterioles in the **renal juxtaglomerular apparatus** (see Plate 5.3) also contain **high-pressure baroreceptors** that regulate **renin** release and, consequently, sodium and water homeostasis, which is important in **long-term regulation** of blood pressure (considered further in Plate 3.23). Low-pressure baroreceptors in the heart and pulmonary circulation respond to changes in volume and modulate **SNS activity** and **vasopressin** release by the posterior pituitary gland. The **cardiac atria** release **ANP** in response to stretch and thus elevated blood volume (see Plate 3.13). In sum, changes in pressure and volume activate a number of systems, producing short-term arterial pressure regulation mainly through the arterial baroreceptor system and longer-term regulation of blood volume through additional mechanisms. Long-term regulation of pressure and volume is the subject of Plate 3.23.

COLOR

- ☐ 1. Afferent pathways from high-pressure baroreceptors to the brainstem's cardiovascular center
- ☐ 2. Afferent pathways from low-pressure baroreceptors in atria to the brainstem
- ☐ 3. Upward and downward arrows illustrating the effect of blood pressure changes on renin release

REVIEW ANSWERS

A. Cardiac atria (especially RA)

B. Arterial baroreceptor reflex

C. Reduced

Plate 3.22   **Cardiovascular Physiology**

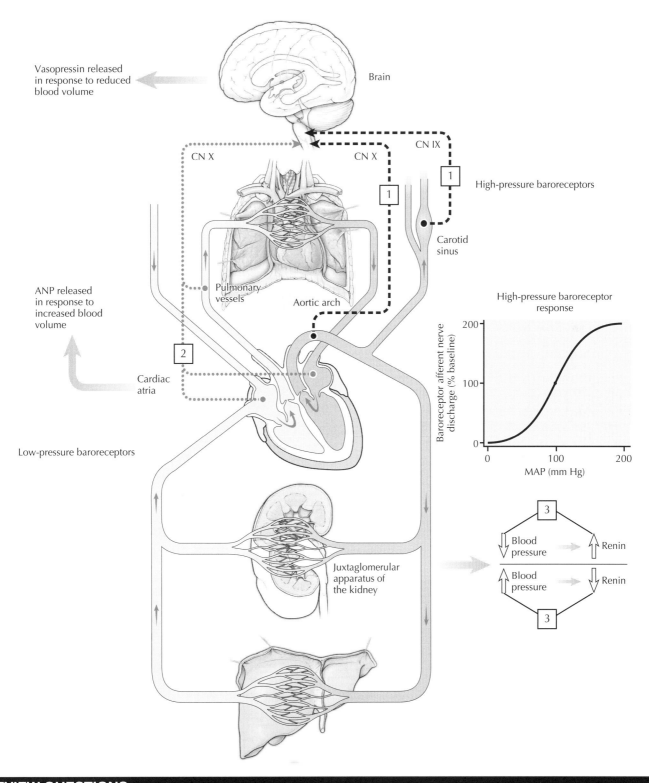

Vasopressin released
in response to reduced
blood volume

Brain

CN X

CN X

CN IX

High-pressure baroreceptors

1

1

Carotid
sinus

ANP released
in response to
increased blood
volume

Pulmonary
vessels

Aortic arch

High-pressure baroreceptor
response

2

Cardiac
atria

Low-pressure baroreceptors

Baroreceptor afferent nerve
discharge (% baseline)

200

100

0

0   100   200

MAP (mm Hg)

Juxtaglomerular
apparatus of
the kidney

3

↓ Blood
pressure   →   ↑ Renin

↑ Blood
pressure   →   ↓ Renin

3

REVIEW QUESTIONS

A. ANP is released into the bloodstream when a rise in blood volume causes stretch of the _____.

B. Rapid, short-term regulation of arterial blood pressure is mainly mediated through the _____.

C. The juxtaglomerular apparatus of the kidney releases renin when arterial blood pressure is _____.

In contrast to the reflexive, moment-to-moment regulation of arterial blood pressure relying mainly on baroreceptor reflexes and adjustment of cardiac and vascular function, **long-term regulation of arterial blood pressure** is accomplished mainly through control of blood volume by neural and humoral mechanisms. Thus changes in blood volume and pressure, in addition to evoking short-term adjustments, will stimulate the **renin-angiotensin-aldosterone system** (**RAAS;** see Part A).

When blood volume and pressure are decreased, and when sympathetic nerve activity to the kidney is activated (as will be the case when pressure is low), the **kidneys** produce **renin** (see Plate 5.5), an enzyme that cleaves plasma **angiotensinogen,** a protein synthesized by the **liver,** to form **angiotensin I.** Angiotensin I is subsequently cleaved to **angiotensin II** by **angiotensin-converting enzyme (ACE),** an enzyme found on the surface of endothelial cells, especially in the **lung** vasculature. Angiotensin II has direct effects on the kidney that cause sodium and water retention. It also acts at the adrenal cortex to stimulate **aldosterone** synthesis. Aldosterone is a steroid hormone that causes sodium (and thus water) retention by the kidney. The sum of these effects causes an increase in blood volume, and thus pressure. Note that decreased blood volume and pressure also cause posterior pituitary release of **antidiuretic hormone** (**ADH,** also known as vasopressin), a peptide hormone that increases renal water reabsorption; simultaneously, thirst is also stimulated and increased water intake contributes to the adjustment of blood volume and pressure.

In contrast, Part B shows the effects of increased blood volume and pressure. Under those circumstances, efferent SNS nerve activity is reduced, ADH secretion by the posterior pituitary is reduced, and the RAAS is inhibited (decreased renin secretion, and thus lower angiotensin I and II, as well as reduced aldosterone synthesis). **ANP** is released by atrial myocytes when the atria are stretched by the elevated blood volume; ANP inhibits aldosterone synthesis and acts directly at the kidney to increase sodium and thus water excretion. These pathways are covered in further detail in Chapter 5, Renal Physiology.

COLOR and **LABEL,** in Part A, the following organs that release enzymes or hormones that are part of the RAAS and contribute to stimulation of renal sodium and water reabsorption:

☐ 1.   Kidneys (release the enzyme renin)

☐ 2.   Liver (produces the protein angiotensinogen, which is cleaved by renin to produce angiotensin I)

☐ 3.   Lungs (major site of angiotensin I conversion to angiotensin II by ACE)

☐ 4.   Adrenal glands (angiotensin II stimulates aldosterone synthesis from the adrenal cortex)

LABEL, in Part B, the following changes in hormone release that contribute to the excretion of renal sodium and water in response to increased blood volume and pressure:

☐ 5.   ADH (ADH release is reduced when volume is elevated, reducing renal water reabsorption; see Plate 5.13)

☐ 6.   ANP (increased atrial stretch causes the release of ANP, which inhibits aldosterone release; it also has direct effects on the kidneys, increasing sodium and water excretion; see Plate 5.5)

TRACE the arrows leading to and from 1 through 4 and 5 and 6 in the above exercises, in **RED TO INDICATE AN INHIBITORY ACTION** or **GREEN TO INDICATE STIMULATORY ACTION.**

Clinical Note

The RAAS presents potential targets for antihypertensive drugs because inhibition of this system is a potential pathway for decreasing blood volume and therefore pressure. Thus ACE inhibitors (e.g., captopril and lisinopril) and angiotensin II receptor blockers (e.g., losartan, candesartan) are often used in treatment of high blood pressure, along with other therapies.

REVIEW ANSWERS

A.   Renin

B.   Increase

C.   Endothelial cells

D.   ANP

E.   Renin

Plate 3.23   **Cardiovascular Physiology**

A. Response to Decreased Blood Volume and Pressure

B. Response to Increased Blood Volume and Pressure

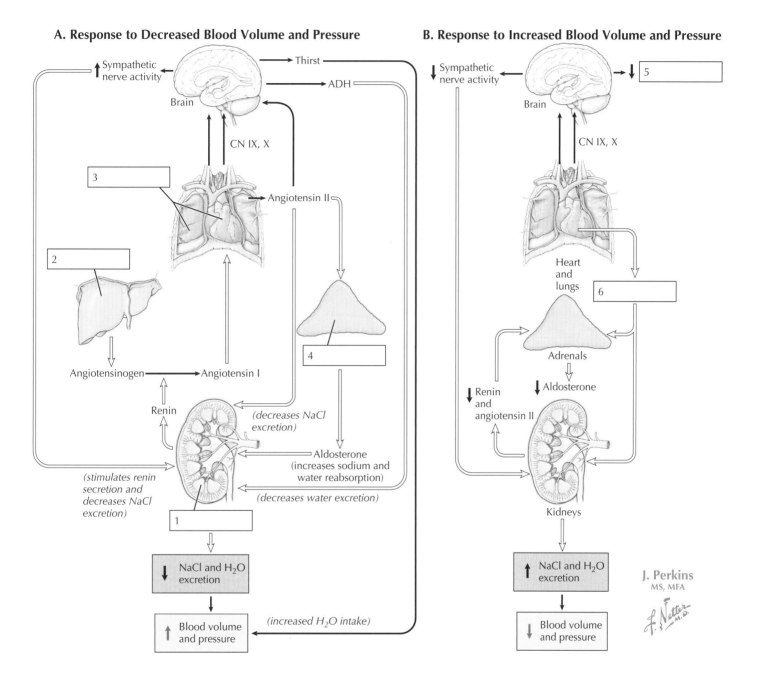

REVIEW QUESTIONS

A. Angiotensinogen is converted to angiotensin I by the action of the enzyme _____.

B. Aldosterone is a hormone that acts at the kidney to _____ salt and water reabsorption.

C. ACE is found on the surface of _____.

D. A significant rise in blood volume will cause release of the hormone _____.

E. Increased sympathetic nerve activity to the kidney will cause renal secretion of _____.

Blood flow to various tissues is regulated by local and extrinsic mechanisms (see earlier plates), but the importance of these mechanisms varies among tissues. In addition, there are unique aspects of blood flow regulation in some tissues. The figure illustrates some of these variations, which reflect the physiological functions and needs of the tissues. The **cerebral circulation** and coronary circulation are two circulations that merit special consideration based on their importance clinically and have some specific features that differ from other circulations (see Plate 3.25 for coronary circulation).

The cerebral circulation is supplied by the arterial **circle of Willis,** which is derived from the internal carotid and vertebral arteries. This circular structure provides a high degree of collateralization between the large arteries that supply blood to the **brain,** allowing continued flow to regions of the brain in case of injury or disease affecting one pathway. Because the brain is housed in a rigid case (the cranium), blood flow must be closely regulated to prevent poor perfusion on the one hand and high intracranial pressure on the other hand, because in either situation neuronal function will be negatively affected. Thus global cerebral blood flow is **autoregulated** (through myogenic regulation; Plate 3.21) at a constant level for mean arterial pressures between 50 and 150 mm Hg. Cerebral blood flow is also controlled by **arterial Pco$_2$.** High arterial Pco$_2$ will cause vasodilation and increased flow in the cerebral circulation, and low Pco$_2$ will have the opposite effect, although under normal conditions arterial Pco$_2$ does not vary greatly except in extreme exercise, hyperventilation, or hypoventilation. In terms of metabolic regulation, it can readily be demonstrated that *regional* blood flow within the brain varies according to the neuronal activity in those regions (remember that global flow is usually constant). However, the exact nature of this functional regulation is yet to be fully defined; it does not appear to be the result of typical metabolic regulation seen in other vascular beds.

In addition, these two related reflexes may affect cerebral blood flow in pathophysiological states:

- **Central nervous system ischemic reflex:** If the vasomotor control center in the medulla becomes ischemic, strong sympathetic outflow acts on the heart and peripheral vessels to elevate arterial blood pressure in a last-ditch attempt to reverse the brain ischemia by increasing cerebral flow (note that cerebral vessels themselves have little or no SNS innervation).
- **Cushing reflex:** Extreme elevation of intracranial pressure (usually associated with traumatic brain injury) will impede cerebral blood flow. A strong sympathetic outflow will result, raising arterial pressure in an attempt to increase blood flow to the brain. Again, this is a last-ditch effort to maintain perfusion of the brain, and this condition is usually fatal.

LABEL the vascular beds:

☐ 1. Brain, which has a dominant autoregulation over a wide range of MAP (brain)

☐ 2. Coronary arteries, which are normally affected by compression of arteries by extravascular forces

☐ 3. Liver and intestines; liver has flow greatly exceeding its metabolic requirements at rest, and lower gastro-intestinal (GI) tract responds to both PNS and ANS.

☐ 4. Kidneys, which also have flow greatly exceeding its metabolic requirements at rest

☐ 5. Skin, which has a prominent role in thermoregulation

☐ 6. Skeletal muscle, which has the greatest increase in flow during exercise, driven by metabolic vasodilation

☐ 7. Lungs, which undergo arterial constriction in a low O$_2$ environment

REVIEW ANSWERS

A. Autoregulation (myogenic regulation)

B. Elevation of intracranial pressure

C. Arterial blood

D. Thermoregulation

E. Metabolic regulation

Plate 3.24   **Cardiovascular Physiology**

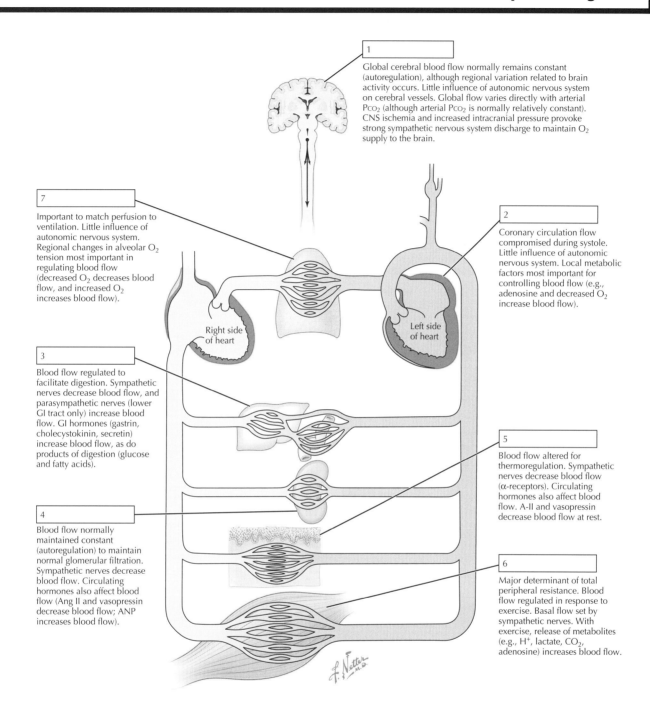

1

Global cerebral blood flow normally remains constant (autoregulation), although regional variation related to brain activity occurs. Little influence of autonomic nervous system on cerebral vessels. Global flow varies directly with arterial P_{CO_2} (although arterial P_{CO_2} is normally relatively constant). CNS ischemia and increased intracranial pressure provoke strong sympathetic nervous system discharge to maintain O_2 supply to the brain.

7

Important to match perfusion to ventilation. Little influence of autonomic nervous system. Regional changes in alveolar O_2 tension most important in regulating blood flow (decreased O_2 decreases blood flow, and increased O_2 increases blood flow).

2

Coronary circulation flow compromised during systole. Little influence of autonomic nervous system. Local metabolic factors most important for controlling blood flow (e.g., adenosine and decreased O_2 increase blood flow).

Right side of heart

Left side of heart

3

Blood flow regulated to facilitate digestion. Sympathetic nerves decrease blood flow, and parasympathetic nerves (lower GI tract only) increase blood flow. GI hormones (gastrin, cholecystokinin, secretin) increase blood flow, as do products of digestion (glucose and fatty acids).

5

Blood flow altered for thermoregulation. Sympathetic nerves decrease blood flow (α-receptors). Circulating hormones also affect blood flow. A-II and vasopressin decrease blood flow at rest.

4

Blood flow normally maintained constant (autoregulation) to maintain normal glomerular filtration. Sympathetic nerves decrease blood flow. Circulating hormones also affect blood flow (Ang II and vasopressin decrease blood flow; ANP increases blood flow).

6

Major determinant of total peripheral resistance. Blood flow regulated in response to exercise. Basal flow set by sympathetic nerves. With exercise, release of metabolites (e.g., H^+, lactate, CO_2, adenosine) increases blood flow.

REVIEW QUESTIONS

A. The most important mechanism for regulating global cerebral blood flow under normal conditions is _____.

B. In the Cushing reflex, the initiating stimulus for increased SNS activity is elevation of _____.

C. Blood flow to the brain will be increased by elevation of CO_2 in _____.

D. Skin blood flow is adjusted as part of the process of _____.

E. In skeletal muscle, resting blood flow is affected by the SNS, but during exercise, flow is mainly affected by

_____.

The **coronary circulation** is of extreme clinical interest, given that **coronary heart disease** is the most common cause of death throughout the world. The coronary circulation is fed by the **right** and **left coronary arteries** originating at the base of the aorta (see illustration). The epicardial arteries on the surface of the heart send branches into the heart wall to form a very extensive microcirculation to serve the highly metabolically active cardiac muscle. The venous drainage of this circulation returns blood to the **coronary sinus,** which empties into the RA. The layers of the heart wall, from inside to out, are the **endocardium** (a single layer of endothelial cells and its basement membrane), the thick, muscular myocardium, and the outer **epicardium** (connective tissue).

Flow to the myocardium is affected by factors that are in some ways different from those regulating other vascular beds. In particular:

- **Compression** of the coronary circulation by **extravascular pressure** generated by contraction of the myocardium
- Powerful **metabolic vasodilation** during diastole

To generate the normal arterial pressure of 120/80 mm Hg, the LV and, in particular, the inner subendocardial third of the myocardium must generate extravascular pressure higher than left ventricular and arterial pressures. This intramyocardial pressure impedes left coronary artery flow during systole. In the lower figure of the illustration, note the sharp drop in left coronary flow just before the rise in arterial pressure. At this time, the heart is in the isometric contraction period and extravascular pressure is being rapidly generated. Left coronary flow remains relatively low for the balance of systole, but at the beginning of diastole, note the large, steep rise in flow. This is caused by two factors: the rapid fall in intramyocardial pressure as the heart undergoes isometric relaxation and the buildup of metabolites during the preceding systole. In the coronary circulation, **adenosine** is particularly important among the metabolites as a **coronary vasodilator.**

In contrast to the high flow in the left coronary during diastole, right coronary flow is highest during systole and follows a pattern similar to arterial pressure curve (top graph). This is because the right ventricular wall does not generate the high pressures seen in the left wall (RVP is 25/0 compared to 120/0 mm Hg in the LV).

Coronary arteries are innervated by sympathetic nerves, but when the SNS is activated, work of the heart is increased and metabolic vasodilation largely overrides vascular sympathetic effects in this circulation.

LABEL and COLOR

- ☐ 1.   Right coronary artery and its branches
- ☐ 2.   Left coronary artery and branches
- ☐ 3.   Coronary sinus and veins feeding into it
- ☐ 4.   Systolic section
- ☐ 5.   Diastolic sections

Clinical Note

Atherosclerosis is the buildup of plaque in the wall of arteries, potentially limiting flow. In coronary arteries, a common site for plaque formation, it may lead to coronary heart disease and even **myocardial infarction** (damage and necrosis of cardiac tissue) and death. Risk factors for atherosclerosis include hypertension, high plasma cholesterol, diabetes, smoking, obesity, poor diet, sedentary lifestyle, and family history. Plaque development begins with fatty streaks in arteries that may occur even in children and progresses asymptomatically for years. Eventually, with significant narrowing of the coronary lumen, symptoms such as angina (chest pain), sweating, breathlessness, and palpitation may occur as a result of myocardial ischemia and its effects. When atherosclerosis culminates in an acute cardiac event such as **unstable angina** (acute, severe chest pain in the absence of significant physical activity) or myocardial infarction, the precipitating cause is often plaque rupture and coronary thrombosis.

REVIEW ANSWERS

A.   Metabolic vasodilation, extravascular compression (intramyocardial pressure effects)

B.   Metabolic vasodilation

C.   Adenosine

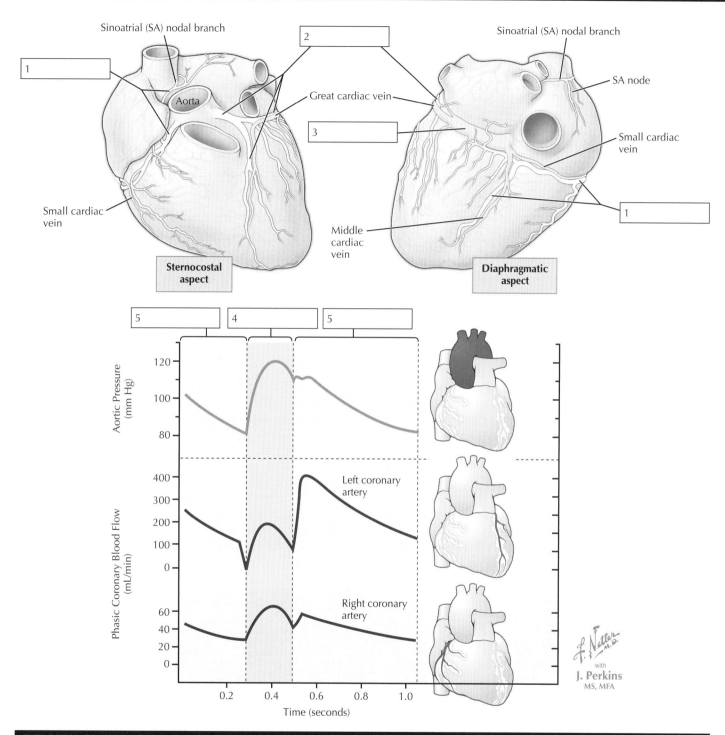

Sinoatrial (SA) nodal branch

1

Aorta

Small cardiac
vein

Sternocostal
aspect

2

Great cardiac vein

3

Middle
cardiac
vein

Sinoatrial (SA) nodal branch

SA node

Small cardiac
vein

1

Diaphragmatic
aspect

5 4 5

Aortic Pressure (mm Hg)

120

100

80

Phasic Coronary Blood Flow (mL/min)

400

300

200

100

0

Left coronary
artery

60

40

20

0

Right coronary
artery

0.2   0.4   0.6   0.8   1.0

Time (seconds)

f. Netter
M.D.

with
J. Perkins
MS, MFA

REVIEW QUESTIONS

A. The two most important factors that affect coronary flow and its regulation, particularly in the left coronary artery, are
_____ and _____.

B. Although the SNS innervates coronary arteries, its effects on those arteries are usually overridden by
_____ when the SNS is activated.

C. Among the typical metabolic products released during tissue metabolism, in the heart, _____ is of special significance as a coronary vasodilator.

3 | Fetal and Neonatal Circulation

The **fetal circulation** has specific features that allow for development of the fetus and its cardiovascular system and for rapid transition to the postnatal environment at birth. It has six structures that are not normally seen in adults:

- **Two umbilical arteries** that branch from the systemic arterial system and carry blood to the placental circulation, where exchange of gases, nutrients, and waste takes place.
- The **umbilical vein** that returns blood to the systemic venous circulation, carrying oxygen and nutrients to the fetus.
- The **ductus venosus,** which is a shunt from the umbilical vein to the **inferior vena cava.** Most of the oxygenated, nutrient-rich blood returning from the placental circulation flows through the liver, but a portion passes through this shunt directly into the venous circulation and back to the RA.
- The **foramen ovale,** a **right-to-left** shunt between the atria, which allows most of the blood from the inferior vena cava to bypass the pulmonary circulation and flow directly to the LA.
- The **ductus arteriosus,** a second right-to-left shunt, which conducts blood from the **PA** to the aorta. Approximately 90% of blood entering the PA bypasses the lungs through this shunt.

At birth, closure of the umbilical vessels occurs because of vasospasm (or physical clamping by the labor and delivery team). As the baby begins breathing, lung inflation and exposure to oxygen-rich air lower resistance of the pulmonary circulation, reducing pulmonary artery pressure and reversing blood flow direction through the ductus arteriosus. Exposure of the ductus to the high oxygen tension in blood from the aorta that has been oxygenated in the lungs initiates its closure. With increased flow of blood to the LA from the pulmonary veins and reduced flow of blood to the RA from the inferior vena cava as a result of loss of the placental circulation, LAP exceeds RAP, causing a flap of tissue (a valve) to functionally close the foramen ovale. Through these processes, the six structures normally become functionally closed, establishing the separation of oxygenated and deoxygenated blood (the series circulation), although complete anatomical closure takes more time. Anatomical remnants of the structures are illustrated in Part B.

LABEL and **COLOR** the structures unique to the fetal circulation and note areas where oxygenated blood is not mixed with venous blood:

- ☐ 1. Two umbilical arteries
- ☐ 2. Umbilical vein, area where oxygenated blood is not mixed with venous blood
- ☐ 3. Ductus venosus, area where oxygenated blood is not mixed with venous blood
- ☐ 4. Foramen ovale
- ☐ 5. Ductus arteriosus

LABEL and **COLOR** the remnants of those structures (above) in postnatal circulation to illustrate what ultimately remains from the fetal circulation:

- ☐ 6. Medial umbilical ligaments
- ☐ 7. Ligamentum teres
- ☐ 8. Ligamentum venosus
- ☐ 9. Fossa ovalis
- ☐ 10. Ligamentum arteriosum

Clinical Note

The ductus arteriosus normally begins to close at birth, attaining complete closure by 3 weeks. **Patent ductus arteriosus (PDA)** is the condition in which the ductus fails to close completely. This condition can be asymptomatic early on but can progress to more serious disease if not eventually treated. One of the common clinical signs leading to diagnosis is a continuous heart murmur that is accentuated during systole.

REVIEW ANSWERS

A. Placental vein (and ductus venosus)

B. Ductus venosus

C. RA, LA

D. PA, aorta (right to left shunt)

Plate 3.26   **Cardiovascular Physiology**

A. Prenatal circulation

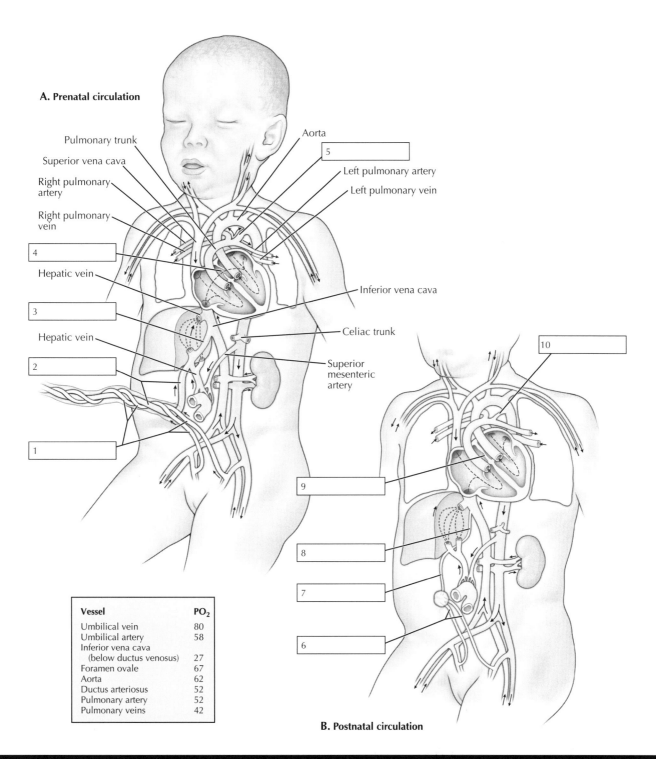

Pulmonary trunk

Superior vena cava

Right pulmonary artery

Right pulmonary vein

4

Hepatic vein

3

Hepatic vein

2

1

Aorta

5

Left pulmonary artery

Left pulmonary vein

Inferior vena cava

Celiac trunk

Superior mesenteric artery

10

9

8

7

6

Vessel	PO_2
Umbilical vein	80
Umbilical artery	58
Inferior vena cava (below ductus venosus)	27
Foramen ovale	67
Aorta	62
Ductus arteriosus	52
Pulmonary artery	52
Pulmonary veins	42

B. Postnatal circulation

REVIEW QUESTIONS

A. In the fetus, the highest oxygen concentration of blood is observed in the _____.

B. The _____ is a shunt between the umbilical vein and the inferior vena cava of a fetus.

C. Blood passes from the _____ to the _____ through the foramen ovale.

D. In the fetus, the direction of blood flow through the ductus arteriosus is from the _____ to the _____.

3 Circulatory Response to Exercise

During **dynamic (aerobic) exercise,** broad changes are required of the cardiovascular system to support the increased performance of work by the body. The regulation of arterial pressure and blood flow during exercise is a complex process, occurring in the face of large changes in **CO** and **regional resistances.** The rhythmic contraction of large skeletal **muscle** groups—for example, during swimming or jogging—requires delivery of proportionally more arterial blood to support oxygen consumption and remove CO_2 and other products of **aerobic metabolism.** In a young, athletic person, CO can rise from the resting level of 5 L/min to as much as 20 to 30 L/min, reflecting increases in both **HR** and **SV.**

SNS activation supports those increases, while producing vasoconstriction and reduced flow (as a proportion of CO) in many vascular beds but not all regional circulations:

- **Skeletal muscle** blood flow increases dramatically as constrictor effects of catecholamines released by the SNS are overridden by metabolic vasodilation (and to some extent by activation of β_2-adrenergic receptors) in the vasculature of working muscle.
- **Coronary** blood flow increases as a result of metabolic vasodilation as the heart performs greater work in pumping more blood. **Adenosine** released by working cardiac cells has a prominent role.
- **Cutaneous** blood flow is initially reduced due to SNS activation, but as exercise progresses, increased core body temperature results in **cutaneous vasodilation** to aid in thermoregulation.

TPR is greatly reduced as a result of the vasodilation in skeletal muscle vascular beds; thus aerobic exercise is associated with high CO and low resistance. The low TPR and SNS-induced **venoconstriction** help support venous pressure and therefore the cardiac filling pressure (preload) necessary in this high output state. Meanwhile, **mean arterial blood pressure** is typically not changed substantially, but the greater SV and low TPR are reflected in the higher systolic arterial pressure and lower diastolic arterial pressures.

CIRCLE the symbol +, −/+, or − (increased, relatively unchanged, decreased) corresponding to the changes occurring during exercise for blood flow in each organ as a percentage of CO.

- ☐ 1. Brain
- ☐ 2. Lung
- ☐ 3. Liver and splanchnic beds
- ☐ 4. Kidneys
- ☐ 5. Skin
- ☐ 6. Muscle

CIRCLE the symbol +, −/+, or −, corresponding to the changes occurring during exercise.

- ☐ 7. HR
- ☐ 8. CO

REVIEW ANSWERS

A. SNS activation

B. Skeletal muscle vasculature

C. Venoconstriction, reduced TPR

D. 25 L/min

E. SNS activation

Plate 3.27

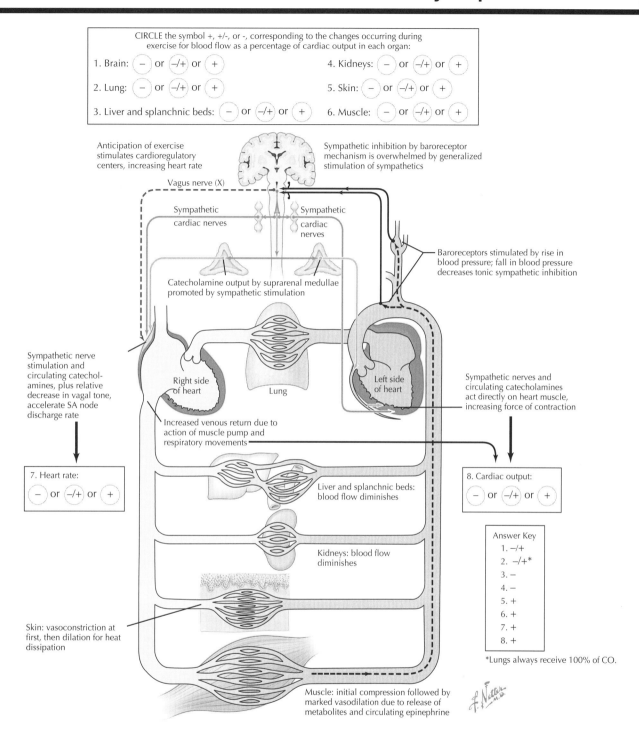

CIRCLE the symbol +, +/-, or -, corresponding to the changes occurring during exercise for blood flow as a percentage of cardiac output in each organ:

1. Brain: (−) or (−/+) or (+)   4. Kidneys: (−) or (−/+) or (+)

2. Lung: (−) or (−/+) or (+)   5. Skin: (−) or (−/+) or (+)

3. Liver and splanchnic beds: (−) or (−/+) or (+)   6. Muscle: (−) or (−/+) or (+)

Anticipation of exercise stimulates cardioregulatory centers, increasing heart rate

Sympathetic inhibition by baroreceptor mechanism is overwhelmed by generalized stimulation of sympathetics

Vagus nerve (X)

Sympathetic cardiac nerves

Sympathetic cardiac nerves

Baroreceptors stimulated by rise in blood pressure; fall in blood pressure decreases tonic sympathetic inhibition

Catecholamine output by suprarenal medullae promoted by sympathetic stimulation

Sympathetic nerve stimulation and circulating catechol-amines, plus relative decrease in vagal tone, accelerate SA node discharge rate

Right side of heart

Lung

Left side of heart

Sympathetic nerves and circulating catecholamines act directly on heart muscle, increasing force of contraction

Increased venous return due to action of muscle pump and respiratory movements

7. Heart rate:

(−) or (−/+) or (+)

8. Cardiac output:

(−) or (−/+) or (+)

Liver and splanchnic beds: blood flow diminishes

Kidneys: blood flow diminishes

Answer Key
1. −/+
2. −/+*
3. −
4. −
5. +
6. +
7. +
8. +

*Lungs always receive 100% of CO.

Skin: vasoconstriction at first, then dilation for heat dissipation

Muscle: initial compression followed by marked vasodilation due to release of metabolites and circulating epinephrine

REVIEW QUESTIONS

A. During exercise, renal blood flow is reduced by what mechanism?

B. The greatest increase in regional blood flow during dynamic exercise occurs in _____.

C. During aerobic exercise, preload to the heart is increased as a result of _____ and _____.

D. If CO rises to 25 L/min during exercise, PA blood flow will be _____.

E. During exercise, contractility of the heart is raised by _____.

Chapter 4 Respiratory Physiology

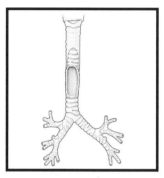
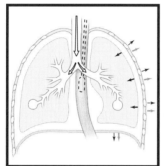
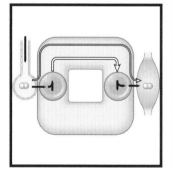
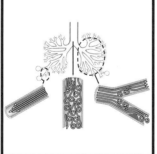

The **respiratory system** consists of the lungs, airways, and muscles of breathing, with its primary function being the exchange of oxygen and carbon dioxide between the body and the atmosphere. It has important roles in a variety of other processes, including acid-base regulation, immune function, temperature regulation, and metabolic functions.

In Part A, review the series circulation of the cardiovascular system. The resting cardiac output of 5 L/min is the same on both sides of the heart. Of the 5 L total blood volume in an average-sized adult, only about 9% is in the pulmonary circulation. The systemic circulation is characterized by high pressure and high resistance, in contrast to **low pressure and low resistance** in the pulmonary system. Resting **pulmonary artery pressure (PAP)** is approximately 25/8 mm Hg, compared to 120/80 mm Hg in the aorta. Likewise, right ventricular pressure is 25/0 mm Hg compared to 120/0 mm Hg for the left ventricle. Because the circulations are in series, any changes in left-side cardiac output must be matched by changes in pulmonary blood flow.

Much of the "control" of **pulmonary vascular resistance (PVR)** is passive. In Part B, the effect of increased pulmonary vascular pressure on PVR is illustrated. When PAP rises—for example, with the increased cardiac output during physical exercise—PVR falls, limiting the extent of the rise in PAP. This fall in PVR is due to **distension** of pulmonary vessels, which are thinner walled than systemic vessels, as well as **recruitment** (opening) of some vessels that were collapsed at lower PAP. This reduction in PVR at higher PAP is important in allowing the series circulation to function smoothly over a range of cardiac output levels.

Another passive factor that affects PVR is **lung volume.** Within the lung, the **alveoli** (the minute air sacs) are surrounded by **alveolar capillaries** (see Plate 4.3) to allow for gas exchange. As the lung is inflated, the expansion of alveoli tends to impinge on blood flow through the alveolar vessels, while the **extra-alveolar vessels** tend to be pulled open as the lung expands. Thus, if the lung is collapsed, resistance is relatively high. As it is inflated from that point, resistance first falls, as extra-alveolar vessels are pulled open, but with overinflation, flow through the alveolar vessels is impeded (see Part C), raising resistance.

As a result, a J-shaped curve is produced, with the **lowest PVR at intermediate volume** when PVR is plotted against lung volume.

PVR can also be affected by various vasoconstrictors (e.g., α-adrenergic agonists, thromboxane, endothelin) and vasodilators (e.g., nitric oxide, prostacyclin), but these actions are usually less important physiologically than passive factors (see previously). One factor that is important in control of resistance in pulmonary vessels is $P_{A_{O_2}}$ **(partial pressure of O_2 in alveolar air).** If $P_{A_{O_2}}$ falls in a region of the lung, vessels exposed to low P_{O_2} constrict, redirecting blood flow to areas of the lung that are better ventilated.

COLOR, in Parts A and B, the blood flowing through the cardiovascular system, noting oxygenation of blood in the pulmonary capillaries:

- ☐ 1. Deoxygenated blood (blue)
- ☐ 2. Oxygenated blood (red)
- ☐ 3. Mixed blood in capillaries (purple)

COLOR in Part C:

- ☐ 4. Alveoli, noting the effect of lung volume (illustrated as alveolar size in the diagram) on alveolar capillaries

---

REVIEW ANSWERS

A. Passive

B. Intermediate

C. $P_{A_{O_2}}$

D. 25/8 mm Hg, 25/0 mm Hg

Plate 4.1 **Respiratory Physiology**

A. Pulmonary and systemic circulations

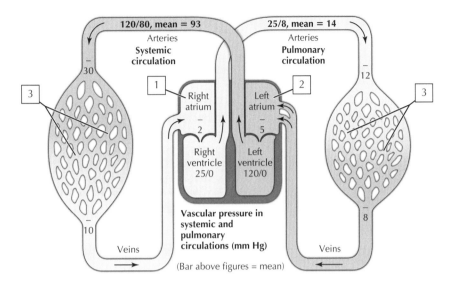

B. Effects of increases in pulmonary blood flow and vascular pressures

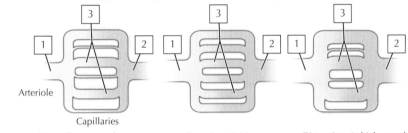

Arteriole

Capillaries

Normally some pulmonary capilliaries are closed and conduct no blood

Recruitment: More capillaries open as pulmonary vascular pressure or blood flow increases

Distension: At high vascular pressures individual capillaries widen and acquire a larger cross-sectional area

C. Effects of lung volume

Extra-alveolar vessels

Alveolar vessels

Low lung volume

High lung volume

As lung volume increases, increasing traction on extra-alveolar capillaries produces distension, and their resistance falls. Alveolar vessels, in contrast, are compressed by enlarging alveoli, and their resistance increases.

REVIEW QUESTIONS

A. Matching of pulmonary to systemic blood flow is mainly accomplished through _____ control of PVR.

B. PVR is lowest at _____ (low, intermediate, or high) lung volume.

C. Normally, the most important factor in active control of pulmonary vascular resistance is _____.

D. Normal resting pulmonary artery pressure is approximately _____, whereas normal right ventricular pressure is approximately _____.

The lungs include the three lobes of the right lung and two lobes of the left lung (Part A). Vessels, bronchi, lymphatics, and nerves enter at the **hilum** of each lung. The **airways include the trachea,** which branches to become the **right and left main bronchi,** which enter the lungs and branch further to become the **smaller bronchi** and eventually **bronchioles** (Parts B and C). Approximately **23 generations** of airways exist, starting with the trachea and leading to the bronchioles, which lead into the alveoli; airways become smaller and more numerous with each generation.

The **conducting zone** of the respiratory system includes airways from the trachea to the terminal bronchioles. Through this zone no gas exchange takes place; thus it is also known as **anatomic dead space** (gas exchange only occurs in the **respiratory bronchioles and alveoli;** see Plate 4.3). The trachea has cartilaginous rings around three-quarters of its circumference, maintaining the patency of the tube but allowing coughing (the other quarter of the circumference is muscle). Plates of **cartilage** exist in bronchi but not in bronchioles.

Most of the conducting system is lined with **ciliated, pseudostratified columnar epithelial cells,** mucus-secreting **goblet cells,** and several other cell types. The ciliated cells and mucus-secreting cells constitute the majority of the lining in large airways, with the mucus protecting against desiccation and trapping inspired particles, and the ciliated cells sweeping trapped particles upward toward the mouth.

In the bronchioles, the epithelium becomes ciliated **cuboidal epithelium,** which constitutes the majority of the lining. Goblet cells diminish and are lost by the terminal bronchioles. **Club cells** (formerly known as Clara cells) in bronchioles secrete various substances that line the bronchioles and play a role in the defense system of the lungs.

The walls of the conducting airways also contain **smooth muscle cells** that are regulated by the autonomic nervous system. The **sympathetic nervous system** dilates airways; the **parasympathetic nervous system** constricts airways.

COLOR and LABEL

- [ ] 1. Pulmonary arteries (blue, indicating deoxygenated blood)
- [ ] 2. Bronchi
- [ ] 3. Superior and inferior pulmonary veins (red, indicating oxygenated blood)
- [ ] 4. Lymph nodes (green)
- [ ] 5. Tracheal cartilage
- [ ] 6. Tracheal mucosa
- [ ] 7. Cartilage
- [ ] 8. Tracheal epithelium
- [ ] 9. Trachealis muscle

REVIEW ANSWERS

- **A.** Terminal bronchioles
- **B.** Cartilage, smooth muscle
- **C.** Goblet cells, ciliary action
- **D.** Parasympathetic, sympathetic

Plate 4.2   **Respiratory Physiology**

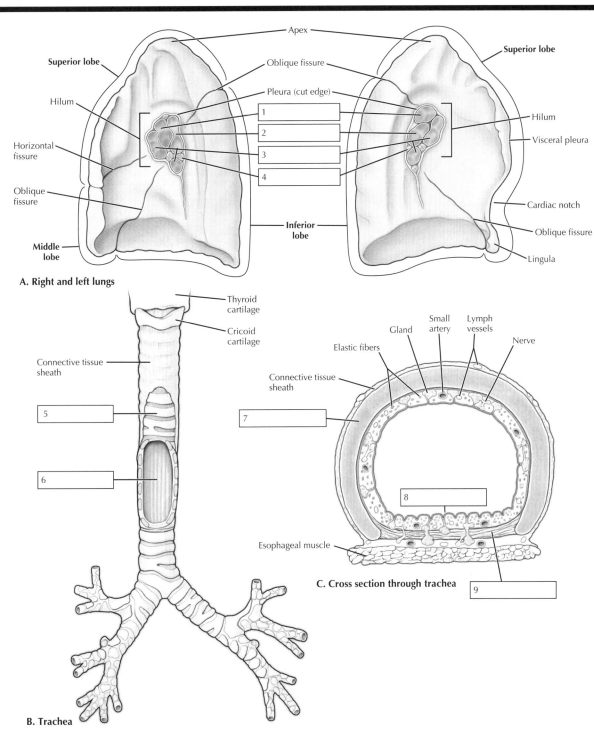

Apex

Superior lobe

Oblique fissure

Pleura (cut edge)

Hilum

Horizontal fissure

Oblique fissure

Middle lobe

Superior lobe

Hilum

Visceral pleura

Cardiac notch

Oblique fissure

Lingula

Inferior lobe

1
2
3
4

A. Right and left lungs

Thyroid cartilage

Cricoid cartilage

Connective tissue sheath

5

6

B. Trachea

Elastic fibers

Connective tissue sheath

Gland

Small artery

Lymph vessels

Nerve

7

8

Esophageal muscle

9

C. Cross section through trachea

REVIEW QUESTIONS

A. Cartilage is found in all segments of the conducting zone except the _____.

B. Three-quarters of the tracheal circumference is _____, and one-quarter of the wall is _____ .

C. Particulate matter in the conducting zone is trapped in mucus secreted by _____ and is swept toward the mouth by _____.

D. Constriction of airways is stimulated by the _____ nervous system, whereas dilation is stimulated by the _____ nervous system.

Netter's Physiology Coloring Book

Plate 4.2

4 Respiratory Zone of the Lungs

Inspired air enters the **conducting zone of the respiratory system** at the trachea, which eventually leads, through many branchings, to the **terminal bronchioles,** which give rise to the **respiratory bronchioles,** the first part of the **respiratory zone.** From there, inspired air enters the **alveolar ducts** and then the **alveolar sacs (alveoli).** The **acini** of the lungs are its functional units and make up the respiratory zone (Part A). There are estimated to be 300 million alveoli in the human lungs, with an area for gas exchange of 50 to 100 m^2. The efficiency of gas exchange in the lungs is a function of this large exchange area, the thinness of the **alveolar-capillary membrane** between the alveoli and capillaries, and the "sheet flow" of blood through the alveolar capillaries, which surround the alveoli.

Alveoli are lined by type I and type II epithelial cells (Part B). **Type I alveolar epithelial cells** constitute more than 90% of the surface area, and their squamous structure contributes to the thinness of the alveolar-capillary membrane. **Gas exchange** occurs across the thin alveolar-capillary membrane composed of the alveolar epithelium, basement membrane, and capillary **endothelium.** **Type II alveolar epithelial cells** secrete **surfactant,** a complex lipoprotein that lines the surface of the alveoli and airways up to the terminal bronchioles, reducing surface tension and increasing lung compliance. **Alveolar macrophages** are also found in the alveoli and perform the important function of removing inhaled particles and microorganisms.

COLOR, in Part A, examples of the following:

- [ ] 1. Smooth muscle
- [ ] 2. Lumenal (inside) surface of alveoli and airways
- [ ] 3. Outside surface of alveoli and airways

COLOR and LABEL in Part B:

- [ ] 4. Surfactant layer
- [ ] 5. Type I alveolar cells
- [ ] 6. Type II alveolar cells
- [ ] 7. Alveolar macrophage
- [ ] 8. Endothelium
- [ ] 9. Interstitium

Clinical Note

Respiratory distress syndrome of the newborn is the most common cause of mortality in premature babies. A baby's first breath always requires great effort to draw air into the collapsed lungs. With lung expansion, surfactant released by type II alveolar epithelial cells forms a monomolecular layer at the air-fluid interface of the alveoli and small airways, and within a few breaths only small negative pressure must be created to inspire. Without surfactant, the negative pressure required for inspiration remains high, and portions of the lung collapse, leading to the syndrome. Treatment consists of ventilatory support with surfactant replacement therapy.

REVIEW ANSWERS

A. Alveoli and small airways

B. Respiratory bronchioles

C. 50 to 100 m^2

D. Alveolar macrophages

E. 300 million

Plate 4.3   **Respiratory Physiology**

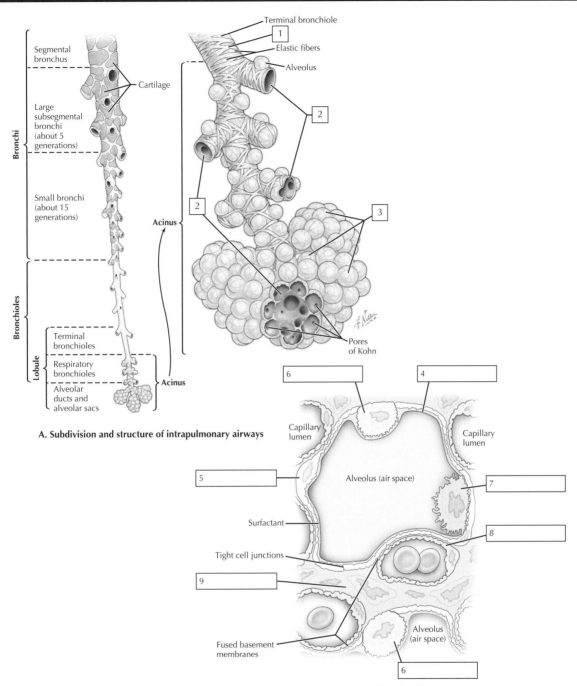

A. Subdivision and structure of intrapulmonary airways

B. Ultrastructure of pulmonary alveoli and capillaries

REVIEW QUESTIONS

A. Surfactant is found in the _____.

B. The respiratory zone begins at the _____.

C. The total area for gas exchange in the human lungs is approximately _____.

D. Dust particles in the alveoli are removed by _____.

E. The estimated number of alveoli in the human lungs is _____.

To understand the process of **ventilation** (the movement of air in and out of the respiratory system), several pulmonary volumes and capacities of the lung must be considered. Four **pulmonary volumes** are the following:

- **Tidal volume (V$_T$):** The volume of air inhaled and exhaled in a breath. Resting V$_T$ is approximately 500 mL.
- **Residual volume (RV):** The volume left in the lung after a maximal exhalation.
- **Expiratory reserve volume (ERV):** The additional volume that *could* be exhaled after a normal, quiet expiration.
- **Inspiratory reserve volume (IRV):** The remaining volume that *could* be inhaled after a normal quiet inspiration.

Four **pulmonary capacities** are the following:

- **Total lung capacity (TLC):** The volume of air in the lung after maximal inspiration. In a healthy adult, TLC is approximately 6 L.
- **Vital capacity (VC):** The volume of air that can be exhaled after maximal inspiration (up to ~5 L).
- **Forced vital capacity (FVC):** The vital capacity during expiration at maximal force.
- **Functional residual capacity (FRC):** The volume remaining in the lung after expiration in normal, quiet breathing.
- **Inspiratory capacity (IC):** The maximum volume that can be inspired after expiration during normal, quiet breathing.

Pulmonary volumes and capacities can be measured by **spirometry** and related techniques. The subject breathes in and out of a **spirometer** (Part A). As air enters and leaves the spirometer, a needle moves up and down, recording changes in volume (Part B). During normal, quiet breathing, V$_T$ is measured as the difference between end inspiratory and end expiratory

volumes. The actual end expiratory and inspiratory volumes within the lung cannot be known directly from this technique, but the machine is calibrated to accurately measure *changes* in volume. ERV can be measured by having the subject exhale maximally and comparing the level reached to that during expiration in quiet breathing; IRV is the difference between the volume attained after maximal inspiration to that after inspiration in quiet breathing (Part B). VC can be measured directly by spirometry by having the subject maximally exhale after maximal inspiration.

To know the values for TLC, FRC, and RV, one of these parameters must be measured indirectly by a technique such as **nitrogen washout, helium dilution,** or **body plethysmography.** Once one of these parameters is measured, the others can be calculated. For example, if FRC is measured by the helium dilution technique, TLC can be calculated as FRC + IC (measured in spirometry), and RV can be calculated as FRC − ERV.

TRACE

- ☐ 1. Spirometer recordings

COLOR and **LABEL** the areas representing:

- ☐ 2. Tidal volume (V$_T$)
- ☐ 3. Inspiratory reserve volume (IRV)
- ☐ 4. Residual volume (RV)

REVIEW ANSWERS

- **A.** 6 L
- **B.** 500 mL
- **C.** FRC
- **D.** TLC

Plate 4.4   **Respiratory Physiology**

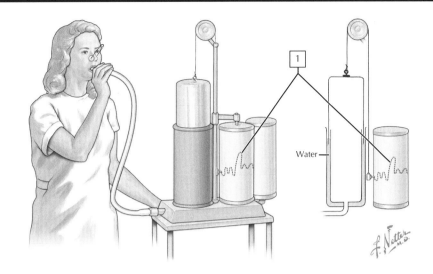

A

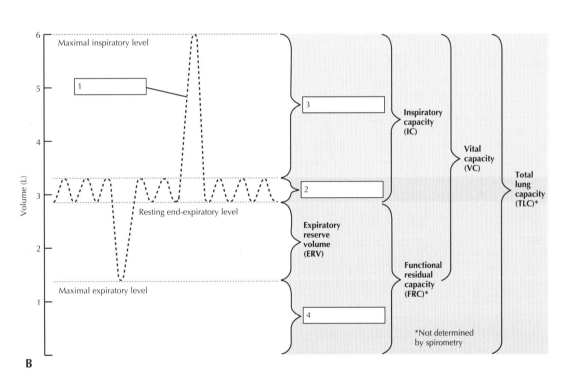

B

REVIEW QUESTIONS

A. Normal TLC is approximately _____.

B. Normal V_T during quiet breathing is approximately _____.

C. The volume remaining in the lung after exhalation in normal, quiet breathing is known as the _____.

D. Of the following, which cannot be measured by spirometry alone?

TLC

IC

EC

V_T

V_T in normal quiet breathing is 500 mL and **respiratory rate (R)** is 12 to 20 breaths/minute. **Minute ventilation ($\dot{V}_E$)** is the volume inspired (or expired) per minute and can be calculated by the formula

$$\dot{V}_E = R \times V_T$$

At resting V_T of 500 mL, when R is 15 breaths/min, the $\dot{V}_E$ is 7500 mL/min. However, 150 mL of the V_T is anatomic dead space in the conducting zone of the lung, where no diffusion occurs. Thus alveolar ventilation ($\dot{V}_A$) in this example is 5250 mL/min (15 breaths/min × 350 mL). Dead space ventilation ($\dot{V}_D$) is 2250 mL/min (15 breaths/min × 150 mL).

The composition of air in the alveoli depends on several factors, including composition of inspired air, $\dot{V}_A$, and the concentration of gases in mixed venous blood. At sea level, assuming dry air, the atmosphere consists of 21% O_2, 79% N_2, and less than 1% other gases. Atmospheric pressure (P_{ATM}) is 760 mm Hg, and according to **Dalton's law,** we can calculate gas concentration:

$$P_{O_2} = 0.21 \times 760 \text{ mm Hg} = 160 \text{ mm Hg}$$

$$P_{N_2} = 0.79 \times 760 \text{ mm Hg} = 600 \text{ mm Hg}$$

Inspired air warms to body temperature and becomes saturated with water, resulting in vapor pressure of 47 mm Hg. Correcting for vapor pressure and applying Dalton's law, in inspired air:

$$P_{IH_2O} = 47 \text{ mm Hg}$$

$$P_{IO_2} = 0.21 \times (760 - 47) \text{ mm Hg} = 150 \text{ mm Hg}$$

$$P_{IN_2} = 0.79 \times (760 - 47) \text{ mm Hg} = 563 \text{ mm Hg}$$

This composition is observed in the conducting zone, but in the respiratory zone, O_2 diffuses from alveolar air to blood and CO_2 diffuses from blood to alveolar air. As a result, in alveolar air,

$$P_{AO_2} = 100 \text{ mm Hg}$$

$$P_{ACO_2} = 40 \text{ mm Hg}$$

The **alveolar gas equation** describes the relationship between partial pressures of O_2 and CO_2 in alveolar air:

$$P_{AO_2} = P_{IO_2} - P_{ACO_2}/R$$

where R is the **respiratory quotient,** which usually has a value of 0.8. P_{AO_2} reflects P_{IO_2} but is lower because of O_2 utilization and return to the lungs as CO_2. The respiratory quotient is the ratio of CO_2 produced by the body to oxygen consumed; it reflects the relative degrees to which carbohydrate, lipid, and protein are being metabolized for energy. The alveolar gas equation can predict P_{AO_2} based on measurement of CO_2 in arterial blood in a healthy person because P_{CO_2} is fully equilibrated between blood and alveolar air in the alveolar capillaries.

Compare the level of O_2 and CO_2 in the atmosphere, inspired air, and alveolar air in Part A and note that P_{O_2} and P_{CO_2} in blood are equilibrated with levels in alveolar air as blood courses through the lungs. Partial pressure of oxygen in mixed venous blood (P_{VO_2}) is 40 mm Hg, and arterial blood has P_{AO_2} of 100 mm Hg (equal to P_{AO_2}). Meanwhile, mixed venous blood enters the lung having P_{VCO_2} of 46 mm Hg, and arterial blood has P_{ACO_2} of 40 mm Hg (equal to P_{ACO_2}). Note that the actual content of gas dissolved in blood is a function of several factors in addition to partial pressure (see Plate 4.6). In Part B, note the changes that occur with hypoventilation.

COLOR the levels of oxygenation of blood in Parts A and B, noting the difference in arterial P_{O_2} during hypoventilation (Part B):

- [ ] 1. P_{O_2} of 100 mm Hg (red)
- [ ] 2. P_{O_2} of 40 or less (blue)
- [ ] 3. P_{O_2} significantly below 100 mm Hg but higher than P_{O_2} in venous blood (purple)

REVIEW ANSWERS

A.   160 mm Hg, 150 mm Hg, and 100 mm Hg

B.   40 mm Hg, 100 mm Hg

C.   46 mm Hg, 40 mm Hg

D.   10,000 mL/min [20/min × 500 mL], 7000 mL/min [20/min × 350 mL], 3000 mL/min [20/min × 150 mL]

Plate 4.5   **Respiratory Physiology**

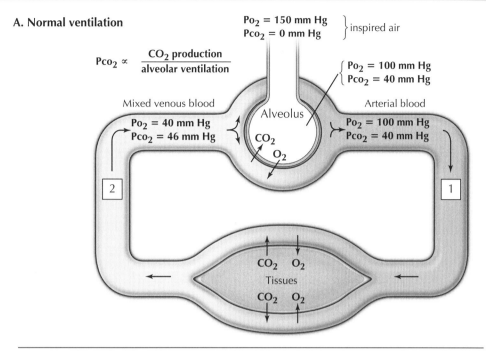

A. Normal ventilation

$$Pco_2 \propto \frac{CO_2 \text{ production}}{\text{alveolar ventilation}}$$

$Po_2 = 150$ mm Hg
$Pco_2 = 0$ mm Hg $\Big\}$ inspired air

$Po_2 = 100$ mm Hg
$Pco_2 = 40$ mm Hg

Mixed venous blood
$Po_2 = 40$ mm Hg
$Pco_2 = 46$ mm Hg

Alveolus

CO_2
O_2

Arterial blood
$Po_2 = 100$ mm Hg
$Pco_2 = 40$ mm Hg

2

1

CO_2 O_2
Tissues
CO_2 O_2

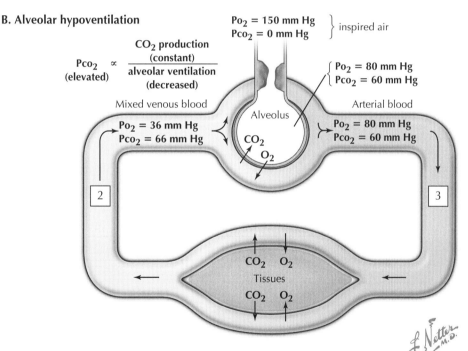

B. Alveolar hypoventilation

$$Pco_2 \atop (\text{elevated})} \propto \frac{CO_2 \text{ production} \atop (\text{constant})}{\text{alveolar ventilation} \atop (\text{decreased})}$$

$Po_2 = 150$ mm Hg
$Pco_2 = 0$ mm Hg $\Big\}$ inspired air

$Po_2 = 80$ mm Hg
$Pco_2 = 60$ mm Hg

Mixed venous blood
$Po_2 = 36$ mm Hg
$Pco_2 = 66$ mm Hg

Alveolus

CO_2
O_2

Arterial blood
$Po_2 = 80$ mm Hg
$Pco_2 = 60$ mm Hg

2

3

CO_2 O_2
Tissues
CO_2 O_2

REVIEW QUESTIONS

A. The partial pressures of O_2 at sea level in dry atmospheric air, inspired air, and alveolar air are, respectively, _____, _____, and _____.

B. The partial pressure of O_2 in mixed venous blood returning to the lung is _____, and the level in arterial blood is _____.

C. The partial pressure of CO_2 in mixed venous blood returning to the lung is _____, and the level in arterial blood is _____.

D. At a respiratory rate of 20 and a tidal volume of 500, $\dot{V}_E$ is _____, $\dot{V}_A$ is _____, and $\dot{V}_D$ is _____.

Diffusion of gas ($\dot{V}_{gas}$) between alveolar air and alveolar capillary blood follows Fick's law,

$$\dot{V}_{gas} = \frac{A \times D\,(P_1 - P_2)}{T}$$

where A is the area of the membrane separating two compartments, T is thickness of the membrane, D is the diffusion constant, and P_1 and P_2 are the gas concentrations in the two compartments. The diffusion constant of a gas is directly related to its solubility and inversely related to the square root of its molecular weight.

At rest, the transit time for blood going through alveolar capillaries is about 0.75 seconds. In healthy lungs at rest, O_2 and CO_2 are equilibrated with alveolar air by one-third of the way through the alveolar capillary, as illustrated in Plate 4.6. Thus, under normal conditions, diffusion of these gases is **perfusion limited,** because the only way to increase gas transfer is to raise perfusion (blood flow) in the lung. The classic example of **perfusion-limited transport** is transport of **nitrous oxide (N_2O),** which is equilibrated in the first fifth of the way through the capillary. During very strenuous aerobic exercise, when cardiac output is greatly increased, or in diseases such as interstitial fibrosis (in which the alveolar capillary membrane is thickened), O_2 transport may be **diffusion limited,** with P_{O_2} not being fully equilibrated between alveolar air and blood leaving the alveolar capillary.

In the bottom panel of Plate 4.6, note the dotted lines that illustrate effects of a diffusion barrier impeding gas exchange, as occurs when membranes are thickened by **pulmonary fibrosis.** The classic example of a diffusion-limited gas is **carbon monoxide (CO).** If a subject breathes CO, it diffuses from alveolar air to blood and is bound to hemoglobin with such high affinity that large amounts of CO diffuse to blood with little change in blood PCO (PCO reflects only the amount of dissolved CO). Thus CO does not fully equilibrate as blood passes through the alveolar capillary, and its transport is limited only by the diffusion capacity of the alveolar membrane.

COLOR

☐ 1. Blood in the pulmonary artery (mixed venous blood) and blood in the first third of the alveolar capillary blue to indicate its partially deoxygenated state.

☐ 2. Blood in the last two-thirds of the alveolar capillary and blood in the pulmonary vein red to indicate its fully oxygenated state.

TRACE

☐ 3. P_{CO_2} (normal healthy diffusion rate)

☐ 4. P_{CO_2} (abnormal diffusion rate)

☐ 5. P_{O_2} (normal healthy diffusion)

☐ 6. P_{O_2} (abnormal diffusion rate)

Clinical Note

Clinically, the **diffusion capacity of the lung for CO (DLCO)** is a pulmonary function test that is administered to assess the ability of the lung to transfer gas from alveolus to lung. DLCO is reduced in several pulmonary disease states, including pulmonary fibrosis, interstitial lung disease, and emphysema.

REVIEW ANSWERS

A. Nitrous oxide

B. Carbon monoxide

C. Interstitial fibrosis

D. Thickness of the membrane

Plate 4.6　　　　　　　　**Respiratory Physiology**

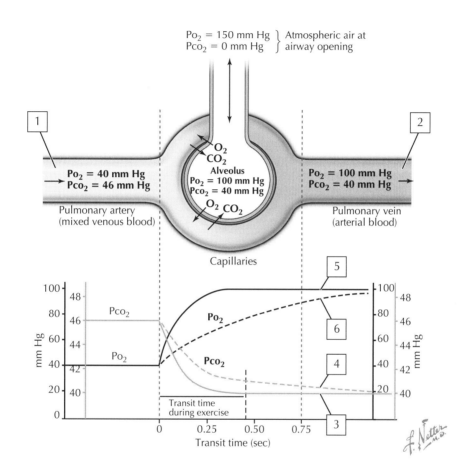

A. A classic example of a perfusion-limited gas is _____.

B. A classic example of a diffusion-limited gas is _____.

C. One disease in which the rate of diffusion of gases across the alveolar capillary membrane is reduced is

_____.

D. According to Fick's law, the diffusion of gas between the alveolar air and capillary blood is inversely related to the

_____.

For the most efficient exchange of gases between the environment and the blood, ventilation within regions of the lung should be properly matched to blood flow. However, neither ventilation nor perfusion of the lung is uniform. In the **standing position,** the weight of the lung stretches alveoli toward the apex. Thus alveoli toward the base of the lung are smaller and more compliant and, as a result, there is an increasing ventilation gradient from the top (less) to the bottom (greater) of the lung (Part B).

In the standing position, the gradient for pulmonary blood flow (perfusion) is much steeper than the ventilation gradient, with perfusion higher toward the bottom of the lung. This is the result of gravitational effects on vascular pressures and the relationship between vascular pressure and alveolar pressure as blood flows through alveolar capillaries. As blood flows through alveolar capillaries, the flow rate is potentially affected by the alveolar pressure on either side of the capillary. In the top of the lung, arterial pressure is low and alveolar pressure may even exceed vascular pressure at times, resulting in a region of low flow, called **zone 1** (Part A). In regions of the lung where alveolar pressure is between the arterial and venous pressure, **zone 2,** the pressure gradient for flow is the difference between arterial pressure and alveolar pressure. Toward the base of the lung, **zone 3,** pulmonary vascular pressures are elevated by the effect of gravity and both arterial and venous pressures are higher than alveolar pressure. This causes distension of vessels and therefore reduced resistance. Thus blood flow is greatest in zone 3.

These gradients in ventilation and perfusion produce a gradient in the $\dot{V}_A/\dot{Q}_C$ (alveolar ventilation/pulmonary capillary blood flow ratio). $\dot{V}_A/\dot{Q}_C$ is lowest at the bottom of the lung and highest at the top (see Part B). With resting pulmonary blood flow (cardiac output) and resting alveolar ventilation both being approximately 5 L/min, $\dot{V}_A/\dot{Q}_C$ is approximately 1 at the vertical midpoint of the lungs, less than 1 at the base, and greater than 1 toward the apex.

Dead space and **shunt** are extremes of $\dot{V}_A/\dot{Q}_C$ imbalance. Alveoli that are ventilated but not perfused constitute **physiological dead space** (as opposed to the anatomic dead space of the conducting zone of the lung). In dead space, $\dot{V}_A/\dot{Q}_C = \infty$. **Shunt flow** in the lungs refers to areas that are perfused but not ventilated; this can be the result of **airway obstruction** producing **physiological shunt.** In shunt flow, $\dot{V}_A/\dot{Q}_C = 0$. Shunt flow can also be **anatomic shunt,** where blood flow serves the conducting zone of the lungs and bypasses the alveoli. The **venous admixture** of oxygenated and deoxygenated blood resulting from anatomic shunt accounts for most of the small **alveolar-to-systemic arterial Po₂ gradient (A–a Po₂ gradient).** In healthy people, this gradient is 6 to 9 mm Hg. $\dot{V}_A/\dot{Q}_C$ imbalances have an important role in pulmonary pathophysiology.

COLOR and note the increase in perfusion toward the bottom of the lung in Part A:

- [ ] 1. Deoxygenated blood (blue, left of the alveoli)
- [ ] 2. Oxygenated blood (red, right of the alveoli)
- [ ] 3. Lung (background of the diagram)

COLOR and **LABEL**, in Part B, the line representing:

- [ ] 4. Ventilation (blue)
- [ ] 5. Perfusion (red)
- [ ] 6. $\dot{V}_A/\dot{Q}_C$ (ventilation/perfusion ratio)

REVIEW ANSWERS

A. Zone 3

B. Infinite

C. 1

D. Abolished (zero)

Plate 4.7   **Respiratory Physiology**

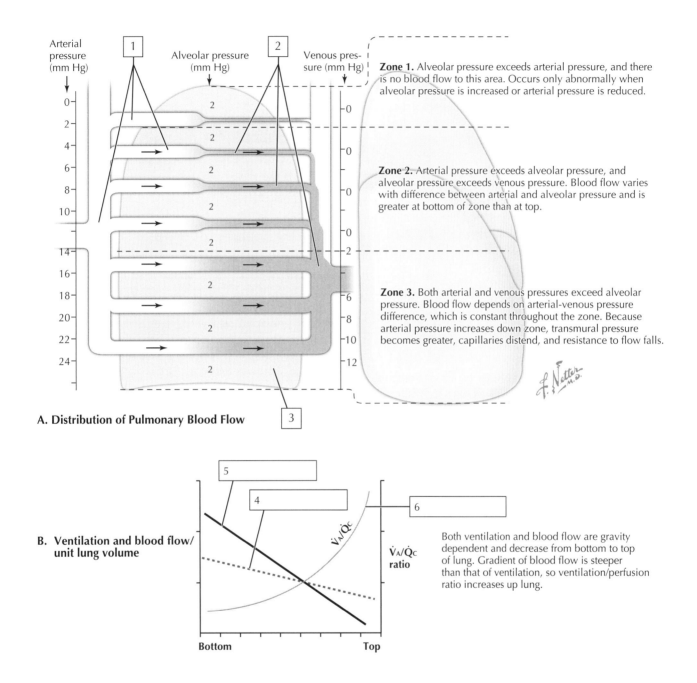

A. Distribution of Pulmonary Blood Flow

Arterial pressure (mm Hg)

Alveolar pressure (mm Hg)

Venous pressure (mm Hg)

Zone 1. Alveolar pressure exceeds arterial pressure, and there is no blood flow to this area. Occurs only abnormally when alveolar pressure is increased or arterial pressure is reduced.

Zone 2. Arterial pressure exceeds alveolar pressure, and alveolar pressure exceeds venous pressure. Blood flow varies with difference between arterial and alveolar pressure and is greater at bottom of zone than at top.

Zone 3. Both arterial and venous pressures exceed alveolar pressure. Blood flow depends on arterial-venous pressure difference, which is constant throughout the zone. Because arterial pressure increases down zone, transmural pressure becomes greater, capillaries distend, and resistance to flow falls.

B. Ventilation and blood flow/ unit lung volume

$\dot{V}_A/\dot{Q}_C$ ratio

Bottom Top

Both ventilation and blood flow are gravity dependent and decrease from bottom to top of lung. Gradient of blood flow is steeper than that of ventilation, so ventilation/perfusion ratio increases up lung.

REVIEW QUESTIONS

A. $\dot{V}_A/\dot{Q}_C$ is lowest in which zone of the lung?

B. In physiological dead space, $\dot{V}_A/\dot{Q}_C$ is _____.

C. For most efficient physiological function, $\dot{V}_A/\dot{Q}_C$ should be _____.

D. In an astronaut orbiting Earth, the gradient in $\dot{V}_A/\dot{Q}_C$ would be _____.

The forces producing ventilation of the lungs are analogous to those producing flow of blood in the cardiovascular system. The pressure gradient for airflow is created by movement of the **chest wall** and diaphragm, and flow occurs against the resistance of the airways:

$$\text{Rate of airflow} = (P_A - P_{ATM}) / R_{aw}$$

where $(P_A - P_{ATM})$ is the pressure gradient from alveolus to atmosphere and R_{aw} is the airway resistance. Of course, the equation for airflow can be expanded to Poiseuille's law (Plate 3.8).

Both the chest wall and lungs are elastic, passively recoiling after distension because of the **elastic recoil pressure** created by the distension. The visceral pleura (outer lining) of the lungs apposes the parietal pleura of the chest wall, and the small, fluid-filled pleural cavity between the pleurae contains only a few milliliters of fluid.

Plate 4.8 illustrates the interactions between forces of the chest wall and lungs during the cycle of normal, quiet breathing (note that in normal, quiet breathing, pleural pressure is always negative).

- In Part A, the system is shown at FRC, where it is at rest after a quiet, passive expiration. Chest wall muscles are relaxed, and the outward elastic recoil pressure of the chest wall is equal to and opposes the inward elastic recoil pressure of the lung. **Alveolar pressure** is zero (atmospheric), and **pleural pressure** (pressure in the pleural cavity) is negative.
- During normal, quiet breathing, the **diaphragm** below the lungs is the major muscle for **inspiration** (Part B). As it contracts and its dome descends, the thoracic space is enlarged, creating negative alveolar pressure and causing **inward flow** of air through the airways (Part B). With active breathing (e.g., during exercise), the **intercostal muscles** become more actively involved in inspiration, elevating the **ribs** and expanding the chest as they contract.
- In normal, quiet breathing, **expiration** is a passive result of recoil of the lungs. During active breathing, muscles of the abdominal wall and intercostal muscles contribute to expiratory force.

COLOR

- [ ] 1. Arrows within the airways indicating inward flow
- [ ] 2. Arrows within the airways indicating outward flow
- [ ] 3. Esophagus
- [ ] 4. Lungs
- [ ] 5. Chest wall
- [ ] 6. Cross sections of the ribs

Clinical Note

The term **pneumothorax** refers to air in the pleural space, potentially resulting in collapse of the lung, usually on one side of the chest. Common symptoms include pain in one side of the chest and shortness of breath. The condition may deteriorate, with falling blood pressure and reduced oxygenation of blood and tissues when not treated. Pneumothorax can be caused by injury to the chest wall or disruption of the integrity of the lung itself, leading in either case to air entering the pleural cavity. In some cases, pneumothorax can lead to death if untreated, but in other cases, pneumothorax may occur spontaneously, in the absence of significant pulmonary disease, and may resolve on its own.

REVIEW ANSWERS

A. Diaphragm

B. Negative

C. Zero (atmospheric)

D. Positive, negative

Plate 4.8 | **Respiratory Physiology**

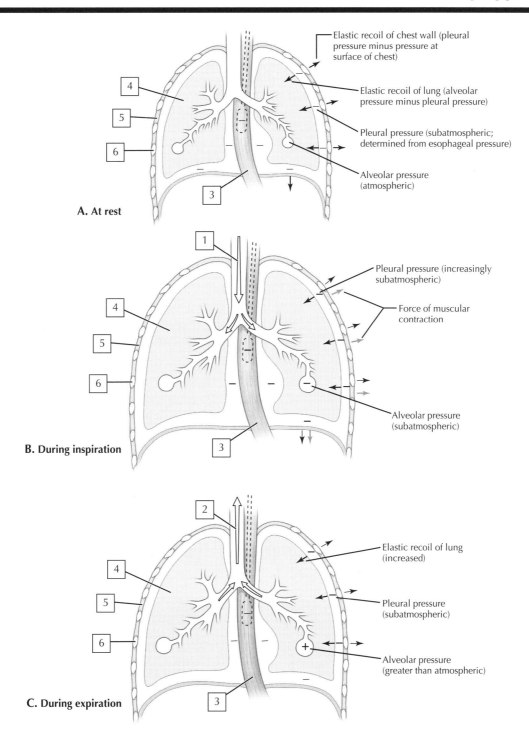

Elastic recoil of chest wall (pleural pressure minus pressure at surface of chest)

Elastic recoil of lung (alveolar pressure minus pleural pressure)

Pleural pressure (subatmospheric; determined from esophageal pressure)

Alveolar pressure (atmospheric)

A. At rest

Pleural pressure (increasingly subatmospheric)

Force of muscular contraction

Alveolar pressure (subatmospheric)

B. During inspiration

Elastic recoil of lung (increased)

Pleural pressure (subatmospheric)

Alveolar pressure (greater than atmospheric)

C. During expiration

REVIEW QUESTIONS

A. In normal, quiet breathing, the work of breathing is performed by the contraction of the _____.

B. In normal, quiet breathing, the pressure in the pleural cavity is always _____.

C. At rest (FRC), the alveolar pressure is _____.

D. During expiration, alveolar pressure is _____, and during inspiration, alveolar pressure is _____.

Elastance, the tendency of a hollow organ to return to its original size when it is distended, can be quantified as **elastic recoil pressure. Lung compliance (CL)** is the inverse of lung elastance and is a measure of the lung's distensibility. In Plate 4.9, the magnitudes of the elastic recoil pressures of the lungs and chest wall are illustrated for various lung volumes from RV to TLC (size and direction of arrows show relative magnitude and direction of recoil force). Starting at RV and proceeding to TLC, **elastic recoil of the chest wall** is at first a large pressure directed **outward;** it diminishes at larger volumes until it reaches zero at approximately 70% of TLC, and at TLC it is directed **inward. Elastic recoil of the lung** is very small at RV and increases as volume increases. For the respiratory system as a whole, when muscles of respiration are relaxed, the combination of these forces results in a net outward force at RV, equilibrium of the forces at FRC, and net inward force at volume above FRC. These forces are quantified and illustrated in the graph, with lung volumes designated A to E in the top diagrams indicated by arrows A to E in the bottom graph. The line for the combined lung and chest wall force represents the sum of the two forces and crosses the origin (0 net elastic recoil pressure) at FRC, where the system is in equilibrium.

The elastic recoil pressure of the lungs and chest wall can be related to pleural pressure:

- Elastic recoil of the lungs is equal to P_A minus pleural pressure.
- Elastic recoil pressure of the chest wall is equal to pleural pressure minus P_{ATM}.

Surface tension is an elastic-like force at the gas-liquid interface caused by intermolecular attraction of the liquid molecules at that surface. In the lung, surface tension reduces C_L and can potentially cause collapse of small airways. The potential problem of surface tension and low C_L is prevented by surfactant produced by type II alveolar epithelial cells. Surfactant is a complex lipoprotein containing dipalmitoyl phosphatidyl choline. It is an amphipathic substance that lines the surface of the alveolar epithelium and small airways; it reduces surface tension and increases C_L, reducing the work of breathing.

COLOR

- ☐ 1.   Arrows indicating outward recoil pressures
- ☐ 2.   Arrows indicating inward recoil pressures

COLOR and **LABEL** the line representing:

- ☐ 3.   Chest wall recoil pressure
- ☐ 4.   Lung recoil pressure
- ☐ 5.   Combined lung and chest wall pressure

REVIEW ANSWERS

A.   Elastance, compliance

B.   TLC (or very high lung volumes)

C.   Negative (outward)

D.   Residual volume

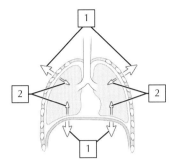

A. At residual volume
Elastic recoil of chest wall directed outward is large; recoil of lung directed inward is very small

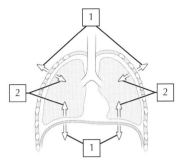

B. At functional residual capacity
Elastic recoils of lung and chest wall are equal but opposite

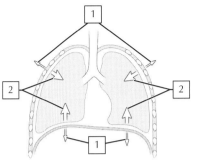

C. At larger lung volume
Elastic recoil of chest wall becomes smaller, and recoil of lung increases

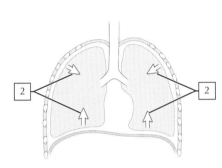

D. At approximately 70% of total lung capacity
Equilibrium position of chest wall (its recoil equals zero)

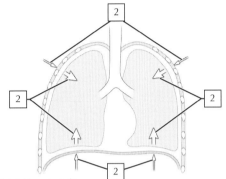

E. At total lung capacity
Elastic recoil of both lung and chest wall directed inward, favoring decrease in lung volume

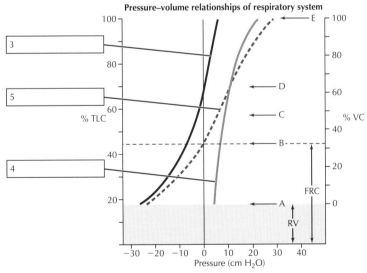

Pressure–volume relationships of respiratory system

F. Elastic recoil pressure of respiratory system is algebraic sum of recoil pressures of lung and chest wall

REVIEW QUESTIONS

A. The tendency of a hollow organ to return to its original size after distension is _____, and _____ is a measure of an organ's distensibility.

B. Elastic recoil of both the chest wall and lungs is positive (inward) at _____.

C. At FRC, elastic recoil of the chest wall is _____.

D. In a normal respiratory system, elastic recoil of the lung is minimal at _____.

Most lung diseases can be classified as either restrictive or obstructive diseases:

- **Restrictive lung diseases** result in reduced functional volume of the lung and include **interstitial lung diseases** such as **idiopathic pulmonary fibrosis, sarcoidosis,** and **asbestosis.**
- **Obstructive lung diseases** are those characterized by reduced flow rate and include **chronic obstructive pulmonary disease (COPD)** and **asthma.**

The dynamic pressure-volume loop that results when lung volume is plotted against intrapleural pressure (top right) is useful in analyzing the work of breathing in the lungs and the possible presence of obstructive or restrictive disease in the lungs. In the normal pressure-volume loop, note the relative area in the **trapezoid EABCD** and compare that area with the areas of the trapezoids in the two subsequent pressure-volume loops. This area is an index of the work performed overcoming elastic forces, and the right half of the **loop (AB′CBA)** indicates the additional work associated with overcoming airway resistance during inspiration.

In **restrictive disease,** the **compliance** of the respiratory system is reduced, resulting in lower TLC and FRC. Note that in Part C (restrictive lung disease), the work of breathing is greater, and the slope of the pressure-volume relationship is reduced compared to the normal lungs. More effort and a greater pressure gradient are required to inflate the lungs.

In **obstructive lung disease,** the work performed during inspiration is increased because of higher airway resistance.

Compare the shape of the pressure-volume loops in the three loops illustrated and note the expansion of the right side of the middle loop (inspiration) resulting from the **increased resistance.** Obstructive disease does not immediately produce a change in C_L but may have an effect over time. For example, in COPD, an important component of the pathophysiology is **emphysema,** the destruction of elastic tissue in the lungs resulting in breakdown of alveolar architecture. This results in lower C_L, but although TLC and FRC are increased, there is less area for gas exchange.

TRACE

☐ 1. EABCD trapezoid and compare the relative areas in the three trapezoids, as an indication of the work of overcoming elastic forces in breathing.

☐ 2. Loop segment AB′CBA and compare those three areas as an indication of the work of overcoming resistance in breathing.

COLOR

☐ 3. Obstructions to air flow to reinforce the point that air-flow resistance is increased compared to the normal lungs.

☐ 4. Darker area around the alveoli, to reinforce the decrease in compliance in restrictive lung disease.

REVIEW ANSWERS

A. Increased

B. Obstructive

C. Increased, reduced

D. Obstructive, restrictive

Plate 4.10   **Respiratory Physiology**

Work of Breathing

A. Normal

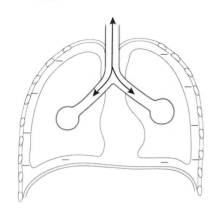

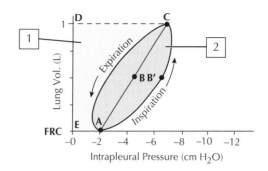

Work performed on lung during breathing can be determined from dynamic pressure–volume loop. Work to overcome elastic forces is represented by area of trapezoid EABCD. Additional work required to overcome flow resistance during inspiration is represented by area of right half of loop AB'CBA.

B. Obstructive disease

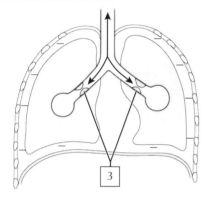

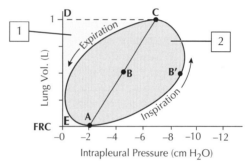

In disorders characterized by airway obstruction, work to overcome flow resistance is increased; elastic work of breathing remains unchanged.

C. Restrictive disease

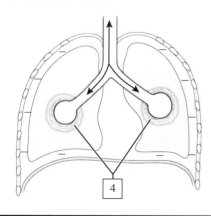

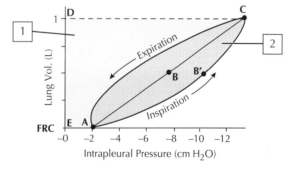

Restrictive lung diseases result in increase of elastic work of breathing; work to overcome flow resistance is normal.

REVIEW QUESTIONS

A. In restrictive lung disease, the work of breathing is _____.

B. Increased airway resistance is a characteristic of _____ lung disease.

C. In emphysema, lung compliance is _____, but the area for gas exchange is _____.

D. Asthma is a(n) _____ (obstructive or restrictive) lung disease, whereas interstitial fibrosis is categorized as an (obstructive or restrictive) _____ lung disease.

Airflow in and out of the lungs is dependent on the pressure gradient between the opening of the mouth and the alveoli. That gradient is zero at the end of inspiration and expiration. Just as it applies to blood flow (Chapter 3), **Poiseuille's law** applies to airflow (Q) through the tubes of the respiratory system:

$$Q = \Delta P \pi r^4 / \eta 8L$$

where ΔP is the pressure gradient in a tube, r^4 is the radius of the tube to the fourth power, η is the viscosity of air, and L is the length of the tube. These relationships are illustrated in the bottom half of Plate 4.11.

In the respiratory system as a whole, the greatest resistance to flow actually occurs in medium-sized airways (generations 4 to 8). Recall from Chapter 3 that in parallel tubes, total resistance is less than the resistance of individual tubes. Considering both the radius and number of tubes at this level, resistance is highest in medium-sized bronchi in aggregate and lower in the larger or smaller airways. Flow is generally **laminar,** although at high flow rates it becomes **turbulent** in the **large airways and trachea;** flow is **transitional** in large airways near branch points and sites of narrowing (see Plate 4.11). Autonomic control of the airways is mainly through the parasympathetic nervous system, with **bronchoconstriction** occurring when parasympathetic nerves are activated; sympathetic activation has the opposite action **(bronchodilation).**

Another factor that affects airway resistance is lung volume. At higher lung volumes, **radial traction** tends to pull airways more open, reducing resistance to air flow.

COLOR and **LABEL** the arrows indicating:

☐ 1. Laminar flow

☐ 2. Turbulent flow

☐ 3. Transitional flow

Clinical Note

Airway tone is normally controlled in large part by the **autonomic nervous system.** When an asthmatic episode results in bronchoconstriction and difficulty breathing, "rescue inhalers" are often used to deliver a short-acting β-adrenergic drug such as albuterol to promote bronchodilation. Stimulation of **β_2-adrenergic receptors** on bronchial smooth muscle promotes relaxation.

REVIEW ANSWERS

A. Large airway diameter

B. Midsized airways

C. β_2-adrenergic receptor

D. Radial traction

Plate 4.11   **Respiratory Physiology**

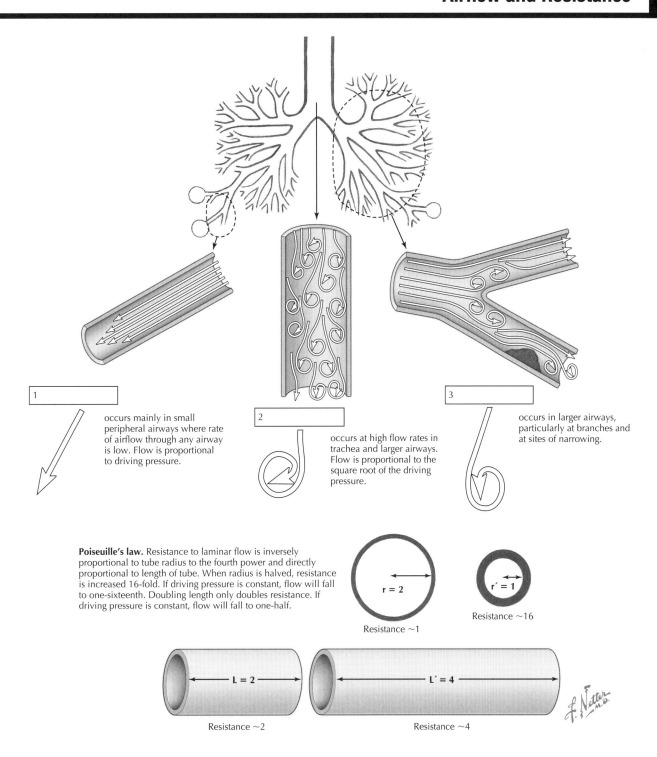

1 [   ]

occurs mainly in small peripheral airways where rate of airflow through any airway is low. Flow is proportional to driving pressure.

2 [   ]

occurs at high flow rates in trachea and larger airways. Flow is proportional to the square root of the driving pressure.

3 [   ]

occurs in larger airways, particularly at branches and at sites of narrowing.

Poiseuille's law. Resistance to laminar flow is inversely proportional to tube radius to the fourth power and directly proportional to length of tube. When radius is halved, resistance is increased 16-fold. If driving pressure is constant, flow will fall to one-sixteenth. Doubling length only doubles resistance. If driving pressure is constant, flow will fall to one-half.

$r = 2$

Resistance ~1

$r' = 1$

Resistance ~16

$L = 2$

Resistance ~2

$L' = 4$

Resistance ~4

REVIEW QUESTIONS

A. In large airways and trachea, when flow becomes turbulent at high flow rates, the turbulence can be attributed to rapid velocity, and in this region, _____.

B. Within the respiratory system, resistance is highest at the level of the _____.

C. Bronchodilation will result when an agonist binds to what specific receptor type in airways?

D. Airway resistance tends to be reduced at high lung volumes by _____ acting on the airways.

In addition to the factors discussed in Plate 4.11, airway resistance is affected by **dynamic compression,** defined as the compression of airways during **forced expiration.** The effects of dynamic compression are revealed in the **expiratory flow-volume curve** (Part A). When a subject performs an **FVC maneuver** by inspiring to TLC and then exhaling with maximum force to RV, a curve like the top solid line is generated. In this curve, the peak (the highest flow rate achieved) is the **peak expiratory flow rate.** Note that the downward slope (the expiratory phase) is **effort independent** (unlike the peak expiratory flow rate) because flow is limited by dynamic airway compression. If less effort is applied (see dotted curve in Part A), lower peak expiratory flow rate is achieved, but the curve converges with that of the **maximal effort** curve on the downslope. This convergence demonstrates the effort independence of expiratory flow rate during active expiration.

In normal, quiet breathing, pleural pressure is always negative, but in active breathing, the contraction of the muscles of breathing results in pleural pressure above zero (above P_{ATM}). Thus, in active breathing, alveolar pressure becomes the sum of pleural pressure and the elastic recoil pressure of the lungs (Part B). At the mouth, P_{ATM} is reached, implying that at some point downstream from the alveolus (toward the mouth), an **equal pressure point** is reached, beyond which airways will be compressed. This dynamic compression of the airways limits the expiratory flow rate and accounts for effort independence of airflow during active expiration. As a result, if greater force is exerted, greater compression takes place and airflow remains the same (Part C).

TRACE

☐ 1. Line representing airflow with maximal effort
☐ 2. Line representing airflow with submaximal effort

COLOR

☐ 3. Alveolus and airway up to the equal pressure point
☐ 4. Narrowed airway segment above the equal pressure point
☐ 5. Equal pressure points
☐ 6. Pleural space

REVIEW ANSWERS

A. Dependent, independent

B. Equal pressure point

C. Elastic recoil pressure of the lungs, pleural pressure

D. Dynamic airway compression

Plate 4.12   **Respiratory Physiology**

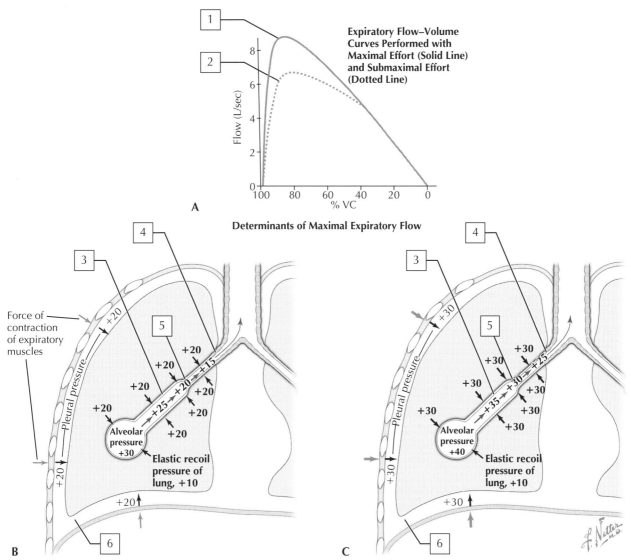

A

Expiratory Flow–Volume Curves Performed with Maximal Effort (Solid Line) and Submaximal Effort (Dotted Line)

Determinants of Maximal Expiratory Flow

B

At onset of maximal airflow, contraction of expiratory muscles at a given lung volume raises pleural pressure above atmospheric level (+20 cm H_2O). Alveolar pressure (sum of pleural pressure and lung recoil pressure) is yet higher (+30 cm H_2O). Airway pressure falls progressively from alveolus to airway opening in overcoming resistance. At equal pressure point of airway, pressure within airway equals pressure surrounding it (pleural pressure). Beyond this point, as intraluminal pressure drops further, below pleural pressure, airway will be compressed.

C

With further increases in expiratory effort, at same lung volume, pleural pressure is greater and alveolar pressure is correspondingly higher. Fall in airway pressure and location of equal pressure point are unchanged, but beyond equal pressure point, intrathoracic airways will be compressed to a greater degree by higher pleural pressure. Once maximal airflow is achieved, further increases in pleural pressure produce proportional increases in resistance of segment downstream from equal pressure point, so rate of airflow does not change.

REVIEW QUESTIONS

A. During active breathing, peak expiratory flow rate is effort _____, and the downward slope of the expiratory flow-volume curve is effort _____.

B. During active breathing, as air flows from the alveolus downstream toward the mouth, the flow-limiting segment is observed beyond the _____.

C. During expiration in active breathing, alveolar pressure is the sum of _____ and _____.

D. The phenomenon responsible for the effort independence of active expiration is _____.

An important part of assessment of **obstructive and restrictive lung diseases** involves measurement and interpretation of flow-volume relationships (see Plate 4.10). In severe COPD, emphysema occurs as a result of lung inflammation, with destruction of alveolar walls and capillaries and thus reduced area for gas exchange and shortness of breath. C_L **is elevated** as a result of this breakdown. The **reduced elastic recoil** of alveoli and airways also produces early formation of the **equal pressure point** (closer to the alveolus) during expiration and, as a result of this dynamic compression, "trapping" of air occurs in the lung. Ultimately, TLC, FRC, and **residual volume (RV)** are elevated.

In the illustration, results of spirometry and related tests are illustrated for **normal lungs** and lungs with obstructive pulmonary disease. In Part A, note that in the top (obstructive disease) tracing, the forced expiratory volume **(FEV)** in the first second of a vital capacity maneuver **(FEV$_1$)** is reduced, as is the expiratory flow rate during the middle portion of a forced expiration **(FEF$_{25-75\%}$).** The **FEV$_1$/FVC ratio** is less than the normal value of 75% (because **FEV$_1$** is reduced, whereas FVC is only slightly below normal or normal).

TRACE and **LABEL**, in Parts A and B, the lines representing:

- ☐ 1. Obstructive lung disease
- ☐ 2. Normal lungs

COLOR and **LABEL** in Part C:

- ☐ 3. Residual volume (RV)
- ☐ 4. Expiratory reserve volume (ERV)
- ☐ 5. Tidal volume (V$_T$)
- ☐ 6. Inspiratory reserve volume (IRV)

REVIEW ANSWERS

A. 4 (elastic recoil pressure of the lung)

B. 2 (lung compliance)

Plate 4.13 **Respiratory Physiology**

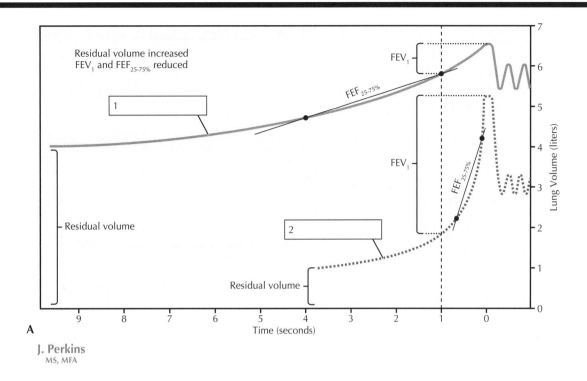

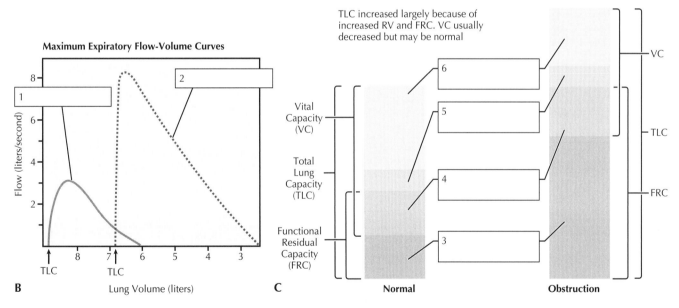

REVIEW QUESTIONS

A. In obstructive lung disease, which of the following parameters is reduced compared to normal?

1. Total lung capacity (TLC)

2. Residual volume (RV)

3. Functional residual capacity (FRC)

4. Elastic recoil pressure of the lung

5. Tidal volume (V_T)

B. In obstructive lung disease, which of the following parameters is elevated compared to normal?

1. $FEF_{25-75\%}$

2. C_L

3. Surface area for gas exchange

4. Peak expiratory flow

5. FEV_1/FVC ratio

4 Pulmonary Function in Restrictive Lung Disease

Measurement of flow-volume relationships in lungs of patients with **restrictive pulmonary diseases** produces markedly different results than those observed in obstructive lung disease. In restrictive diseases such as **interstitial fibrosis,** thickening of alveolar walls occurs, with higher elastic recoil pressure of the lung and **lower** C_L as a result. Plate 4.14 illustrates an FVC maneuver in an individual with **normal lungs** compared to an individual with **restrictive lung disease** (Part B); note the lower volumes with restrictive disease, including TLC, FVC, and **residual volume (RV).** While the subject is breathing in a normal, quiet manner before the maneuver, note the lower FRC and **tidal volume (V_T)** with restrictive disease. During the maneuver, FEV_1 is reduced, but because FVC is also lower, the **FEV_1/FVC ratio is usually normal or elevated** in restrictive disease. The $FEF_{25-75\%}$, a measure of flow rate during the middle portion of the forced expiration, may be reduced or normal in patients with restrictive lung disease. Examining the **maximum expiratory flow-volume curves** (Part C), it is apparent that in restrictive disease, peak expiratory flow rate is reduced and the curve is shifted rightward.

REVIEW ANSWERS

A. 4 (elastic recoil pressure of the lung)

B. 5 (FEV_1/FVC ratio)

Plate 4.14   **Respiratory Physiology**

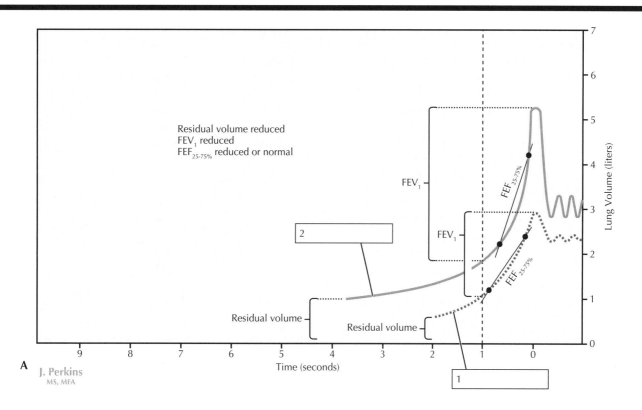

Residual volume reduced
FEV$_1$ reduced
FEF$_{25-75\%}$ reduced or normal

A

J. Perkins
MS, MFA

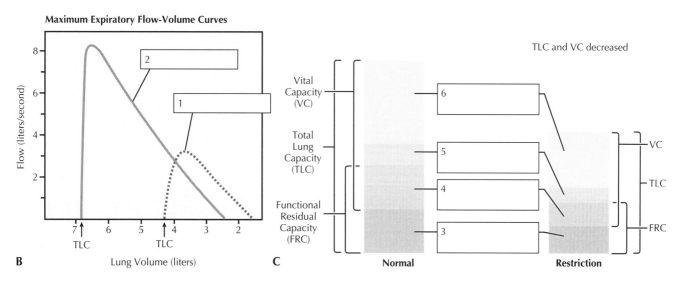

Maximum Expiratory Flow-Volume Curves

TLC and VC decreased

B

C

Normal   Restriction

REVIEW QUESTIONS

A. In restrictive lung disease, which of the following parameters is elevated compared to normal?

1. Total lung capacity (TLC)

2. Residual volume (RV)

3. Functional residual capacity (FRC)

4. Elastic recoil pressure of the lung

5. Vital capacity (VC)

B. In restrictive lung disease, which of the following parameters is likely to be elevated compared to normal?

1. FEF$_{25-75\%}$

2. C_L

3. Surface area for gas exchange

4. Peak expiratory flow

5. FEV$_1$/FVC ratio

Diffusion of gases between air and blood through the alveolar-capillary membrane follows Fick's law (Plate 4.6), but the actual content of gas in blood and its transport depends on many other factors. In fact, our resting, **average oxygen consumption rate of 250 mL O_2/min** cannot be accomplished simply by diffusion and delivery of dissolved gas to tissues, illustrating the importance of these other factors.

According to **Henry's law,** the concentration of dissolved gas in a liquid is directly proportional to the partial pressure of the gas in the atmosphere to which the liquid is exposed and the solubility of the gas in that particular solvent. In the case of oxygen, for each mm Hg P_{O_2}, only 0.003 mL O_2/mL Hg O_2 will dissolve in blood at body temperature. Given that $P_{A_{O_2}}$ is normally about 100 mm Hg, the concentration of dissolved O_2 in arterial blood is only 0.3 mL O_2/100 mL blood. Obviously, this alone would be grossly insufficient for supplying 250 mL O_2/min to the body. In fact, the actual concentration of O_2 in arterial blood is approximately 20.4 mL/100 mL blood, a result of **binding of oxygen to hemoglobin (Hb)** in red blood cells. The normal concentration of hemoglobin in blood is approximately 15 g/100 mL blood, and because 1.34 mL O_2 binds to 1 g hemoglobin at 100% saturation, blood can carry 20.4 mL O_2/100 mL blood (0.3 mL of dissolved O_2 plus 20.1 mL of O_2 bound to hemoglobin). Putting this in the form of equations,

$$O_2 \text{ binding capacity} = 1.34 \text{ mL } O_2/\text{g Hb}/100 \text{ mL blood}$$

For normal hemoglobin concentration of 15 g/100 mL blood, O_2 binding capacity

$$= 13.5 \text{ mL } O_2/\text{gHb} \times 15 \text{ g Hb}/100 \text{ mL blood}$$
$$= 20.1 \text{ mL } O_2/100 \text{ mL blood}$$

$$\text{Oxygen content of blood} = \% \text{ saturation} \times O_2 \text{ binding capacity} + \text{dissolved oxygen}$$

For normal hemoglobin content of 15 g hemoglobin/100 mL blood and approximately **100% saturation of arterial blood** at 100 mm Hg P_{O_2}, **arterial oxygen content**

$$= 100\% \times (1.34 \text{ mL } O_2/\text{g Hb}) \times (15 \text{ g Hb}/100 \text{ mL blood})$$
$$+ (0.003 \text{ mL } O_2/100 \text{ mL blood/mm Hg}) \times (100 \text{ mm Hg})$$
$$= 20.4 \text{ mL } O_2/100 \text{ mL blood}$$

Compared to normal arterial blood, which is nearly 100% saturated with O_2 and carries 20.4 mL O_2/100 mL blood, **venous blood is approximately 75% saturated.** Thus normal **venous oxygen content**

$$= 75\% \times (1.34 \text{ mL } O_2/\text{g Hb}) \times (15 \text{ g Hb}/100 \text{ mL blood})$$
$$\times (0.003 \text{ mL } O_2/100 \text{ mL blood/mm Hg}) \times (40 \text{ mm Hg})$$
$$= 15.2 \text{ mL } O_2/100 \text{ mL blood}$$

Based on these calculations, each deciliter (100 mL) of blood delivers approximately 5 mL of O_2 to the tissues as it passes through the systemic circulation, and given that systemic blood flow (cardiac output) at rest is 5 L/min or 50 deciliters/min, **O_2 consumption is approximately 250 O_2 mL/min:**

$$O_2 \text{ consumption} = [a - v]_{O_2} \times \text{cardiac output}$$
$$= (5 \text{ mL } O_2/100 \text{ mL}) \times 5000 \text{ mL/min}$$
$$= 250 \text{ mL } O_2/\text{min}$$

COLOR and LABEL

☐ 1. Oxygen molecules

☐ 2. Red blood cells

☐ 3. Plasma

☐ 4. Alveoli of lung

☐ 5. Body tissue

Note the relative contributions of dissolved O_2 and O_2 combined with hemoglobin to the transport of oxygen to the tissues where O_2 is actually consumed.

TRACE the lines indicating relative contribution of dissolved vs. hemoglobin-bound O_2 to oxygen transport to tissues:

☐ 6. O_2 in solution in blood

☐ 7. O_2 combined with hemoglobin (Hb)

Clinical Note

CO is a colorless and odorless gas produced during combustion of fossil fuels and other organic matter. Prolonged exposure to levels as low as 0.04% can be lethal. Because CO binds to hemoglobin at very high affinity, it displaces oxygen and reduces the oxygen-carrying capacity of blood. Thus the sigmoidal oxyhemoglobin dissociation curve will plateau at lower O_2 content. CO poisoning is treated by breathing 100% O_2 and, under some conditions, hyperbaric O_2.

REVIEW ANSWERS

A. 1.5% (0.3/20.4)

B. 25% (5/20.4)

C. Solubility of the gas in that liquid

D. 100, 75

Plate 4.15
Respiratory Physiology

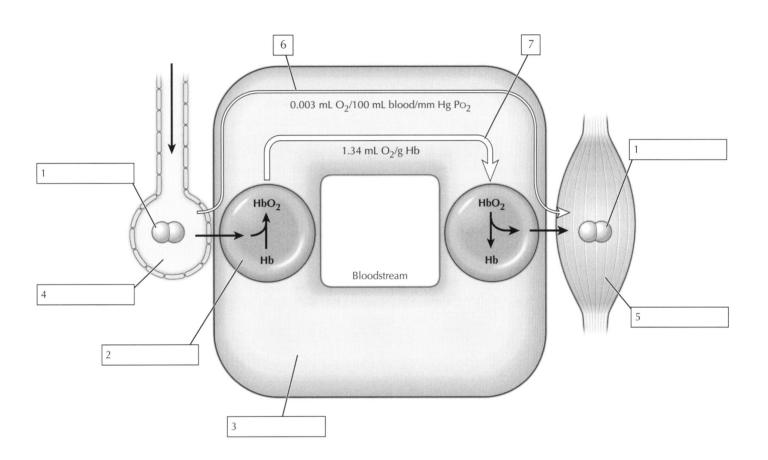

0.003 mL O_2/100 mL blood/mm Hg P_{O_2}

1.34 mL O_2/g Hb

HbO$_2$

Hb

HbO$_2$

Hb

Bloodstream

REVIEW QUESTIONS

A. Approximately what percent of oxygen in arterial blood is dissolved oxygen under normal circumstances?

B. What percent of oxygen in arterial blood is actually delivered to the tissues under normal, resting circumstances?

C. Content of a gas in a liquid is directly related to the partial pressure of the gas in the atmosphere with which the fluid has equilibrated and the _____.

D. Under normal, resting conditions, arterial blood is _____% saturated with O_2 in contrast to venous blood, which is _____% saturated.

As noted in Plate 4.15, at a P_{O_2} of 100 mm Hg, the P_{O_2} of alveolar air and arterial blood, hemoglobin is almost 100% saturated with O_2, whereas at a P_{O_2} of 40 mm Hg, the P_{O_2} of mixed venous blood, hemoglobin is 75% saturated with O_2. In Plate 4.16, the **oxyhemoglobin dissociation curve** in Part A illustrates this relationship between P_{O_2} and **%S$_{O_2}$, the percent saturation of hemoglobin with oxygen.** Based on the sigmoidal curve, a high level of O_2 saturation with hemoglobin occurs as blood passes through the lungs, and a significant level of dissociation of O_2 from hemoglobin occurs as blood passes through systemic capillaries. On the right side of the graph, the O_2 content values assume a blood hemoglobin concentration of 15 g/100 mL blood. Note that the O_2 in solution (dissolved O_2, dotted line) is quite low across the whole range of illustrated P_{O_2} values, highlighting the importance of hemoglobin in O_2 transport.

In addition to the basic sigmoidal curve illustrated in Part A, **the curve can be shifted to the right or left based on changes in P_{CO_2}, pH, and temperature.** More specifically, the curve shifts to the right with increased P_{CO_2}, low pH, and high temperature, conditions associated with tissue hypoxia and increased metabolism: For example, during exercise (Parts B, C, and D). With the rightward shift of the oxyhemoglobin dissociation curve, affinity of hemoglobin for O_2 is reduced, enhancing O_2 delivery to tissues. 2,3-Diphosphoglycerate (2,3-DPG) also shifts the oxyhemoglobin curve to the right. Notably, 2,3-DPG is a product of red blood cell glycolysis, and its levels are elevated during hypoxia.

TRACE

- ☐ 1. Sigmoidal oxyhemoglobin dissociation curve
- ☐ 2. Shallow dissolved O_2 line
- ☐ 3. Basic oxyhemoglobin dissociation curve
- ☐ 4. Rightward shifted curve at high P_{CO_2}, low pH, or high temperature
- ☐ 5. Leftward shifted curve at low P_{CO_2}, high pH, or low temperature

Clinical Note

By far, the most common form of hemoglobin in adult blood is **hemoglobin A (HbA),** constituting more than 95% of the Hb in normal blood. The **genetic variant hemoglobin, HbS,** is responsible for **sickle cell disease,** conferring changes in the physical properties of Hb that result in sickling of red blood cells. **HbF (fetal hemoglobin)** is the main form of the oxygen-binding protein in the fetus; it is nearly completely absent in adults except in some diseases (e.g., sickle cell disease). Finally, **HbA1c is glycated hemoglobin** and is considered an indicator of blood glucose level over the past 3 months. HbA1c is used in the **diagnosis of diabetes and the evaluation of glucose control** in people with diabetes.

REVIEW ANSWERS

- A. Left
- B. Right
- C. Left
- D. Right

Plate 4.16   **Respiratory Physiology**

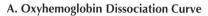

A. Oxyhemoglobin Dissociation Curve
(at pH 7.4, P_{CO_2} 40 mm Hg, 37°C)

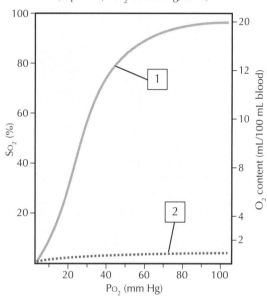

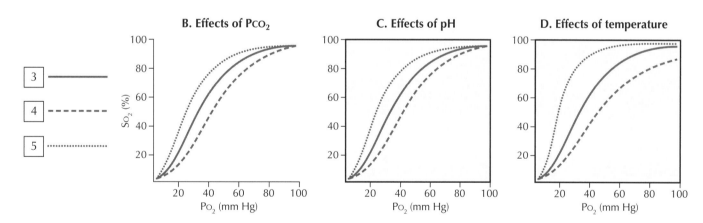

B. Effects of P_{CO_2}

C. Effects of pH

D. Effects of temperature

REVIEW QUESTIONS

For each condition, indicate whether the oxyhemoglobin dissociation curve would be shifted to the right or to the left:

A. A reduction in 2,3-DPG level

B. Acidemia (low blood pH)

C. Low body temperature

D. High P_{CO_2}

Carbon dioxide is transported in blood in a very different manner than oxygen. CO_2 dissolved in blood reacts with H_2O to form **carbonic acid, H_2CO_3,** which dissociates to form H^+ **and HCO_3^-** (see Plate 4.17). This reaction is catalyzed by the enzyme **carbonic anhydrase** within red blood cells. As the bicarbonate anion is formed, it diffuses out of the red blood cell in exchange for Cl^- (maintaining electrochemical equilibrium), a process known as the **chloride shift.** Much of the H^+ formed is buffered within the red blood cells by binding to hemoglobin (as **carbaminohemoglobin**). Overall, the transport of CO_2 is accomplished by transport as:

- HCO_3^-, 70%
- Carbaminohemoglobin, 23%
- **Dissolved CO_2,** 7%

Note in Plate 4.17 that unlike the oxyhemoglobin dissociation curve in Plate 4.16, the **CO_2 equilibrium curve is linear and steep,** accounting for the small difference in P_{CO_2} between mixed **venous blood** (left curve) and **arterial blood** (45 mm Hg vs. 40 mm Hg). Note also that the curve is shifted to the left when hemoglobin is in the deoxygenated state, increasing the affinity for CO_2. This is known as the **Haldane effect.** As blood is deoxygenated in systemic capillaries, as a result of the Haldane effect, the **affinity of hemoglobin for CO_2 increases,** facilitating its transport to the lungs. At the same time, affinity for H^+ is also increased. In contrast to the higher affinity for CO_2 when oxygen is off-loaded in systemic capillaries, in alveolar capillaries, as hemoglobin binds O_2, affinity for CO_2 falls, facilitating off-loading of CO_2.

Interestingly, although the P_{CO_2} of venous blood is roughly the same as P_{O_2}, the content of CO_2 is much higher because of the large amount of HCO_3^-. In addition, the amount of dissolved CO_2 in venous blood is much higher than that of dissolved O_2 because of the greater solubility of CO_2.

TRACE the transport of CO_2 from tissues to lungs, noting the relative contribution of each pathway:

☐ 1. H_2CO_3/HCO_3^-
☐ 2. Carbaminohemoglobin
☐ 3. Dissolved CO_2

TRACE the CO_2 equilibrium curves, reinforcing the Haldane effect:

☐ 4. Arterial blood
☐ 5. Venous blood, noting the higher affinity of hemoglobin for CO_2 in the deoxygenated state

REVIEW ANSWERS

A. Oxyhemoglobin, bicarbonate anion (HCO_3^-)

B. Deoxyhemoglobin

C. Carbonic acid, carbonic anhydrase

D. 40 mm Hg, alveolar P_{CO_2}

A. CO$_2$ equilibrium curves
(for normal arterial and venous blood)

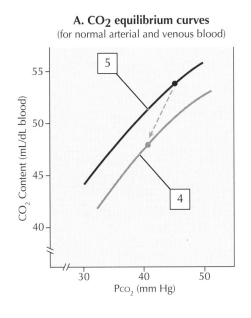

B. Carbon dioxide transport

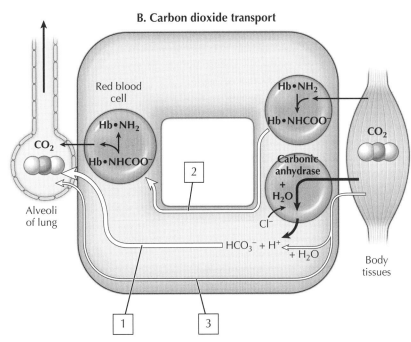

REVIEW QUESTIONS

A. Although most oxygen is transported in blood as _____, most carbon dioxide is transported as

_____.

B. Binding affinity of hemoglobin for CO$_2$ is elevated when hemoglobin is in the form of _____.

C. CO$_2$ dissolved in blood is converted to _____ by the enzyme _____.

D. The P$_{CO_2}$ of arterial blood is normally _____ and reflects its equilibration with _____ .

Blood pH is normally tightly regulated, in the range of 7.35 to 7.45, by the **lungs, kidneys,** and buffers in the body fluids (see Plate 4.18 and Chapter 5). This tight regulation is necessary because significant disturbance in pH affects enzyme activity, protein structure, and nearly all other bodily processes, resulting in death when not corrected. CO_2 transport has critical importance in maintaining the **acid-base equilibrium.**

Acid in the body includes **volatile acid,** which is CO_2 in its various forms. CO_2 produced by oxidative metabolism of carbohydrates and fats can readily be eliminated through respiration in the lungs to maintain pH balance. **Nonvolatile acids,** such as lactic acid and phosphoric acid, are buffered by various intra- and extracellular processes, including the important **bicarbonate buffering system** in blood and other extracellular fluids. As nonvolatile acids are buffered by bicarbonate anion, the kidneys replenish the bicarbonate anion and excrete acid. H^+ is also secreted in urine as bicarbonate is regenerated.

When a metabolic disease or abnormal renal function results in a change in pH, it is described as a **metabolic acidosis or alkalosis.** Intra- and extracellular buffering systems (primarily involving protein and bicarbonate, respectively) provide the immediate compensation, along with rapid adjustment of volatile acid (CO_2) elimination through altered respiratory rate. Over a longer period, the kidneys compensate by adjusting acid excretion and bicarbonate regeneration rate. On the other hand, when the original acid-base disturbance is caused by respiratory issues, it is **respiratory acidosis or alkalosis,** and the primary compensation is through kidney mechanisms.

COLOR

☐ 1. Pathway for elimination of volatile acid (CO_2)

☐ 2. Pathway for elimination of CO_2 derived from buffering of nonvolatile acid

☐ 3. Pathways for renal handling of excess acid

☐ 4. Lungs

☐ 5. Kidney

☐ 6. Blood

REVIEW ANSWERS

A. 7.35, 7.45

B. Nonvolatile

C. Renal mechanisms

D. The kidneys

Plate 4.18   **Respiratory Physiology**

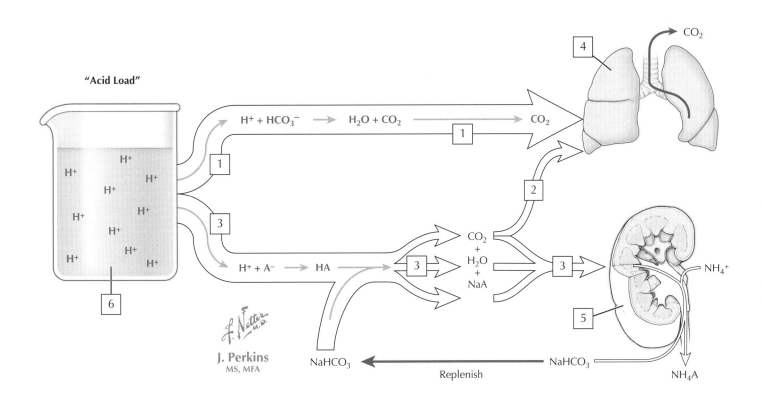

"Acid Load"

$H^+ + HCO_3^-$ → $H_2O + CO_2$ → CO_2

1

1

3

$H^+ + A^-$ → HA

3

CO_2
+
H_2O
+
NaA

2

3

6

CO_2

4

NH_4^+

5

J. Netter
M.D.

J. Perkins
MS, MFA

$NaHCO_3$ ← $NaHCO_3$

Replenish

NH_4A

REVIEW QUESTIONS

A. Normal blood pH is in the range of _____ to _____.

B. Bicarbonate and proteins are most important in buffering of _____ acids.

C. The primary compensation for respiratory acid-base disturbances is through _____.

D. Bicarbonate depletion through buffering of nonvolatile acids is replenished by _____.

Netter's Physiology Coloring Book **Plate 4.18**

4 Control of Respiration

Although we can control breathing voluntarily by holding our breath or hyperventilating, it is fundamentally an involuntary process that closely regulates Pa_{O_2} and Pa_{CO_2} (arterial O_2 and CO_2). Control of respiration is accomplished primarily by:

- Brainstem respiratory centers
- Peripheral and central chemoreceptors
- Mechanoreceptors in lungs and joints

Signals from these areas are integrated in the **medullary respiratory center,** which regulates V_T and breathing pattern by affecting activity of respiratory muscles.

Central chemoreceptors located on the ventral surface of the medulla respond indirectly to changes in Pa_{CO_2} (they respond directly to changes in cerebrospinal fluid pH, which reflects Pa_{CO_2}). When Pa_{CO_2} falls or rises, respiratory rate is decreased or increased, respectively. **Peripheral chemoreceptors** in the aortic and carotid bodies (see Chapter 3), unlike the central chemoreceptors, respond to changes in Pa_{O_2} and pH, as well as Pa_{CO_2}. A fall in Pa_{O_2} (especially below 60 mm Hg), a rise in Pa_{CO_2}, or a fall in pH will stimulate respiration when detected by peripheral chemoreceptors. Respiration is inhibited when the opposite changes in these parameters are detected. The chemical control of respiration is illustrated in Plate 4.19 (the pulmonary vein is drawn for effect rather than anatomic correctness).

Respiration is controlled by a number of other mechanisms as well. **Pulmonary mechanoreceptors** terminate inspiration when the lung is inflated, preventing overinflation. This response is known as the **Hering-Breuer reflex. Joint and muscle mechanoreceptors** detect movement of muscles and joints and respond by increasing respiratory rate, which plays a part in the respiratory adjustments in exercise (see later). **Irritant receptors** in the large airways respond to particulate matter and noxious gases by activating signals to the CNS, resulting in reflexive bronchoconstriction and coughing. Last, **juxtacapillary receptors (J receptors)** in alveoli are stimulated by hyperinflation of the lungs and various chemical stimuli, producing reflexive rapid, shallow breathing.

An integrated respiratory response occurs during exercise. During maximal aerobic exercise, oxygen consumption can rise from the normal, average rate of 250 mL O_2/min to as high as 4 L O_2/min, without substantial change in Pa_{O_2} or Pa_{CO_2}. The rapid, initial rise in respiration is largely a result of neural and reflexive mechanisms, but with continued exercise, feedback mechanisms become more important. Body temperature and blood pH play an important role. Although Pa_{O_2} and Pa_{CO_2} do not change substantially, respiratory control systems may become more sensitive to changes during exercise. Once exercise is terminated, neural and reflexive systems rapidly diminish respiratory rate, but respiration does not return to the resting level until metabolic alterations are reversed and feedback systems are no longer activated.

COLOR the following structures and note the pathway by which chemoreceptor signals result in adjustment of breathing:

- [ ] 1. Alveolus
- [ ] 2. Aortic body
- [ ] 3. Carotid body
- [ ] 4. Medulla
- [ ] 5. Phrenic nerve
- [ ] 6. Intercostal nerves
- [ ] 7. Intercostal muscles
- [ ] 8. Diaphragm

REVIEW ANSWERS

A. Pa_{CO_2}

B. Overinflation of the lungs

C. Neural, reflexive, feedback

D. Lung irritant receptors

Plate 4.19   **Respiratory Physiology**

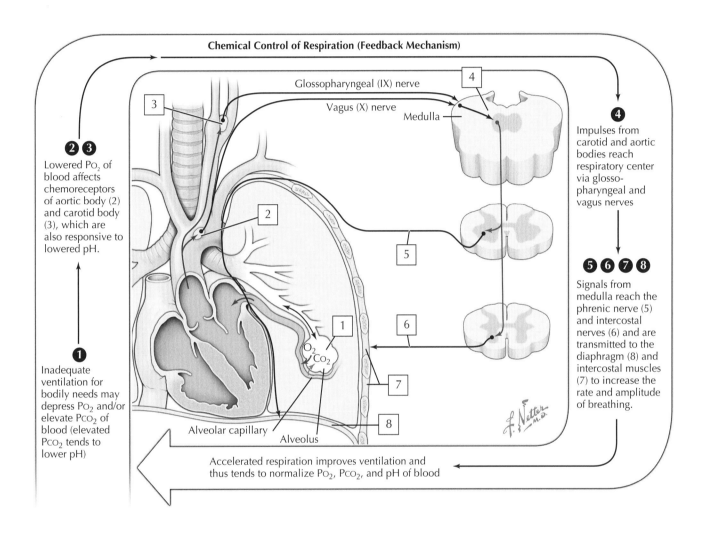

Chemical Control of Respiration (Feedback Mechanism)

Glossopharyngeal (IX) nerve

Vagus (X) nerve

Medulla

4

② ③

Lowered P_{O_2} of blood affects chemoreceptors of aortic body (2) and carotid body (3), which are also responsive to lowered pH.

3

2

5

6

1

O_2
CO_2

7

8

❶

Inadequate ventilation for bodily needs may depress P_{O_2} and/or elevate P_{CO_2} of blood (elevated P_{CO_2} tends to lower pH)

Alveolar capillary
Alveolus

④

Impulses from carotid and aortic bodies reach respiratory center via glosso-pharyngeal and vagus nerves

⑤ ⑥ ⑦ ⑧

Signals from medulla reach the phrenic nerve (5) and intercostal nerves (6) and are transmitted to the diaphragm (8) and intercostal muscles (7) to increase the rate and amplitude of breathing.

Accelerated respiration improves ventilation and thus tends to normalize P_{O_2}, P_{CO_2}, and pH of blood

REVIEW QUESTIONS

A. Although peripheral chemoreceptors respond to Pa_{O_2}, Pa_{CO_2}, and pH, central chemoreceptors respond mainly to

_____.

B. In the Hering-Breuer reflex, respiration is terminated to prevent _____.

C. The rapid respiratory response at the initiation of exercise is stimulated through _____ and _____ mechanisms, whereas the longer-term response is accomplished through _____ mechanisms.

D. Reflexive coughing and bronchoconstriction are produced by stimulation of _____.

Chapter 5 Renal Physiology

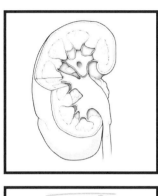
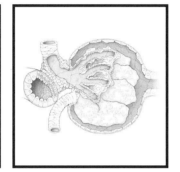
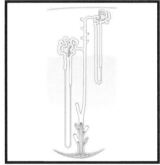
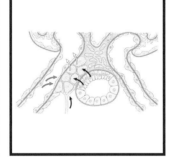

The kidneys are bilateral organs that filter blood supplied by the renal arteries. The filtered blood leaves the kidneys through the **renal veins** (Part B). The kidneys perform a host of functions that help maintain homeostasis, including the following:

- **Regulation of fluid and electrolyte balance:** The kidneys regulate the volume of extracellular fluid (ECF) through reabsorption and excretion of NaCl and water. They are also the site of regulation of the plasma levels of other key substances (Na^+, K^+, Cl^-, HCO_3^-, H^+, Ca^{2+}, and phosphates).
- **Regulation of plasma osmolarity:** "Opening" and "closing" of specific water channels (aquaporins) in the renal collecting ducts (CDs) produce concentrated and dilute urine (respectively), regulating plasma osmolarity and volume.
- **Elimination of metabolic waste products:** Urea (from protein metabolism), creatinine (from muscle metabolism), bilirubin (from breakdown of hemoglobin), uric acid (from breakdown of nucleic acids), metabolic acids, and foreign substances such as drugs are excreted in urine.
- **Production/conversion of hormones:** The kidney produces **erythropoietin** (a hormone that stimulates red blood cell production in bone marrow) and **renin** (a proteolytic enzyme that converts liver angiotensinogen to angiotensin I, covered in Plate 5.15). The renal tubules also convert 5-hydroxyvitamin D to the active **1,25-dihydroxyvitamin D,** which can act on kidney, intestine, and bone to regulate calcium homeostasis.
- **Metabolism:** The renal production of ammonia through **ammoniagenesis** has an important role in acid-base homeostasis (covered in Plate 5.17). The kidney, like the liver, has the ability to produce glucose through **gluconeogenesis.**

Each kidney in an adult is approximately the size of a fist and is surrounded by a **fibrous capsule.** The parenchyma is divided into the **cortex** and **medulla.** The renal cortex contains **renal corpuscles,** which are **glomerular capillaries** surrounded by **Bowman's capsules.** The corpuscles are connected to renal tubules, together forming the **nephrons,** the functional units of the kidneys that remove waste in the form of urine (covered in Plate 5.2). The renal medulla has outer and inner stripes that contain portions of the **loops of Henle** and **CDs,** and these structures form a pyramidal shape, as seen in Part A.

After the tubular fluid is processed in the nephron, the remaining fluid flowing through the CDs (urine) exits the medullary pyramids into the **minor calyces.** The minor calyces combine to form the **major calyces,** which empty into the **ureter.** The ureters lead to the bladder, where the urine is stored until excretion.

COLOR and **LABEL** the following structures:

- [ ] 1. Cortex
- [ ] 2. Medulla
- [ ] 3. Papilla of pyramid
- [ ] 4. Minor calyces
- [ ] 5. Major calyces
- [ ] 6. Renal pelvis
- [ ] 7. Ureter
- [ ] 8. Renal artery
- [ ] 9. Renal vein

REVIEW ANSWERS

A. They regulate the amount of water and electrolytes (especially Na^+) that is reabsorbed from the collecting ducts during urine formation.

B. Renin

C. Ammoniagenesis, gluconeogenesis

D. Loops of Henle, collecting ducts

E. Urine

Plate 5.1 | **Renal Physiology**

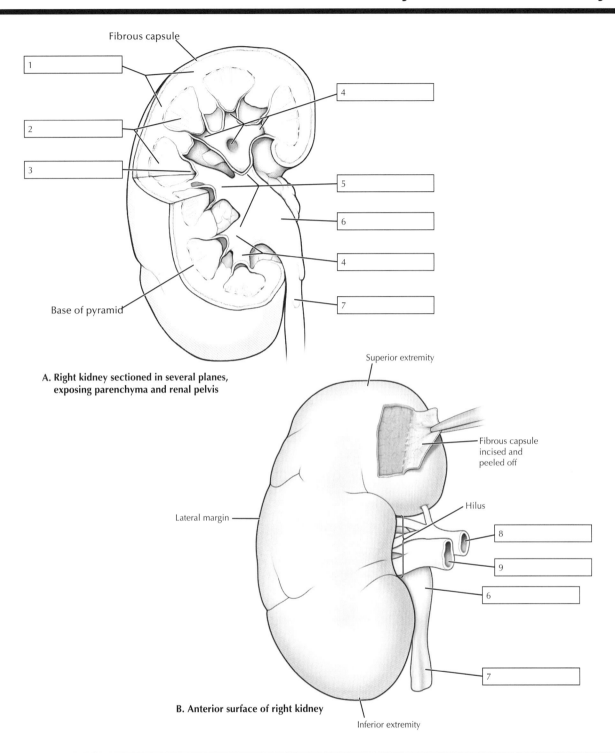

Fibrous capsule

1

2

3

4

5

6

4

7

Base of pyramid

**A. Right kidney sectioned in several planes,
exposing parenchyma and renal pelvis**

Superior extremity

Fibrous capsule
incised and
peeled off

Hilus

Lateral margin

8

9

6

7

B. Anterior surface of right kidney

Inferior extremity

REVIEW QUESTIONS

A. How do the kidneys help regulate plasma osmolarity and volume?

B. The kidneys produce the proteolytic enzyme _____, which converts angiotensinogen secreted by the liver to angiotensin I.

C. Metabolic functions of the kidneys include _____ and _____.

D. The renal medulla contains _____ and _____.

E. Tubular fluid flowing from the collecting ducts into the minor calyces is called _____.

The functional units of the kidney are the nephrons, which are the **renal corpuscles,** composed of the glomerular capillaries surrounded by Bowman's capsules, and the **renal tubules** and **collecting ducts (CDs)** to which they are connected. The renal tubule can be divided into the proximal tubule (PT), the loop of Henle, and the distal tubule (DT). Each kidney contains more than one million nephrons, and there are two populations of nephrons: cortical (also called *superficial,* or short, ~80% of total) and juxtamedullary (also called *deep,* ~20% of total). Note that the juxtamedullary nephrons have very long loops of Henle, which extend through the medulla and allow for concentration and dilution of urine; the cortical nephrons have very short loops of Henle, and they can dilute, but not concentrate, urine. The importance of the juxtamedullary nephrons in the renal concentrating mechanism is discussed in Plate 5.13. Also note that in each nephron, the distal convoluted tubule nears its parent glomerulus; this site forms the juxtaglomerular apparatus, which helps regulate filtration through the glomerulus (discussed in Plate 5.3).

The structure of both nephron populations is illustrated. A portion of the blood plasma is filtered at the glomerular capillaries through Bowman's capsule and takes the following path through the nephron:

1. Proximal convoluted tubule (S1 segment)
2. Proximal straight tubule (S2 and S3 segments)
3. Thin descending limb of Henle
4. Thin ascending limb of Henle
5. Thick ascending limb of Henle (TALH)
6. Distal convoluted tubule
7. CD

The CDs empty urine into the **calyces** and, ultimately, the ureter, which leads to the bladder, where urine is stored until excreted.

The following key nephron processes are involved in the regulation of circulating substances:

- **Filtration** of fluid and solutes from the plasma into the nephrons
- **Reabsorption** of fluid and solutes from the renal tubules into the peritubular capillaries and vasa recta
- **Secretion** of select substances into the tubular fluid, which facilitates their excretion; both endogenous (e.g., K^+, H^+, creatinine, norepinephrine, and dopamine) and exogenous (e.g., para-aminohippurate [PAH], salicylic acid, and penicillin) substances diffuse from peritubular capillaries and are subsequently secreted into the tubular fluid and excreted in the urine
- **Excretion** of excess fluid, electrolytes, and other substances (e.g., urea, bilirubin, and acid [H^+])

The nephron sites contributing to these processes are addressed in later plates.

COLOR and **LABEL** the nephron structures, illustrating the path through the nephron, while noting their location in the cortical and juxtamedullary nephron zones:

☐ 1. Proximal convoluted tubule (S1 segment)
☐ 2. Proximal straight tubule (S2 and S3 segments)
☐ 3. Thin descending limb of Henle
☐ 4. Thin ascending limb of Henle
☐ 5. Thick ascending limb of Henle (TALH)
☐ 6. Distal convoluted tubule
☐ 7. Collecting duct (CD)

REVIEW ANSWERS

A. Glomerular capillaries and Bowman's capsule

B. Cortical (superficial) and juxtamedullary (deep), the juxtamedullary nephrons

C. The renal cortex

D. Filtration, reabsorption, secretion, and excretion

Plate 5.2

Renal Physiology

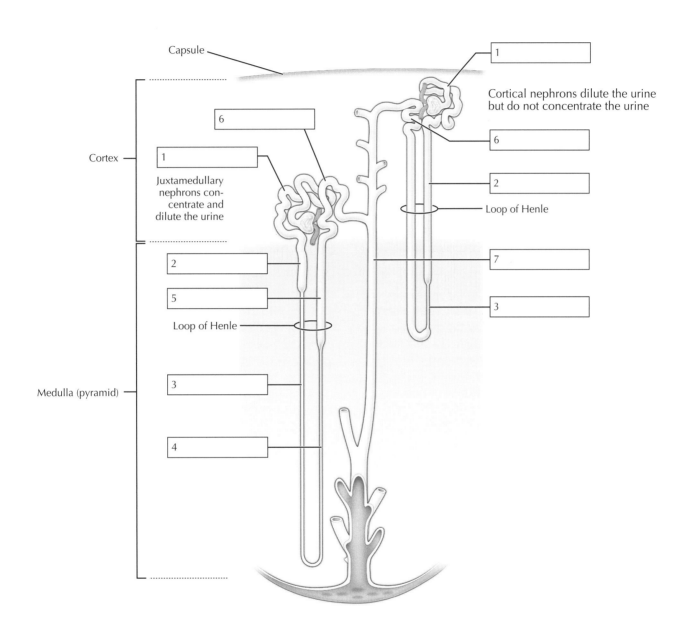

Capsule

1

Cortical nephrons dilute the urine but do not concentrate the urine

6

Cortex

6

1

2

Juxtamedullary nephrons con-centrate and dilute the urine

Loop of Henle

2

7

5

Loop of Henle

3

Medulla (pyramid)

3

4

A. What structures make up the renal corpuscle?

B. What names are given to the two populations of nephrons, and which population contributes to urine concentration?

C. Where are the renal corpuscles located?

D. What are the four main functions of the nephrons?

The glomerulus is a capillary system that filters blood to form the **ultrafiltrate** of plasma that flows into Bowman's space (in Bowman's capsule). The glomerular capillary has a **fenestrated endothelium** that allows filtration but keeps blood cells, proteins, and most macromolecules out of the glomerular ultrafiltrate. The **glomerular capillaries** are surrounded by a single layer of epithelial cells **(podocytes);** this layer of podocytes contributes to the filtration barrier. Filtration by the glomerulus occurs according to size and charge. Because the basement membrane and podocytes are negatively charged, most proteins (which are also negatively charged) cannot be filtered. **Mesangial cells** are also present; they support the glomerulus but can also contract, decreasing the surface area for filtration.

The glomerular capillaries arise from the **afferent arterioles,** and the plasma and blood elements that are not filtered leave the capillaries through the **efferent arterioles.** These vessels contribute to the local control of the glomerular filtration rate (GFR, the flow from the capillaries into Bowman's space to the tubules). GFR is discussed in Plate 5.4.

Another important structural and functional element is the **juxtaglomerular apparatus,** which is the area where the **distal convoluted tubule** returns to abut its "parent" glomerulus. At this site, specialized **macula densa cells** in the distal convoluted tubule are in contact with the **juxtaglomerular (JG) cells** of the afferent arteriole, forming the juxtaglomerular apparatus. The macula densa cells of the juxtaglomerular apparatus are important in sensing tubular fluid flow and sodium delivery to the **distal nephron** (portion of the nephron from the thick ascending loop of Henle to the collecting ducts), and because of their proximity to the afferent arteriole, macula densa cells can regulate renal plasma flow and GFR. Macula densa cells also participate in the regulation of the release of the enzyme renin from JG cells adjacent to the afferent arterioles. The renin secretion aids in fluid and electrolyte homeostasis through the renin-angiotensin-aldosterone system (RAAS, see Plates 5.15 and 5.16). Macula densa cells also receive input from adrenergic nerves through β_1-receptors.

COLOR and **LABEL** the structures associated with the glomerulus:

- ☐ 1. Afferent arteriole (abuts the juxtaglomerular cells)
- ☐ 2. Juxtaglomerular cells (part of the juxtaglomerular apparatus)
- ☐ 3. Macula densa cells (part of the juxtaglomerular apparatus)
- ☐ 4. Distal convoluted tubule
- ☐ 5. Glomerular capillaries
- ☐ 6. Efferent arteriole
- ☐ 7. Proximal tubule

COLOR and **LABEL** the components of the glomerular capillary membrane (from capillary lumen to Bowman's space):

- ☐ 8. Fenestrated endothelium
- ☐ 9. Capillary basement membrane
- ☐ 10. Podocytes

Clinical Note

Chronic **glomerular inflammation** (e.g., associated with diabetes) can result in thickened basement membranes, swollen epithelial cells, and narrowing of the capillary lumen. This damage permanently disrupts the filtration barrier, decreasing the GFR and increasing solutes and fluid in the blood; the disruption can also allow passage of red blood cells (RBCs) and normally unfiltered substances such as proteins, which then appear in the urine. **Chronic glomerulonephritis** can lead to renal failure.

REVIEW ANSWERS

A. Glomeruli

B. Large elements (e.g., RBCs) and negatively charged substances (e.g., proteins; under normal conditions)

C. Flow rate, sodium concentration

D. Afferent arteriole, efferent arteriole

E. Epithelial cells on the glomerular basement membrane that contribute to the filtration barrier

Plate 5.3 | **Renal Physiology**

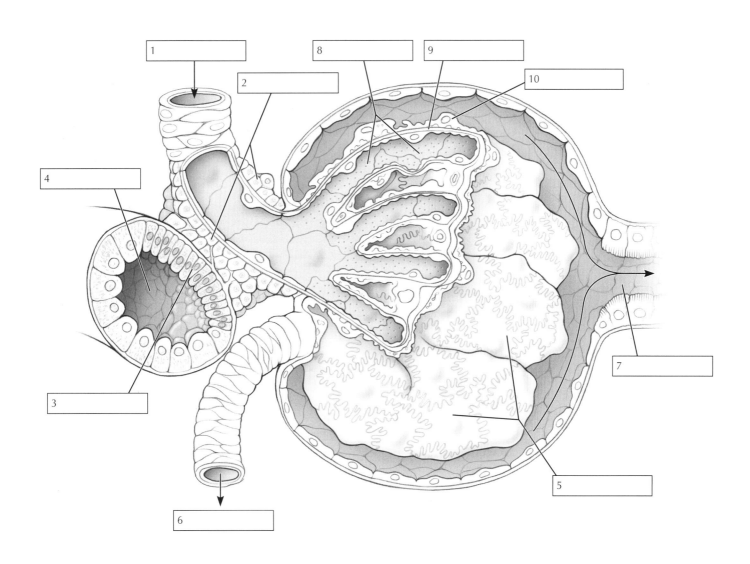

1

8

9

10

2

4

3

7

6

5

REVIEW QUESTIONS

A. What structures filter the blood?

B. What are examples of blood elements that are not filtered?

C. Macula densa cells in the distal tubule sense tubular fluid _____ and _____.

D. Blood enters the glomerulus from the _____ and leaves the glomerulus through the _____.

E. What are podocytes?

The **GFR** is determined by the **Starling forces** and the permeability of the **glomerular capillary membrane** to the solutes in the plasma. As stated previously, with the exception of most proteins, protein-bound substances, and formed elements, plasma is freely filtered at the glomerular capillaries. Because the molecules must travel through several barriers to move from the capillary lumen to Bowman's space, there are size limitations. Small molecules such as water, glucose, creatinine, and urea are freely filtered. As molecule size increases, or net negative charge of molecules increases, filtration becomes increasingly restricted.

Starling forces (described in Plate 1.13) govern fluid movement into or out of the capillaries. The pressures determining glomerular filtration are **glomerular capillary hydrostatic pressure (HP_{GC})** favoring fluid filtration of the capillary, **glomerular capillary oncotic pressure (π_{GC})** attracting fluid into the glomerular capillary, **Bowman's space hydrostatic pressure (HP_{BS})** opposing HP_{GC}, and **Bowman's space oncotic pressure (π_{BS})** attracting fluid into Bowman's space (typically negligible, because proteins are not normally filtered). Assuming π_{BS} is zero,

$$\text{Net filtration pressure} = HP_{GC} - (HP_{BS} + \pi_{GC})$$

Glomerular capillaries are different from other capillaries (which have significantly reduced pressures at the distal end of the capillary) because the **efferent arteriole** can constrict and maintain pressure in the glomerular capillary. Thus there is very little reduction in HP_{GC} through the capillary and filtration can be maintained along its entire length. **Afferent and efferent arteriolar resistance** can be controlled by **sympathetic nerves,** circulating hormones (e.g., **angiotensin II**), **myogenic regulation,** and **tubuloglomerular feedback signals,** allowing regulation of glomerular filtration by both intrarenal and extrarenal mechanisms.

The GFR is an important measure of renal function. It is the volume of plasma filtered across all of the glomeruli in the kidneys, per unit time. In a healthy adult, GFR is approximately 100 to 125 mL/min, with men having a higher GFR than women. Many factors help maintain GFR at a fairly constant rate, over a wide range of mean arterial pressure (MAP, between 80 and 180 mm Hg). GFR is determined by the net filtration pressure (see the previous equation) and the permeability coefficient K_f (mL/min × mm Hg; a function of water permeability of the glomerular capillary membrane and its total surface area, which reflects nephron number and size). The equation is

$$GFR = K_f [HP_{GC} - (HP_{BS} + \pi_{GC})]$$

Significant alteration of any of the parameters in the above equation can affect the GFR, and hence fluid and electrolyte homeostasis.

LABEL the forces involved in glomerular filtration and **TRACE** the arrows showing direction of the force:

☐ 1. HP_{GC} (glomerular capillary hydrostatic pressure)

☐ 2. HP_{BS} (Bowman's space hydrostatic pressure)

☐ 3. π_{GC} (capillary oncotic pressure)

LABEL the site associated with the K_f (filtration coefficient):

☐ 4. Glomerular capillary membrane

Clinical Note

The GFR is a common diagnostic tool that is useful in determining decreases in renal function that can arise from acute or chronic disturbances. For example, a hemorrhage that reduces MAP below 80 mm Hg may decrease HP_{GC} enough to dramatically decrease or stop filtration, resulting in acute renal failure. Decreases in GFR can also result from kidney stones blocking flow and increasing HP_{BS}, or a reduction in *Kf,* which occurs with **glomerulosclerosis.**

REVIEW ANSWERS

A. Starling forces, the permeability of the capillaries to solutes in the plasma

B. False; there are intrarenal and extrarenal mechanisms to regulate glomerular filtration.

C. Glomerular filtration rate (GFR)

D. Decrease

E. No, normal GFR is maintained over a wide range of mean arterial pressures.

Plate 5.4   **Renal Physiology**

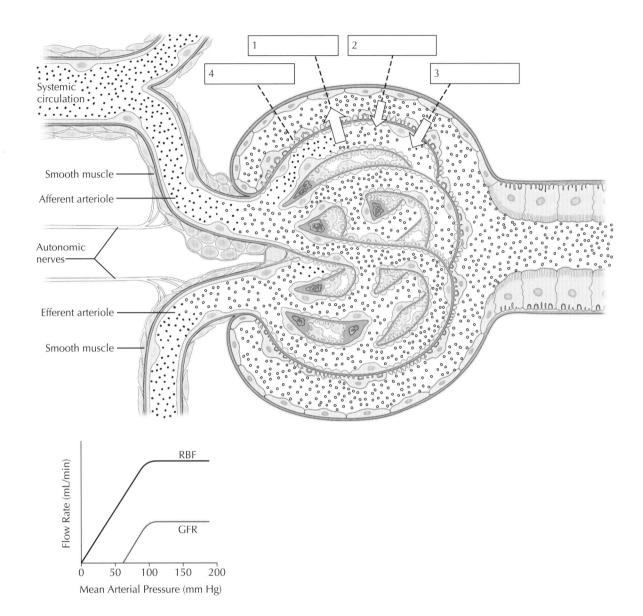

A. Glomerular filtration rate is determined by the _____ and _____.

B. True/False: Glomerular filtration is controlled only through extrarenal mechanisms.

C. The volume of plasma filtered across all of the glomeruli in the kidneys per unit time is called the _____.

D. An increase in only glomerular capillary oncotic pressure (π_{GC}) would _____ the net filtration pressure.

E. Do changes in MAP (within approximately 80 to 180 mm Hg) ordinarily have an effect on the GFR?

Intrinsic feedback systems, hormones, vasoactive substances, and **renal sympathetic nerves** regulate the GFR through effects on **renal hemodynamics** (flow, resistance, and pressure). Intrinsic systems include the **myogenic mechanism** and **tubuloglomerular feedback (TGF).** Using the myogenic mechanism, the renal arteries and arterioles respond directly to increases in local hydrostatic pressure (reflecting changes in systemic blood pressure) by constricting, thereby maintaining constant filtration pressure in the glomerular capillaries. TGF is a regulatory mechanism that involves the macula densa cells of the juxtaglomerular apparatus. The kidney is unique in that the glomerular capillaries have arterioles (resistance vessels) at *either end* of the capillary network. Constriction of the afferent or efferent arterioles can produce immediate effects on the HP_{GC}, controlling GFR. Because the juxtaglomerular apparatus functionally couples the DT with the **afferent arteriole,** the concentration of NaCl passing the macula densa in the DTs can control afferent arteriolar resistance. Decreases in NaCl concentration in the DT will decrease afferent arteriolar resistance and increase GFR in that nephron; conversely, if distal tubular NaCl concentration is high, TGF will increase afferent arteriolar resistance, decreasing GFR. A decrease in concentration of NaCl passing the macula densa will also stimulate renin release from the juxtaglomerular cells.

The main factors that regulate renal hemodynamics include the following:

1. **RAAS** (see Plate 3.23): In response to low renal blood flow, the reduced stretch of renal vascular baroreceptors stimulates **renin** secretion by **the juxtaglomerular cells.** Renin activates the RAAS and, ultimately, angiotensin II production.
2. **Angiotensin II:** Angiotensin II has direct and indirect effects on the GFR. It constricts the renal arteries and arterioles (with a greater effect on the efferent arteriole), and it constricts mesangial cells, decreasing K_f. These effects contribute to the complex regulation of GFR, generally favoring maintenance of or a decrease in GFR.
3. **Atrial natriuretic peptide (ANP):** ANP is secreted from cardiac atria in response to stretch from increased atrial volume. It acts on the kidneys to dilate the afferent arterioles and constrict the efferent arterioles, increasing HP_{GC} and thus GFR. This results in a diuresis (increased urine excretion) and natriuresis (increased sodium excretion), reducing fluid volume.
4. **Sympathetic nerves and catecholamines** (epinephrine and norepinephrine) **secretion:** The sympathetic nervous system (SNS) is stimulated in response to decreased systemic blood pressure and causes constriction of the renal artery and arterioles, reducing GFR.
5. **Intrarenal prostaglandins:** PGE_2 and prostacyclin are vasodilators and act at the level of the arterioles and glomerular mesangial cells to counteract the effects of angiotensin II vasoconstriction, which helps to prevent loss of filtration during extreme constriction of the kidneys.

COLOR and **LABEL** in Part A:

☐ 1. Afferent arteriole

☐ 2. Juxtaglomerular cells

COLOR in Part B:

☐ 3. Arrows, on left side, showing stimulation of the renin-angiotensin system (beginning with an increase in renin), leading to an increase in vasoconstriction in the renal vasculature

☐ 4. Arrows, on right side, showing inhibition of the renin-angiotensin system, leading to a decrease in vaso-constriction in the renal vasculature

REVIEW ANSWERS

A. Myogenic mechanism, tubuloglomerular feedback

B. Macula densa, tubuloglomerular

C. ANP is released from cardiac atria in response to elevated volume. It dilates the afferent arterioles and constricts the efferent arterioles.

Plate 5.5 **Renal Physiology**

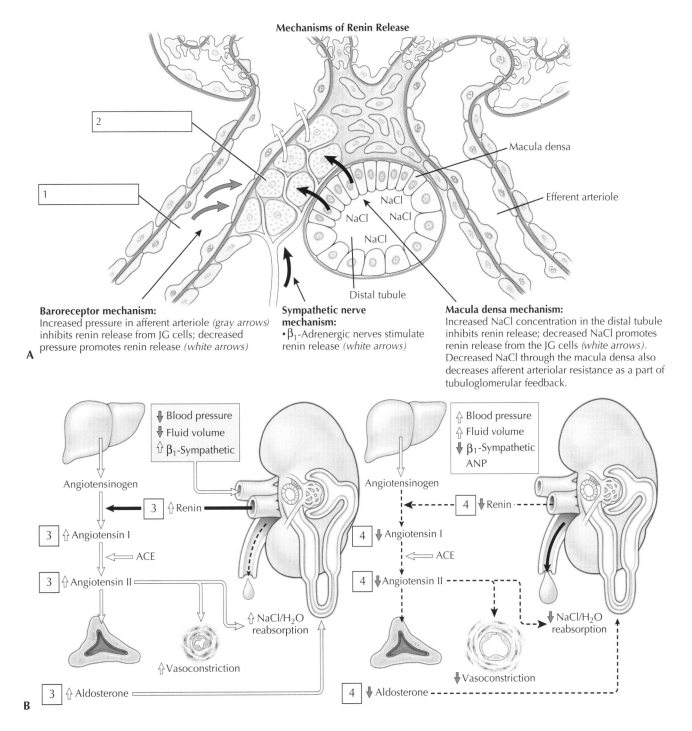

Mechanisms of Renin Release

Macula densa

Efferent arteriole

NaCl
NaCl
NaCl
NaCl

Distal tubule

Baroreceptor mechanism:
Increased pressure in afferent arteriole (gray arrows) inhibits renin release from JG cells; decreased pressure promotes renin release (white arrows)

Sympathetic nerve mechanism:
• β_1-Adrenergic nerves stimulate renin release (white arrows)

Macula densa mechanism:
Increased NaCl concentration in the distal tubule inhibits renin release; decreased NaCl promotes renin release from the JG cells (white arrows). Decreased NaCl through the macula densa also decreases afferent arteriolar resistance as a part of tubuloglomerular feedback.

A

⬇ Blood pressure
⬇ Fluid volume
⬆ β_1-Sympathetic

Angiotensinogen

3 ⬆ Renin

3 ⬆ Angiotensin I

⬅ ACE

3 ⬆ Angiotensin II

⬆ NaCl/H₂O reabsorption

⬆ Vasoconstriction

3 ⬆ Aldosterone

⬆ Blood pressure
⬆ Fluid volume
⬇ β_1-Sympathetic
ANP

Angiotensinogen

4 ⬇ Renin

4 ⬇ Angiotensin I

⬅ ACE

4 ⬇ Angiotensin II

⬇ NaCl/H₂O reabsorption

⬇ Vasoconstriction

4 ⬇ Aldosterone

B

REVIEW QUESTIONS

A. Intrinsic regulation of renal hemodynamics occurs through the _____ and _____.

B. Changes in NaCl concentration in the distal tubule can be sensed by the _____ cells and cause changes in glomerular filtration; this mechanism is called _____ feedback.

C. When is ANP released from cardiac myocytes, and what effect does the peptide have on the afferent and efferent renal arterioles?

GFR is an important measure of kidney health, and it can be assessed using the principle of **renal clearance** (see Clinical Note). Renal clearance (C_x) is the **volume of plasma cleared of a substance (X) per unit time.** The clearance equation incorporates the urine and plasma concentrations of a substance, along with the urine flow rate and is usually reported in mL/min or L/day.

$$C_x = (U_x \times \dot{V})/P_x$$

This equation can be used to determine the clearance of any filtered substance (X) and the principle can also be used to determine the GFR. If a substance is **freely filtered but not reabsorbed or secreted,** its clearance can be equated to the GFR; in this case, the filtered amount of the substance will equal the amount **excreted** (F = E), and thus C_x = GFR. The exogenous substance inulin (which can be infused intravenously) meets these requirements but is not routinely used in patients. Although no endogenous substance exactly meets these requirements (freely filtered, but not reabsorbed or secreted), **creatinine** (a by-product of muscle metabolism) is freely filtered and not reabsorbed, although 10% is secreted into the renal tubule. Thus, the clearance of creatinine overestimates the GFR by approximately 10% (see Clinical Note).

The renal clearance of any substance found in the blood can be determined by taking a timed urine collection (to determine urine flow rate, $\dot{V}$), obtaining a blood sample, measuring the plasma and urine concentrations of the substance, and applying the clearance equation. The **net handling of substances** by the kidneys can be estimated by comparing the clearance of any freely filtered substance (X) to the GFR; if the clearance of X is greater than the GFR, there is net secretion of X and, conversely, if the clearance of X is less than the GFR, there is net reabsorption of X.

COLOR and **LABEL**, on the simplified nephron diagram, the arrows that depict the four major processes for renal handling of solutes and indicate whether the processes are relevant for inulin, creatinine, both, or neither:

☐ 1. Filtration/both

☐ 2. Reabsorption/neither

☐ 3. Secretion/creatinine

☐ 4. Excretion/both

Clinical Note

Plasma creatinine (P_{Cr}) is used clinically to estimate GFR. In most cases, the body produces creatinine at a constant rate, and therefore the excretion rate is also constant. GFR is approximately equal to the clearance of creatinine [GFR = $(U_{Cr} \times \dot{V})/P_{Cr}$]; thus, if the GFR decreases, Cr clearance decreases, and plasma creatinine increases. Therefore the **GFR is proportional to 1/P_{Cr}.** As a clinical application, this allows a rapid approximation of the GFR by simply analyzing the P_{Cr}. P_{Cr} is normally approximately 1 mg%, so GFR is approximately 1/1 (normal: 100%). If P_{Cr} rises to 2, GFR is ½, or 50% of normal, and so on.

REVIEW ANSWERS

A. Plasma

B. Freely filtered and not reabsorbed or secreted, so F = E

C. Creatinine

D. GFR is proportional to 1/P_{Cr}

Plate 5.6 | **Renal Physiology**

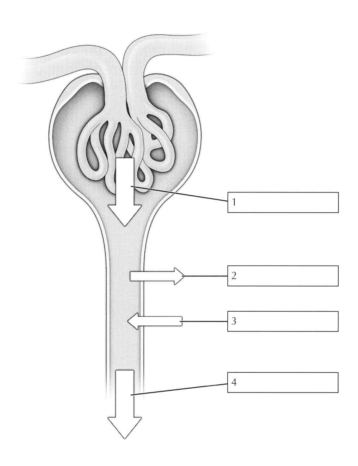

1

2

3

4

REVIEW QUESTIONS

A. The renal clearance of a substance is the volume of _____ cleared of the substance per unit time.

B. Clearance of the exogenous substance inulin can be equated to the GFR because inulin is _____.

C. The endogenous substance that can be used to estimate GFR is _____.

D. A plasma creatinine sample can be used to determine renal function because _____.

Nephrons are associated with **filtration, reabsorption, secretion,** and **excretion.** The following definitions and relationships hold true for freely filtered substances and will help your understanding of how the kidney is working:

- For all filtered substances, the filtration rate (F_x) will equal the sum of the reabsorption rate (R_x) and excretion rate (E_x), minus the secretion rate (S_x):

$$F_x = (R_x + E_x) - S_x$$

- The **filtered load (FL$_x$)** of a substance (i.e., the amount of a specific substance filtered per unit time) is the product of the plasma concentration of the substance (P_x) times the GFR:

$$FL_x = P_x \times GFR$$

- The **urinary excretion rate (E$_x$)** of a substance is the urine concentration of the substance (U_x) times the volume of urine produced per unit time ($\dot{V}$):

$$E_x = U_x \times \dot{V}$$

- The **reabsorption rate** of a substance **(R$_x$)** is equal to the FL of the substance minus the urinary excretion rate of the substance:

$$R_x = FL_x - E_x$$

- Certain substances are secreted (e.g., creatinine, PAH, K^+), and the **secretion rate (S$_x$)** is equal to the excretion rate minus the FL of the substance:

$$S_x = E_x - FL_x$$

The stylized nephron illustrated can be used to visualize the basic concepts above.

COLOR the arrows for:

- ☐ 1. Filtration
- ☐ 2. Reabsorption
- ☐ 3. Secretion
- ☐ 4. Excretion

FILL IN the equations for:

- ☐ 5. Filtered load ($FL_x = P_x \times GFR$)
- ☐ 6. Reabsorption rate ($R_x = FL_x - E_x$)
- ☐ 7. Secretion rate ($S_x = E_x - FL_x$)
- ☐ 8. Urinary excretion rate ($E_x = U_x \times \dot{V}$)

REVIEW ANSWERS

A. S_x

B. E_x

C. Reabsorbed

Plate 5.7   **Renal Physiology**

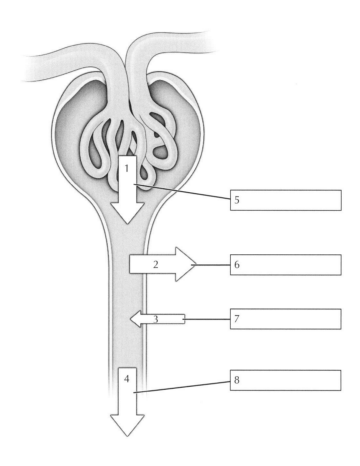

REVIEW QUESTIONS

A. $FL_x = (R_x + E_x) - \underline{\quad}$?

B. $U_x \times \dot{V} = \underline{\quad}$?

C. A substance X is freely filtered, but its excretion rate is less than the FL_x. This implies that some of X is _____.

When the plasma filtered into Bowman's space enters the **proximal tubule (PT),** the process of reabsorption begins. In general, nephrons reabsorb the majority of the fluid and solutes that pass through them, with the PT having the greatest reabsorptive capacity and the distal sites fine-tuning the process. In addition, certain substances (creatinine, PAH, and penicillin) are secreted into various segments of the renal tubule.

Each segment of the nephron has important basic functions. The PT has a brush border membrane, which increases the surface area for absorption facilitating the bulk reabsorption of fluid and solutes. **The thin descending limb of Henle** is permeable to water but impermeable to solutes, allowing concentration of tubular fluid (see Plate 5.13). The **thick ascending limb of Henle (TALH)** is permeable to sodium and other solutes, but impermeable to water, allowing dilution of the tubular fluid (the loop of Henle is integral for establishing a medullary interstitial concentration gradient that is necessary for concentration of urine; see Plate 5.13). The **distal tubule (DT)** and **early collecting duct** are the last of sites of sodium reabsorption, and the **collecting duct (CD)** is the site of H$^+$ secretion and excretion and urine concentration.

Sodium ion concentration is a major driving force for the renal reabsorption of fluid, electrolytes, and a variety of other solutes. The FL of Na$^+$ through the glomeruli is high (~25,000 milliequivalents [mEq]/day), and to maintain body fluid homeostasis, more than 99% of the FL$_{Na}$ must be reabsorbed back into the blood. This reabsorption is accomplished by luminal (apical) secondary active transport of sodium down a concentration gradient established by the basolateral **Na$^+$/K$^+$ ATPase** pumps. As sodium transporters reabsorb sodium (and other solutes), they generate the driving force for **water reabsorption.** When the water leaves the tubule, the concentration of electrolytes and solutes remaining in the tubular fluid increases, providing higher gradients for their diffusion into the cell. Approximately **65% to 70%** of the water in tubular fluid is reabsorbed from the PT into the peritubular capillaries, primarily driven by sodium reabsorption. The table in Plate 5.8 indicates the amount of the FL of sodium (and thus water) that is reabsorbed in the segments. Plate 5.8 illustrates the primary sites and transporters for sodium reabsorption along different segments of the nephron.

COLOR the different segments of the nephron in the center of the diagram and the corresponding transporters and channels for sodium reabsorption at these sites:

Proximal tubule (PT):
- [ ] 1. Cotransporter (symporter) with Na$^+$ (i.e., glucose, amino acids, organic acids, phosphate)
- [ ] 2. Na$^+$/H$^+$ antiporter (exchanger)

Thick ascending limb of Henle (TALH):
- [ ] 3. Na$^+$-K$^+$-2Cl$^-$ cotransporter (NKCC-2)
- [ ] 4. Na$^+$/H$^+$ antiporter

Distal tubule (DT):
- [ ] 5. Na$^+$-Cl$^-$ cotransporter (thiazide-sensitive)
- [ ] 6. Epithelial sodium channels (ENaC)

Collecting duct (CD):
- [ ] 7. Epithelial sodium channels (ENaC)

COLOR

- [ ] 8. Basolateral Na$^+$/K$^+$ ATPase (sodium pump) in each cell type (green), reinforcing that the active sodium pump sets up the gradient for luminal sodium to enter the cells down its concentration gradient

Clinical Note

To help control extracellular volume in patients with hypertension or congestive heart failure, drugs that target renal sodium transporters can be used to increase excretion of sodium and water. **Loop diuretics** such as furosemide and bumetanide inhibit the NKCC-2 transporters in the TALH, whereas thiazide diuretics act on the Na$^+$Cl$^-$ transport in the DT. Extended use of these diuretics can result in urinary potassium loss, and plasma potassium must be monitored when these drugs are used. Amiloride is a **potassium-sparing diuretic** that targets ENaC in the late DT and CDs.

REVIEW ANSWERS

A. Proximal tubule

B. 30 to 35

C. Proximal tubule and thick ascending limb of Henle

D. Thick ascending limb of Henle

E. Secondary

Plate 5.8 | **Renal Physiology**

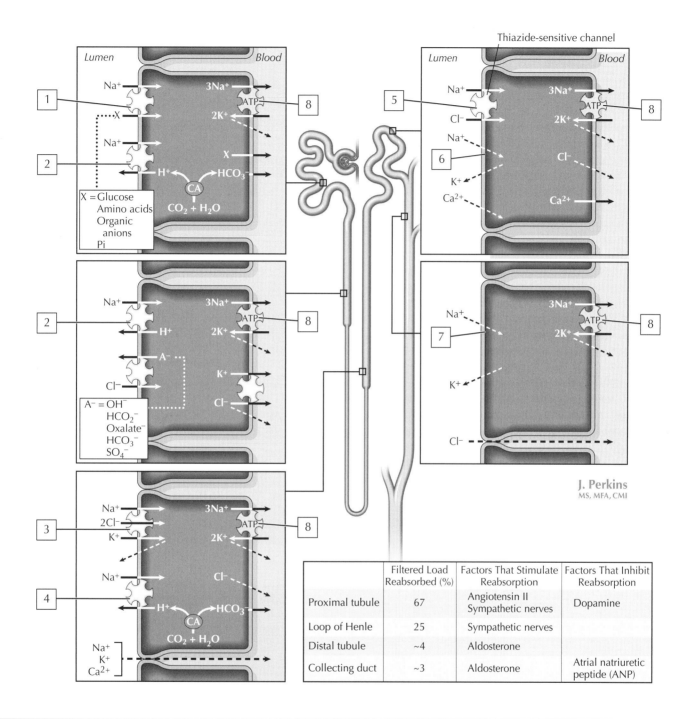

	Filtered Load Reabsorbed (%)	Factors That Stimulate Reabsorption	Factors That Inhibit Reabsorption
Proximal tubule	67	Angiotensin II Sympathetic nerves	Dopamine
Loop of Henle	25	Sympathetic nerves	
Distal tubule	~4	Aldosterone	
Collecting duct	~3	Aldosterone	Atrial natriuretic peptide (ANP)

J. Perkins
MS, MFA, CMI

REVIEW QUESTIONS

A. Which part of the renal tubule reabsorbs the most sodium?

B. The amount of water entering the descending thin loop of Henle is approximately _____% of the amount filtered at the glomerulus.

C. Where are Na^+/H^+ exchangers found in the renal tubule?

D. Where are NKCC-2 transporters found in the renal tubule?

E. Are luminal sodium transporters primary or secondary active transporters?

Glucose is freely filtered at the glomeruli, is reabsorbed in the **proximal tubules** via **insulin-independent** sodium-glucose transporters (SGLTs) and exits the basolateral membranes into the peritubular capillaries via GLUT-2 facilitated transporters.

Because of the large FL of sodium, the reabsorption of sodium is not a rate-limiting step in the absorption of glucose and other co-transported solutes. For many solutes, including glucose, the **rate-limiting step** is the number of specific transporters available for the solute. Renal SGLTs have a **transport maximum (TM)** that is far higher than necessary. Under normal conditions, the FL of glucose is low enough that the transporters can carry all of the solute back into the blood, leaving none in the tubular fluid and urine (Part A). Thus the renal clearance of glucose is normally **zero.**

However, if the plasma glucose level is high (as in persons with diabetes), the FL of glucose will increase and the glucose in the tubular fluid may saturate the carriers. The **renal threshold** for glucose is the plasma concentration at which glucose reaches its TM and above which excess glucose will be excreted in the urine **(glucosuria).** Thus, when the plasma glucose (hence FL of glucose) is under the renal threshold for reabsorption, all of the glucose in the tubular fluid will be reabsorbed (Parts A and B). However, if the FL increases and *exceeds* the threshold, the transporters can become saturated (TM, Part B) and the excess glucose continues past the PT and is excreted in the urine, resulting in glucosuria (Part C). The graph illustrates the relationship between **filtered, reabsorbed,** and **excreted glucose.** The point where glucose reabsorption plateaus and excretion increases is the TM.

COLOR

- [ ] 1. Filtered glucose molecules
- [ ] 2. Reabsorbed glucose molecules
- [ ] 3. Unabsorbed glucose molecules (noting glucose ends up in the urine)

TRACE and LABEL the following lines:

- [ ] 4. Filtered glucose (dashed line)
- [ ] 5. Reabsorbed glucose (dotted line)
- [ ] 6. Excreted glucose (solid line)
- [ ] 7. Transport maximum (TM, arrows)

REVIEW ANSWERS

A. Proximal tubule (PT), SGLT

B. Independent

C. Rate-limiting

D. Renal threshold

Plate 5.9   **Renal Physiology**

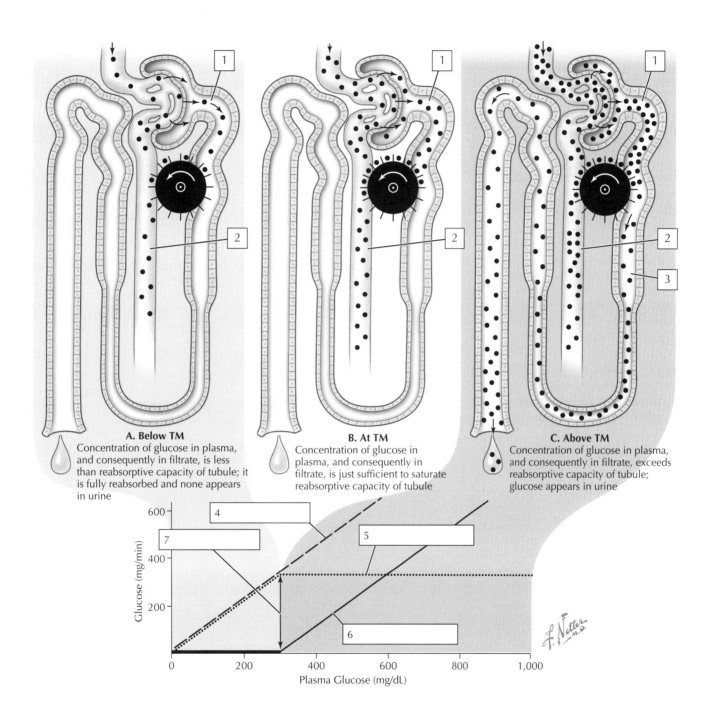

A. Below TM
Concentration of glucose in plasma, and consequently in filtrate, is less than reabsorptive capacity of tubule; it is fully reabsorbed and none appears in urine

B. At TM
Concentration of glucose in plasma, and consequently in filtrate, is just sufficient to saturate reabsorptive capacity of tubule

C. Above TM
Concentration of glucose in plasma, and consequently in filtrate, exceeds reabsorptive capacity of tubule; glucose appears in urine

REVIEW QUESTIONS

A. Under normal conditions, 100% of filtered glucose is reabsorbed in the _____ via _____ transporters.

B. Glucose transport in the kidneys is insulin _____.

C. The number of luminal glucose transporters is the _____ step in glucose reabsorption.

D. The concentration at which glucose reaches its TM and above which it will begin to appear in the urine is called the _____.

5   Renal Bicarbonate Reabsorption

Adequate plasma bicarbonate is necessary for acid-base homeostasis (see Plate 5.17), and to accomplish this, the kidneys **reabsorb 100%** of the filtered bicarbonate (HCO_3^-). However, this reabsorption occurs **indirectly** and involves the secretion of H^+ (through **Na^+/H^+ exchangers** and active **H^+ pumps**) in multiple nephron segments.

In the tubular lumen, filtered HCO_3^- and secreted H^+ form CO_2 and H_2O (a reaction catalyzed by brush border **carbonic anhydrase [CA]**), which diffuse into the tubular cells. Within the cell the CO_2 and H_2O are converted back to carbonic acid (by intracellular CA), which dissociates to HCO_3^- and H^+; the HCO_3^- is transported out of the cell via **basolateral HCO_3^-/ Cl^- exchangers** or **Na^+-HCO_3^- cotransporters,** depending on the nephron segments. The H^+ generated from this process is secreted back into the tubular lumen via the Na^+/H^+ exchangers or active H^+ pumps (depending on the nephron segments) and can be used to reabsorb more HCO_3^-. In the **CDs** the H^+ can be buffered and excreted (see Plate 5.18). This mechanism is present in three segments of the nephron, facilitating reabsorption of filtered bicarbonate in the **PT** (80% of FL), **TALH** (15%), and **CD** (5%).

Under normal conditions, the renal clearance of HCO_3^- is **zero**, meaning that there is no HCO_3^- in the urine. The regulation of bicarbonate handling is an integral part of acid-base homeostasis and will be discussed in Plate 5.19.

COLOR the following transporters in the PT, TALH, and CD cells:

☐ 1. Na^+/H^+ exchangers

☐ 2. H^+ pumps

COLOR the sites of HCO_3^- reabsorption:

☐ 3.   PT

☐ 4.   TALH

☐ 5.   CD

REVIEW ANSWERS

A.   False; HCO_3^- is indirectly reabsorbed

B.   PT, TALH, and CD

C. H^+

D.   Bicarbonate is important in acid-base homeostasis because it is the major extracellular acid buffer.

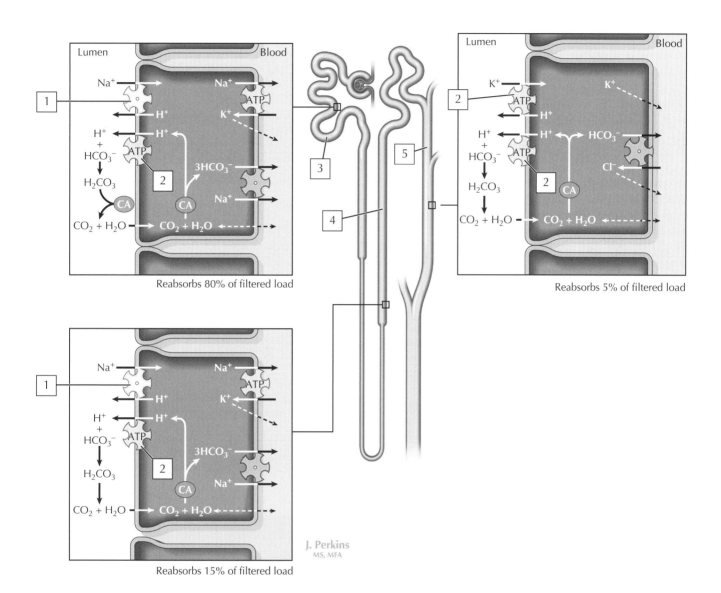

Reabsorbs 80% of filtered load

Reabsorbs 5% of filtered load

Reabsorbs 15% of filtered load

J. Perkins
MS, MFA

REVIEW QUESTIONS

A. True/False: HCO_3^- is reabsorbed directly into the tubular cells.

B. In which nephron segments is bicarbonate reabsorbed?

C. When bicarbonate is transported out of the tubular cells and into the blood, _____ is secreted into the tubular lumen.

D. Why is bicarbonate reabsorption important?

Potassium is another electrolyte that is important to overall homeostasis. In adults, the dietary intake must be matched by urinary and fecal excretion. As discussed in Plate 1.5, plasma K+ concentration must be maintained at relatively low levels (3.5 to 5 mEq/L), and the kidneys regulate K+ reabsorption and secretion to maintain homeostasis. Plate 5.11 illustrates potassium ion handling through the nephron and the effects of dietary K+ intake.

In general, potassium reabsorption in the PT (~67% of the FL) and TALH (20% of the FL) is fairly constant, and the response to low- or high-K+ diets (increased reabsorption or increased secretion, respectively) occurs in the distal segments (DT and CD).

- **Proximal tubule (PT):** K+ reabsorption occurs by **paracellular** movement (between cells). This is driven by "solvent drag": As the PT actively reabsorbs much of the filtered Na+, water follows, creating a concentration gradient for K+ diffusion.
- **Thick ascending limb of Henle (TALH):** The NKCC-2 transporters reabsorb Na+, K+, and 2 Cl− ions into the cells
- **Late distal tubules (DTs):** In response to an **elevation** in plasma K+ concentration, aldosterone is secreted from the adrenal cortex and acts at principal cells of the late DT to increase basolateral **Na+/K+ ATPases**, as well as **luminal K+ (and Na+) channels.** By this process, K+ is actively transported into the tubular cell and then passively diffuses through the K+ channels into the tubular lumen.
- **Collecting ducts (CDs):** As in the late DT, K+ is secreted into the CD from the principal cells through aldosterone-sensitive **K+ channels** (as described in DT). In addition, in the **α-intercalated cells** of the CD, a luminal **H+/K+ ATPase** reabsorbs K+ in exchange for H+ secreted into tubular fluid.

Renal potassium handling is influenced by the following factors:

- **Dietary K+ intake:** High K+ intake will stimulate aldosterone secretion, increasing Na+/K+ ATPases in the late DT and CD principal cells, causing secretion of K+ into the tubule and excretion in the urine. Low K+ intake will decrease secretion from the distal DT and CDs, and the K+ reabsorption from the α-intercalated cells of the CDs will predominate.
- **Plasma volume:** Decreased plasma volume will activate the RAAS, elevating aldosterone and thus facilitating K+ secretion by principal cells in the late DT and CDs.
- **Tubular fluid flow rate:** When tubular flow rate is high (as during volume expansion), the concentration gradient for K+ from cells to lumen is elevated, and K+ secretion increases in the DT and CD.
- **Acid-base status:** To maintain normal acid-base balance, excess acid must be buffered and excreted in the urine (see Plates 5.17 and 5.18). To facilitate acid excretion, the H+/K+ ATPases in the α-intercalated cells of the CDs secrete H+ into the tubular fluid while reabsorbing K+ (the K+ leaves the cells via K+-Cl− symports).

COLOR the arrows illustrating reabsorption or secretion of K+ in normal and high-K+ diets (Part A) and low-K+ diets (Part B) and the nephron segments involved:

- ☐ 1. Proximal tubule (PT)
- ☐ 2. Thick ascending limb of Henle (TALH)
- ☐ 3. Late distal tubules (DTs)
- ☐ 4. Collecting ducts (CDs)

REVIEW ANSWERS

A. Urinary and fecal

B. Late DT and CD, by principal cells

C. Aldosterone, secretion (or excretion)

D. Dietary K+, plasma volume, tubular fluid flow rate, the RAAS, and acid-base status

E. K+ channels, epithelial sodium channels (ENaC, in DT), and Na+/K+ ATPases in the principal cells of the late DT and CDs

Plate 5.11   **Renal Physiology**

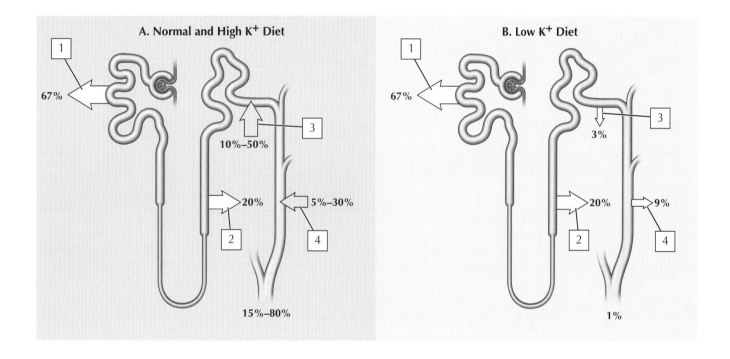

A. Normal and High K⁺ Diet

1

67%

3

10%–50%

20%

5%–30%

2

4

15%–80%

B. Low K⁺ Diet

1

67%

3

3%

20%

9%

2

4

1%

REVIEW QUESTIONS

A. Under normal conditions, K⁺ dietary intake matches _____ K⁺ losses.

B. In which nephron segments can K⁺ secretion occur?

C. When dietary K⁺ increases, the hormone _____ is secreted from the adrenal cortex and increases K⁺ _____.

D. Name factors that can alter renal K⁺ handling.

E. What transporters or channels does aldosterone affect?

Plasma **calcium (Ca^{2+})** and **inorganic phosphate (Pi)** are critical for bone development and health. Most Ca^{2+} and Pi are found in bone matrix, and continual remodeling of bone is facilitated by active vitamin D$_3$ and **parathyroid hormone (PTH).**

About 40% of plasma Ca^{2+} is bound to proteins, leaving **60% free** for filtration at the glomeruli. The kidneys reabsorb ~99% of filtered Ca^{2+} at the following sites (Part A):

- **Proximal tubule (PT):** As the PT actively reabsorbs filtered Na$^+$, associated solvent drag is responsible for ~70% of Ca^{2+} reabsorption (through the **paracellular** space).
- **Thick ascending limb of Henle (TALH): Paracellular** reabsorption (~20% of reabsorption)
- **Distal tubule (DT):** PTH (released in response to low plasma Ca^{2+}) increases **luminal Ca^{2+} channels** and **basolateral Ca^{2+} ATPase pumps** and **Na$^+$/Ca^{2+} exchangers** (~8%–9% of reabsorption).

Phosphates are also required for bone matrix formation, as well as for intracellular respiration and high-energy mechanisms (i.e., ATP formation and utilization). The majority of Pi is filtered (>90%), and Pi reabsorption and excretion are highly dependent on dietary intake. Pi reabsorption can occur at the following sites:

- **Proximal convoluted tubule:** Under normal dietary conditions, ~75% of the filtered Pi is reabsorbed by luminal **Na$^+$-Pi cotransporters,** and the balance is excreted in urine.
- **Proximal straight tubule (PST)** and **DT:** When diet is low in Pi, resulting in low plasma Pi, Na$^+$-Pi cotransporters are increased in the PST and DT, contributing to reabsorption of up to 90% of the FL (see Part B).

Control of renal Pi reabsorption occurs primarily in response to plasma Pi concentration and **PTH,** both of which affect the number of Na$^+$-Pi cotransporters in the luminal membranes.

- Diets high in Pi will elevate plasma Pi and reduce Na$^+$-Pi cotransporters in the PT, increasing Pi excretion; conversely, diets low in Pi increase Na$^+$-Pi cotransporters in the PST and DT.
- In addition to responding to low plasma Ca^{2+}, **PTH** is secreted in response to **high plasma Pi concentration,** decreasing luminal Na$^+$-Pi cotransporters and reducing Pi reabsorption.

Plasma Ca^{2+} and Pi regulation are intertwined because of constant bone remodeling, involving matrix resorption and deposition. In response to low plasma Ca^{2+}, vitamin D$_3$ increases intestinal Ca^{2+} and Pi absorption, and PTH stimulates bone resorption; both actions increase Ca^{2+} and Pi in ECF. At the kidneys, PTH increases Ca^{2+} reabsorption but compensates for the excess ECF Pi by decreasing Pi reabsorption and thus increasing Pi excretion to maintain Ca^{2+}-Pi homeostasis.

COLOR, in Part A, Renal Ca^{2+} handling, illustrating the sites of Ca^{2+} reabsorption, and note that overall ~99% of the filtered Ca^{2+} is reabsorbed:

- ☐ 1. Proximal tubule (PT)
- ☐ 2. Thick ascending limb of Henle (TALH)
- ☐ 3. Distal tubule (DT)
- ☐ 4. Collecting ducts (CDs)

COLOR, in Part B, renal Pi handling, illustrating the sites of Pi reabsorption:

- ☐ 5. Proximal convoluted tubule
- ☐ 6. Proximal straight tubule (green, indicating reabsorption only when plasma Pi concentration is low)
- ☐ 7. Distal tubule (DT, green, indicating reabsorption only when plasma Pi concentration is low)

Clinical Note

Solid aggregates of minerals can form in the kidneys **(nephrolithiasis)** or ureters **(urolithiasis).** These kidney stones, or calculi, can obstruct flow, and if they grow large enough (2–3 mm), they can block the ureter and cause intense pain and vomiting. The most common stones are **calcium oxalate.** Treatment depends on the size of the stone(s): Small stones can pass without intervention, whereas larger stones may require laser or ultrasound treatment to break them up.

REVIEW ANSWERS

A. Bone

B. Ca^{2+}, Pi

C. Distal tubule (DT)

D. Proximal convoluted tubule

E. Proximal straight tubules and distal tubules (DTs)

Plate 5.12　　　　　　**Renal Physiology**

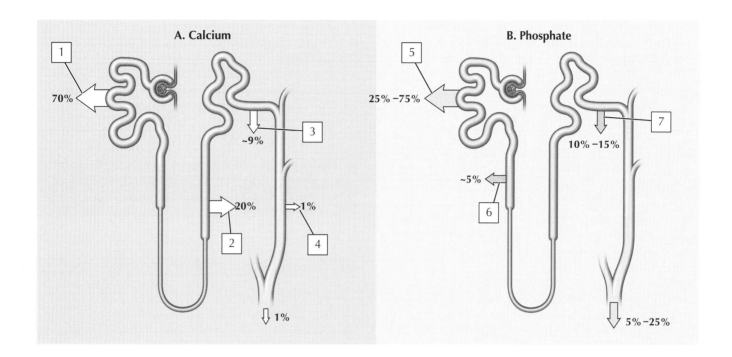

A. Calcium

1

70%

~9%

3

20%

2

1%

4

1%

B. Phosphate

5

25% –75%

10% –15%

~5%

6

7

5% –25%

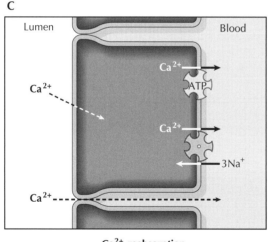

C

Lumen   Blood

Ca^{2+}

Ca^{2+} Ca^{2+}
ATP

Ca^{2+} $3Na^+$

Ca^{2+}

Ca^{2+} reabsorption

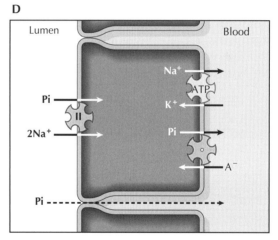

D

Lumen   Blood

Pi Na^+
II   ATP
$2Na^+$ K^+

Pi

Pi

A^-

Pi

Pi reabsorption

REVIEW QUESTIONS

A. Plasma calcium and phosphorous are important in _____ resorption and remodeling.

B. PTH will be increased in response to either low plasma _____ or high plasma _____.

C. PTH acts at the _____ to increase Ca^{2+} reabsorption.

D. PTH acts at the _____ to decrease Pi reabsorption.

E. What nephron sites will increase Na^+-Pi cotransporters in response to a low-Pi diet?

The kidneys maintain extracellular osmolarity and volume homeostasis by regulating the concentration and dilution of urine. This is made possible by the loops of Henle of the juxtamedullary nephrons and **the vasa recta capillaries,** which allow the formation of a medullary interstitial osmotic concentration gradient that facilitates solute-free water reabsorption when needed.

The descending and ascending limbs of the loops of Henle have specific permeability characteristics:

- The thin descending limbs of Henle *concentrate* the tubular fluid, because they are permeable to **water**, but not solutes.
- The TALH *dilute* the tubular fluid, because they are permeable to solutes, but not water. The **NKCC-2** and **Na⁺-Cl⁻ cotransporters** reabsorb the electrolytes, diluting the tubular fluid before it enters the DT. In addition, **urea** can diffuse into the TALH from the medullary interstitium (part of urea recycling [see Plate 5.14]).

Through this mechanism the tubular fluid entering the DT has an osmolarity of ~100 mOsm/L. After this point, whether the urine will be dilute or concentrated will depend on mechanisms within the **collecting ducts (CDs).** If the ECF volume is expanded and osmolarity is reduced, the dilute tubular fluid will continue through the CDs and be excreted as dilute urine, returning the ECF to homeostasis. However, if the **ECF osmolarity is high,** or the ECF volume is low, **antidiuretic hormone (ADH)** is secreted from the posterior pituitary gland into the blood and stimulates the insertion of **aquaporin (AQP)-2 water channels** into the luminal membranes of the CD cells (ADH also stimulates urea reabsorption from the CDs, which contributes to the medullary interstitial osmolarity). This action allows **solute-free water reabsorption** and produces concentrated urine. However, this can only occur if an interstitial osmotic gradient exists to draw the water from the tubular lumen to the interstitial space. **AQP-1** is always present in the thin descending limb of Henle and basolateral membranes of the CDs; **AQP-2** is inserted in CDs when ADH is elevated.

Plate 5.13 illustrates the medullary interstitial concentration gradient. In this generalized interstitial gradient, the osmolarity is ~300 mOsm/L at the corticomedullary border and rises to ~1200 mOsm/L in the deepest part of the medullary interstitium by the bottom of the loop of Henle and the lower CDs (explained in Plate 5.14). With this gradient in place, if AQP-2 water channels are present in the luminal membranes, water from the tubular fluid readily diffuses into the hyperosmotic interstitium, and then into the **vasa recta network of capillaries,** and into the systemic circulation.

TRACE the numbers representing the interstitial osmolar gradient (285–1200 mOsm/L) from the cortex through the medulla, noting the large gradient in the medulla.

COLOR

☐ 1. Vasa recta

☐ 2. Collecting duct, the site of ADH action

Clinical Note

The concept of **free-water clearance** is useful in quantifying water excretion during diuresis. It is defined as the water excretion in excess of the water required for iso-osmotic excretion of the solutes present in the urine. Free-water clearance is determined by subtracting the osmolar clearance from the urine flow rate: $C_{H_2O} = \dot{V} - [(U_{osm}/P_{osm}) \times \dot{V}]$. Thus a dilute urine will have a positive C_{H_2O}, a concentrated urine will have a negative C_{H_2O}, and iso-osmotic urine will have a C_{H_2O} of zero.

REVIEW ANSWERS

A. Water, concentrates

B. Solutes, dilutes

C. Osmolarity, volume

D. Bottom of the loops of Henle and the lower CDs

Plate 5.13   **Renal Physiology**

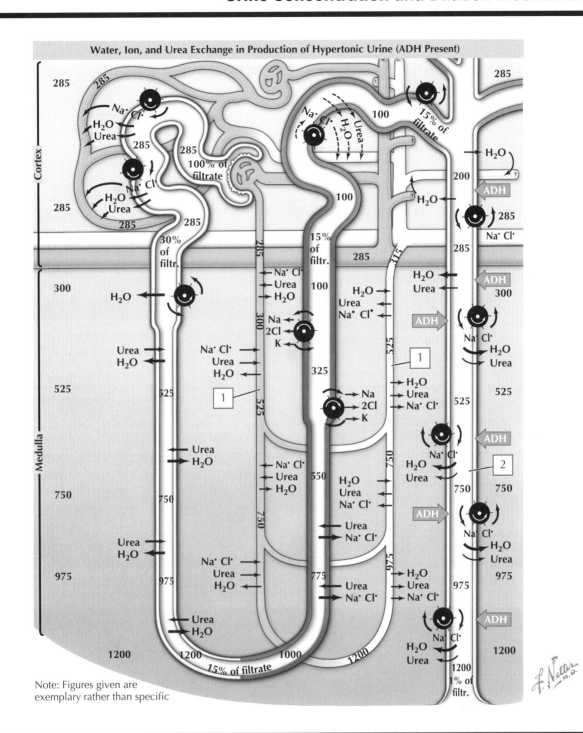

Water, Ion, and Urea Exchange in Production of Hypertonic Urine (ADH Present)

Note: Figures given are exemplary rather than specific

REVIEW QUESTIONS

A. The thin descending limb of Henle is impermeable to solutes but permeable to _____. As a result, it _____ the tubular fluid.

B. The thick ascending limb of Henle is impermeable to water but permeable to _____. As a result, it _____ the tubular fluid.

C. ADH is released from the posterior pituitary gland in response to an increase in plasma _____ or a decrease in plasma _____.

D. The osmolar concentration in the medullary interstitium is highest near what structure(s)?

The **countercurrent multiplier mechanism** establishes an **interstitial osmolar gradient** from the cortex to the inner medulla. It depends on the coordinated effects of the ascending and descending limbs of the loop of Henle and their selective permeability to solutes and water (see Plate 5.13). Plate 5.14 illustrates the repeated cycle in which solutes are transported out of the TALH, raising the osmolar concentration of the interstitial fluid and providing a gradient for water to be reabsorbed from the thin descending limb. This cycle is repeated until the full interstitial gradient (from 300 mOsm/L in the cortex to 1200 mOsm/L in the deep medulla) is established.

Creation of the gradient occurs through the following processes:

- The **NKCC-2 transporters in the TALH** transport solutes into the interstitium. This process can produce a gradient of 200 mOsm/L between tubular fluid and interstitial fluid (Step 2 in Plate 5.14).
- The **increased interstitial osmolarity promotes free water reabsorption** (via AQP-1) out of the descending limb of Henle until osmolar equilibrium is reached between the tubular fluid in the descending limb and that area of the interstitium (Step 3). The reabsorption of water in the descending limb continually increases osmolarity of the tubular fluid as it moves into the ascending limb. The 200 mOsm/L gradient between the interstitium and the ascending limb is maintained by the continued transport of solutes out of the ascending limb.
- As the tubular fluid moves forward, a more **concentrated tubular fluid now flows** from the descending limb into the ascending limb (Step 4). With the higher concentration of solutes entering the ascending limb, more solutes can be transported into the interstitium, further increasing interstitial fluid osmolarity (Step 5), which draws more water from the descending limb into the interstitium (Step 6). This further concentrates the tubular fluid entering the thick ascending limb. This cycle is repeated until the full interstitial gradient

is established (hence, "countercurrent multiplier"). The final osmolar concentration is dependent on the length of the loops of Henle, and in humans the concentration at the bottom of the medullary loops of Henle can reach **1200 mOsm/L.**

- Last, **urea recycling** contributes to developing and maintaining the interstitial osmolar gradient because ADH increases both **water and urea reabsorption** in the medullary (not cortical) CDs. Thus a portion of the urea is reabsorbed into the medullary interstitium. Some of the urea diffuses back into the thin limbs of Henle and can be again absorbed in the CDs. This cycle continues and effectively "traps" urea in the medullary interstitium, contributing to the interstitial concentration gradient.

COLOR

☐ 1. NKCC-2 transporters in the ascending limb in Step 2, noting the 200 mOsm/L difference between tubular fluid and interstitial fluid

☐ 2. Dashed arrows indicating solute-free water movement from the descending limb into the interstitium in Step 3

☐ 3. 400 mOsm/L tubular fluid concentration moving from the descending limb into the ascending limb in Step 4

☐ 4. NKCC-2 transporters in the ascending limb in Step 5, illustrating the further movement of solutes into the interstitium, while maintaining the 200 mOsm/L difference between tubular fluid and interstitial fluid

☐ 5. Arrows indicating more solute-free water movement from the descending limb into the interstitium in Step 6

REVIEW ANSWERS

A. Descending, ascending

B. NKCC-2

C. 200

D. Water

E. In the presence of ADH in the CDs, urea is reabsorbed into the interstitium and adds to the osmolar concentration.

Plate 5.14   **Renal Physiology**

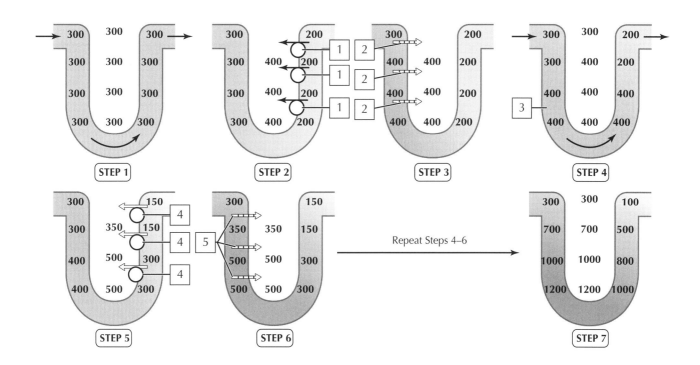

STEP 1 STEP 2 STEP 3 STEP 4

STEP 5 STEP 6 Repeat Steps 4–6 STEP 7

REVIEW QUESTIONS

A. The countercurrent multiplier depends on the selective permeability of the _____ and _____ limbs of Henle.

B. The _____ transporters in the ascending limb of Henle transport solutes into the interstitium.

C. There is a _____ mOsm/L gradient from the tubular fluid to the interstitial fluid, which is produced by the solute transport out of the ascending limb of Henle.

D. Elevated interstitial osmolarity allows _____ reabsorption from the descending limb of Henle.

E. How does urea recycling contribute to the medullary interstitial concentration gradient?

5 Regulation of Sodium and Water Reabsorption: Local and Neurohumoral Mechanisms

Renal sodium handling is closely regulated because of its importance in ECF homeostasis. A number of intrarenal factors can alter sodium (and thus fluid) reabsorption in response to changes in ECF. Several of these mechanisms have been discussed in Plate 5.5 in relation to renal hemodynamics.

- **GFR:** There is a tendency for Na$^+$ excretion to mirror changes in the GFR. An elevation in GFR increases the FL of Na$^+$, and the tubule reabsorbs the Na$^+$ less effectively, increasing Na$^+$ excretion. Conversely, a decrease in GFR reduces the FL of Na$^+$, and the tubules reabsorb the Na$^+$ load more completely, reducing Na$^+$ excretion.
- **Baroreceptors:** When blood pressure decreases, baroreceptors in the walls of the afferent arterioles stimulate the juxtaglomerular (JG) cells to release **renin** into the afferent arterioles (see RAAS, below).
- **Medullary blood flow:** If vasa recta blood flow increases, the medullary concentration gradient will not be maintained, reducing the reabsorption of sodium in the thick ascending limb and limiting water reabsorption in the CDs. This will result in natriuresis and diuresis.

In addition to the intrarenal controls listed above, there are also neural and hormonal mechanisms affecting sodium and water reabsorption (Plate 5.15):

- **Sympathetic nerves** innervate afferent and efferent arterioles (via α-adrenergic receptors). During sympathetic stimulation the arterioles constrict, decreasing GFR. In addition, the SNS directly stimulates Na$^+$ reabsorption in several nephron sites and stimulates renin secretion.
- The **RAAS:** In response to low tubular fluid sodium concentration or low tubular fluid flow rate the JG cells produce the proteolytic enzyme renin and secrete it into the circulation (Plate 5.5). Renin hydrolyzes angiotensinogen (a plasma protein produced by the liver) to **angiotensin (Ang) I,** which is converted to Ang II by **angiotensin-converting enzyme (ACE)** in the lung (and other tissues); Ang II stimulates release of the mineralocorticoid **aldosterone** from the adrenal cortex. In the kidney, Ang II directly stimulates **luminal Na$^+$/H$^+$ antiporters** in the proximal tubule (increasing sodium and water reabsorption) and has **vasoconstrictor** effects on the afferent and efferent arterioles, lowering GFR and increasing sodium and water retention.

- **Aldosterone** stimulates Na$^+$ and water reabsorption (and K$^+$ secretion) by the principal cells of the DTs and CDs through effects on Na$^+$/K$^+$ ATPase and epithelial Na$^+$ channels (ENaC).
- ANP is discussed in Plates 3.22 and 5.5. ANP opposes the actions of Ang II by increasing GFR (by dilating the afferent arteriole and constricting the efferent arteriole) and inhibiting Na$^+$-Cl$^-$ cotransport in the DT, thus causing natriuresis and diuresis.
- **Urodilatin** is an **intrarenal natriuretic peptide** that is produced in medullary DT and CD cells in response to an elevation in blood volume or pressure.

COLOR, in Part A, illustrating stimulation of sodium- and water-retaining mechanisms, the arrows indicating factors **STIMULATING** the RAAS:

- ☐ 1. Decreased blood pressure, downward arrow
- ☐ 2. Decreased fluid volume, downward arrow
- ☐ 3. Increased β$_1$-adrenergic receptor activation through the SNS, upward arrow

---

COLOR and LABEL, in Part A, the arrows illustrating the activation pathway of the RAAS:

- ☐ 4. Renin (from kidney), upward arrow
- ☐ 5. Angiotensinogen (color arrow coming from the liver)
- ☐ 6. Angiotensin I, upward arrow
- ☐ 7. Angiotensin II, upward arrow
- ☐ 8. Aldosterone, upward arrow

COLOR, in Part B, illustrating inhibition of sodium-and water-retaining mechanisms, arrows indicating factors **INHIBITING** the RAAS:

- ☐ 9. Increased blood pressure, upward arrow
- ☐ 10. Increased fluid volume, upward arrow
- ☐ 11. Decreased β$_1$-adrenergic receptor activation through SNS, downward arrow

---

REVIEW ANSWERS

A. Increase

B. Stimulating

C. Aldosterone

D. ANP and urodilatin; urodilatin is produced by the kidney

Plate 5.15　　　　　　　　　　　　　　　　　　　　　**Renal Physiology**

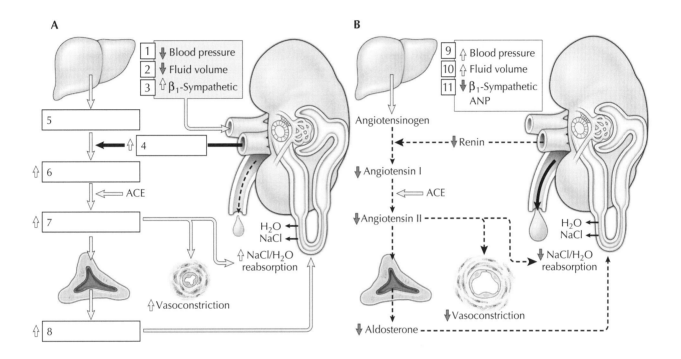

A

1	⬇ Blood pressure
2	⬇ Fluid volume
3	⬆ β₁-Sympathetic

5

4 ⬆

6 ⬆

⬅ ACE

7 ⬆

⬆ Vasoconstriction

8 ⬆

H₂O ⬅
NaCl ⬅

⬆ NaCl/H₂O reabsorption

B

9	⬆ Blood pressure
10	⬆ Fluid volume
11	⬇ β₁-Sympathetic ANP

Angiotensinogen

⬇ Renin

⬇ Angiotensin I

⬅ ACE

⬇ Angiotensin II

⬇ Aldosterone

⬇ Vasoconstriction

H₂O ⬅
NaCl ⬅

⬇ NaCl/H₂O reabsorption

REVIEW QUESTIONS

A. An increase in tubular fluid flow rate will _____ sodium and water excretion in urine.

B. Baroreceptors in the afferent arteriole respond to a decrease in pressure by _____ the release of renin.

C. The activity of basolateral Na⁺/K⁺ ATPase and luminal ENaC (epithelial Na⁺ channels) in the principal cells of the DT and CD is increased by _____.

D. Which two peptides cause a natriuresis and diuresis? Which peptide is secreted by the DT and CD in the kidney?

Control of ECF is a continual process, with changes in plasma osmolarity and volume signaling multiple neural and humoral systems to regulate the renal concentration and dilution of the urine. The integration of these systems in the response to ECF volume contraction and expansion is illustrated in Plate 5.16.

When **plasma volume is contracted,** fluid and sodium **conservation** systems are activated. The kidneys respond to the following mechanisms:

- An increase in **sympathetic nervous system activity** (1) increases renal vascular resistance and decreases GFR; (2) directly stimulates sodium reabsorption in several segments of the renal tubule; and (3) stimulates **renin** secretion.
- The **RAAS** is activated and increases **angiotensin II** and **aldosterone,** increasing sodium (and water) reabsorption in the proximal tubules (via angiotensin II) and in the DTs and CDs (via aldosterone).
- **ADH** is released, stimulating the insertion of **AQP-2** water channels in the luminal membranes of the principal cells of the CDs, enhancing solute-free water reabsorption.

These systems limit further volume contraction by reducing urinary losses of fluid and sodium (Part A).

When **plasma volume is expanded,** the mechanisms above are reversed, resulting in the elimination of fluid and reduction of plasma volume and ECF (Part B). In addition, ANP (secreted from the right cardiac atrium in response to stretch) has a key role in producing **natriuresis** and **diuresis** by the following:

- Decreasing ADH secretion
- Inhibiting aldosterone synthesis
- Increasing GFR
- Decreasing sodium (and water) reabsorption in the CDs by reducing aldosterone-sensitive Na⁺ channels (ENaC)

COLOR and **LABEL,** in Part A, illustrating response to volume contraction, the organs and then the arrows indicating the role of each factor in the elevation of sodium- and fluid-conserving mechanisms/pathways:

☐ 1. Sympathetic nerve activity
☐ 2. Renin
☐ 3. Angiotensin I
☐ 4. Angiotensin II
☐ 5. Aldosterone
☐ 6. ADH

COLOR, in Part B, illustrating the response to volume expansion, the organs and then the arrows indicating elevation of natriuretic/diuretic peptides:

☐ 7. ANP
☐ 8. Urodilatin

REVIEW ANSWERS

A. Activated

B. Released (by atrial myocytes)

C. Volume contraction, AQP-2 (or water channels)

Plate 5.16   **Renal Physiology**

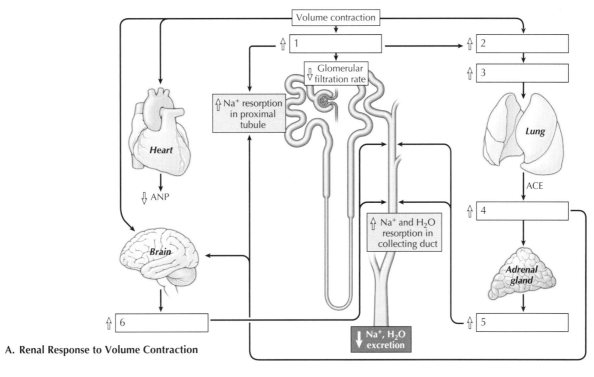

A. Renal Response to Volume Contraction

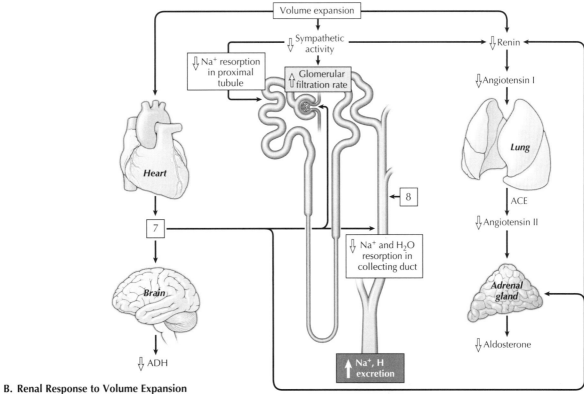

B. Renal Response to Volume Expansion

REVIEW QUESTIONS

A.   In response to volume contraction, the RAAS is _____.

B.   In response to volume expansion, ANP is _____.

C.   ADH is elevated during _____ and inserts _____ into the luminal membranes of the CDs.

The importance of maintaining extracellular pH within a narrow physiologic range (7.35–7.45) has been discussed previously (Plate 4.18), with the focus on how the **lungs** handle volatile acid (carbonic acid) in the blood. Now we will finish the discussion and describe how the **kidneys** excrete excess nonvolatile acid load.

On average, we ingest and produce ~40–80 millimoles of acid each day. This is a huge amount in the context of the ~40 *nanomolar* concentration (at pH 7.4) that is maintained in the ECF. The excess acid must be:

- **Buffered** in the ECF (and cells), to prevent a fall in pH to below physiological levels (i.e., below 7.35)
- **Secreted** into the renal tubules, buffered in the tubular fluid, and excreted in the urine (Plate 5.18)

The body handles the excess acid using extracellular and intracellular buffers in a continuous regulatory "dance," escorting acid in and out of cells and through the blood to the kidneys for excretion.

The major ECF buffer is **bicarbonate** (HCO_3^-), which exists at a relatively high concentration in the ECF (24 mM) and thus is available for consuming H^+ through the following reaction:

$$HCO_3^- + H^+ \rightleftharpoons H_2CO_3 \overset{CA}{\rightleftharpoons} CO_2 + H_2O$$

The carbonic acid (H_2CO_3) can be converted to CO_2 and H_2O in the presence of CA, a reaction that occurs in tissues and ECF. The CO_2 can be breathed off by the lungs.

Intracellular buffering is also important. H^+ enters and leaves the cells through H^+/K^+ and Na^+/H^+ exchangers, respectively, and is buffered **by intracellular phosphates** (and, to a lesser degree, proteins).

In addition, the kidneys generate new HCO_3^- to replenish the ECF HCO_3^-. Remember, there is a 1:1 relationship between bicarbonate reabsorbed or excreted and H^+ transported in the opposite direction, and thus when an H^+ is excreted, an HCO_3^- is retained.

COLOR

- ☐ 1. Lungs
- ☐ 2. Kidney

TRACE the following pathways:

- ☐ 3. Nonvolatile acid pathway to the kidneys
- ☐ 4. New HCO_3^- pathway from the kidney back to the ECF

REVIEW ANSWERS

A. Kidneys and lungs

B. Bicarbonate

C. Phosphate

D. Excreted

Plate 5.17   **Renal Physiology**

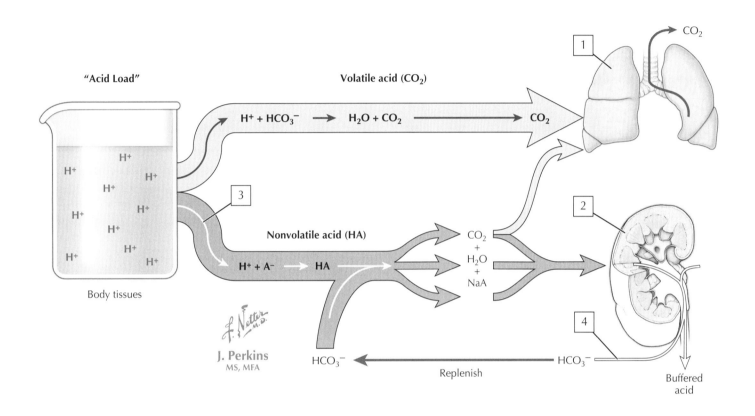

"Acid Load"

Volatile acid (CO_2)

$$H^+ + HCO_3^- \longrightarrow H_2O + CO_2 \longrightarrow CO_2$$

Body tissues

Nonvolatile acid (HA)

$$H^+ + A^- \longrightarrow HA$$

CO_2 + H_2O + NaA

$HCO_3^- \longleftarrow$ Replenish $\longleftarrow HCO_3^-$

CO_2

Buffered acid

J. Perkins
MS, MFA

1

2

3

4

REVIEW QUESTIONS

A. Which two organs handle the removal of acid from the body?

B. What is the major ECF buffer?

C. What is the major ICF buffer?

D. When a bicarbonate ion is retained, an H+ is _____.

As discussed in Plate 5.10, bicarbonate reabsorption occurs in the PT, TALH, and CD and is dependent on the secretion of H^+ into the tubular lumen. In the CDs, H^+ is secreted in *excess* of filtered bicarbonate, with significant secretion occurring from the **α-intercalated cells** of the CDs (Parts B and C). These cells have luminal H^+ ATPases and H^+/K^+ ATPases that actively secrete H^+ into the tubular fluid. The H^+ in the tubular fluid of the CDs is then buffered via the following mechanisms:

- **Production of titratable acids (TAs):** Basic phosphate (HPO_4^{2-}) is a strong buffer, and thus the phosphate entering the CD can buffer the secreted H^+, producing phosphoric acid ($H_2PO_4^-$), the primary form of TA in the urine. TA is a main form of acid excreted, and although TA production can increase to buffer additional acid that is secreted, the maximal rate of formation of TA is limited by the amount of HPO_4^{2-} entering the CDs (refer to phosphate handling, Plate 5.12). (Remember, bicarbonate cannot be used to buffer H^+ for excretion because bicarbonate is completely reabsorbed.)
- **Ammoniagenesis:** In the PT cells, **glutamine,** from tubular fluid and the peritubular capillary blood, is metabolized, generating **ammonia (NH_3)** and HCO_3^-. The bicarbonate ions are absorbed into the peritubular capillaries as new HCO_3^-. In the CDs, the NH_3 buffers H^+, forming **ammonium (NH_4^+)** for excretion in the urine. Unlike TAs, which are limited by the amount of basic phosphate available in the CDs, ammoniagenesis can rapidly increase to allow excretion of high loads of acid as NH_4^+.

Net acid excretion (NAE) describes the amount of acid that is excreted in the urine (see equation below):

$$NAE = TA + NH_4^+ - HCO_3^-$$

Under most conditions, **urinary HCO_3^- is zero,** because all the HCO_3^- is reabsorbed. However, when HCO_3^- appears in the urine, it is a loss of base and is subtracted from the excreted acid to calculate NAE. HCO_3^- excretion reflects renal tubular acidosis or the renal response to alkalosis, and in both conditions there is an equimolar gain of H^+ for the HCO_3^- excreted.

COLOR, in Part A:

☐ 1. Na^+/H^+ and Na^+/NH_4^+ exchangers in the luminal membranes of the proximal tubules, reinforcing the transport of H^+ and NH_4^+ into the tubular fluid, and the reabsorption of HCO_3^-.

COLOR, in Parts B and C:

☐ 2. H^+ ATPase and H^+/K^+ ATPase in the luminal membranes of the α-intercalated cells of the collecting ducts, reinforcing the secretion of H^+ in this late segment, and buffering by phosphates (Part C) and ammonia (Part B). Note the paracellular diffusion of NH_3 into the tubular fluid in Part B.

REVIEW ANSWERS

A. $NAE = TA + NH_4^+ - HCO_3^-$

B. Na^+/H^+ exchangers

C. α-Intercalated cells

D. Proximal tubule cells

Plate 5.18 | **Renal Physiology**

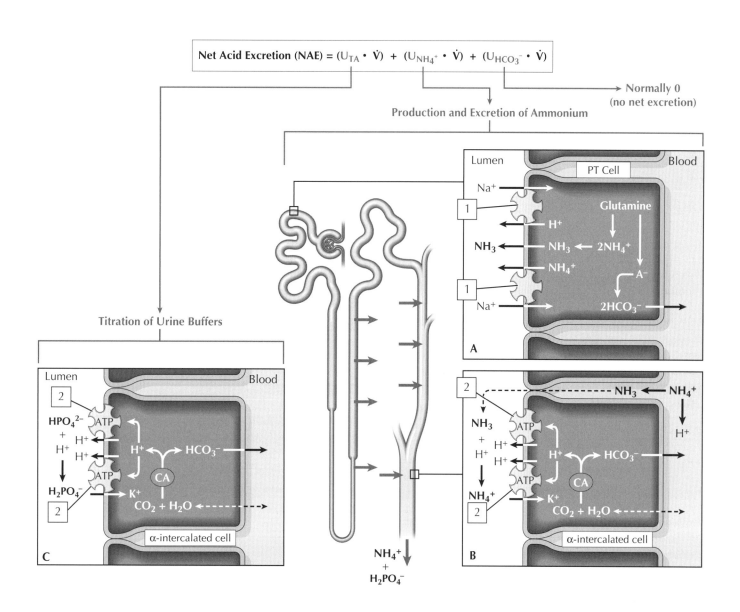

Net Acid Excretion (NAE) = $(U_{TA} \cdot \dot{V}) + (U_{NH_4^+} \cdot \dot{V}) + (U_{HCO_3^-} \cdot \dot{V})$

Normally 0
(no net excretion)

Production and Excretion of Ammonium

Titration of Urine Buffers

PT Cell

Lumen — Blood

Na^+
1
H^+

$NH_3 \leftarrow NH_3 \leftarrow 2NH_4^+$

Glutamine

NH_4^+

A^-

1
Na^+
$2HCO_3^-$

A

Lumen — Blood

2

HPO_4^{2-}
+
H^+

ATP

H^+
H^+
H^+
HCO_3^-

CA

$H_2PO_4^-$

ATP

K^+
$CO_2 + H_2O$

2

α-intercalated cell

C

2
$NH_3 \leftarrow NH_4^+$

NH_3
+
H^+

ATP

H^+
H^+
H^+
HCO_3^-

H^+

CA

NH_4^+

ATP

K^+
$CO_2 + H_2O$

2

α-intercalated cell

B

NH_4^+
+
$H_2PO_4^-$

REVIEW QUESTIONS

A. Net acid excretion = _____.

B. H+ secretion into the tubular fluid in the proximal tubule occurs through which transporters?

C. Which cells in the collecting ducts secrete H+ into tubular fluid?

D. Where in the nephron does ammoniagenesis occur?

Acid-base status is assessed by examining the plasma values of pH, P_{CO_2}, and HCO_3^-. Under normal conditions in arterial blood these values will be approximately:

- pH = 7.4
- P_{CO_2} = 40 mm Hg
- $[HCO_3^-]$ = 24 mM

When the pH of the ECF falls outside the normal physiological range, acidosis (i.e., pH <7.35) or alkalosis (i.e., pH >7.45) results. The primary disturbance is identified by which component (P_{CO_2} or HCO_3^-) is altered in the direction consistent with the change in pH. Thus, if the **pH is decreased,** the disturbance is designated as follows:

- **Respiratory acidosis** if the P_{CO_2} is increased, or
- **Metabolic acidosis** if the HCO_3^- is decreased

If the **pH is increased,** the disturbance is designated as:

- **Respiratory alkalosis** if P_{CO_2} is decreased (see Plate 4.18), or
- **Metabolic alkalosis** if HCO_3^- is increased

The compensation for metabolic acidosis or alkalosis includes an early adjustment of respiratory rate (hyperventilation to blow off excess **CO_2** in acidosis or hypoventilation to retain CO_2 in alkalosis). For metabolic and respiratory disturbances, the **renal compensation** occurs over several hours through the excretion of acid (in acidosis) or bicarbonate (in alkalosis), returning the pH toward normal.

Acidosis can result from a **gain of acid** or a **loss of** HCO_3^-. Net acid gain can arise from either decreased respiration (e.g., chronic obstructive pulmonary disorder), which increases CO_2 (respiratory acidosis), or from the **accumulation of acids** from metabolic sources (metabolic acidosis), including the following:

- **Keto acids,** which are generated by β-oxidation of fatty acids (in starvation or poorly controlled diabetes)
- **Phosphoric acid,** which accumulates during renal failure
- **Lactic acid,** which is released from damaged tissues during hypoxia or heart failure
- **Ingested substances** such as ethylene glycol (antifreeze) and methanol

Bicarbonate losses can result from diarrhea, insufficient HCO_3^- reabsorption in the PT, or proximal (type 2) renal tubular acidosis.

REVIEW ANSWERS

A. If the low pH is consistent with arterial P_{CO_2} (elevated), it is respiratory. If consistent with the plasma HCO_3^- (reduced), it is metabolic.

B. Plasma pH, P_{CO_2}, and HCO_3^-

C. Either acid loading or base loss

D. Vomiting or bicarbonate overdose

E. β-Intercalated cells and HCO_3^-/Cl^- exchangers

Whether from acid load or HCO_3^- loss, the excess acid must be buffered systemically and then excreted by the kidneys. The excess acid is secreted into the renal CDs and combines with HPO_4^{2-} or ammonia to form TA and ammonium, respectively, for excretion (Plate 5.18).

Alkalosis results from the **loss of acid or gain of** HCO_3^-. Chronic hyperventilation will cause the loss of acid and result in **respiratory alkalosis;** this can be alleviated by breathing in and out of a bag (to raise CO_2). **Metabolic alkalosis** can result from the following:

- **Vomiting** (loss of H+ as HCl) and volume contraction
- **Sodium bicarbonate overdose**
- **Chronic diuretic usage,** causing hypokalemia, volume contraction, aldosterone excess, and chloride depletion

During alkalosis, **HCO_3^-/Cl^- exchangers** in the **β-intercalated cells** of the renal CDs are activated, secreting bicarbonate, which is excreted in urine until normal pH is attained.

COLOR the CO_2 and HCO_3^- in each diagram, noting their relative sizes in each of the acid-base disturbances:

☐ 1. CO_2
☐ 2. HCO_3^-

TRACE the balance beam line in each diagram, reinforcing whether the primary disturbance is acidosis or alkalosis:

☐ 3. Acid-base balance
☐ 4. Respiratory acidosis
☐ 5. Metabolic acidosis
☐ 6. Respiratory alkalosis
☐ 7. Metabolic alkalosis

Clinical Note

Examples of causes of respiratory and metabolic acid-base disorders are listed on the left side of Plate 5.19. In each case, when the primary cause of the disturbance is addressed, the pH should return to normal values.

Plate 5.19

Renal Physiology

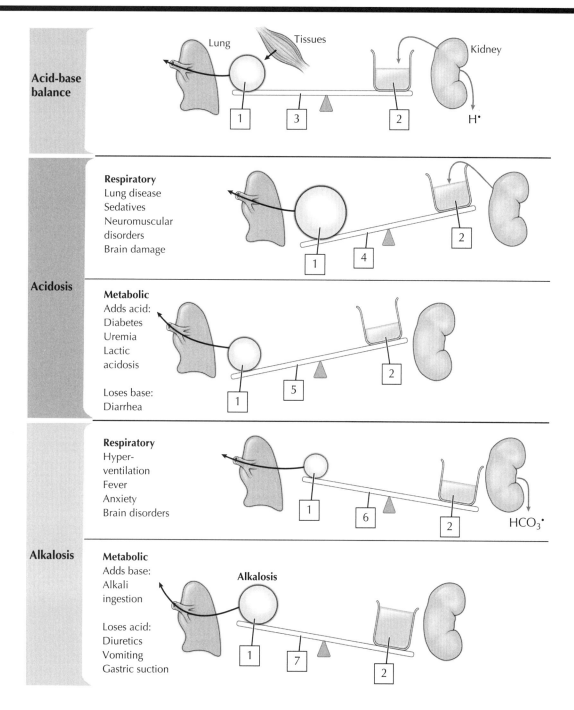

Acid-base balance

Lung | Tissues | Kidney

1 | 3 | 2 | H˙

Acidosis

Respiratory
Lung disease
Sedatives
Neuromuscular disorders
Brain damage

1 | 4 | 2

Metabolic
Adds acid:
Diabetes
Uremia
Lactic acidosis

Loses base:
Diarrhea

1 | 5 | 2

Alkalosis

Respiratory
Hyper-ventilation
Fever
Anxiety
Brain disorders

1 | 6 | 2 | $HCO_3^{\cdot}$

Metabolic
Adds base:
Alkali ingestion

Loses acid:
Diuretics
Vomiting
Gastric suction

Alkalosis

1 | 7 | 2

REVIEW QUESTIONS

A. How would you determine if a pH of 7.32 was a respiratory or metabolic acidosis?

B. What three plasma values are used to assess acid-base status?

C. Metabolic acidosis can result from what two changes in acid-base status?

D. Name some causes of metabolic alkalosis.

E. What cell type and transporter in the CDs are involved in the renal response to metabolic alkalosis?

Metabolic acidosis results from acid gain or base loss (Plate 5.19). The **anion gap (AG)** is a diagnostic tool used to differentiate between the two possible causes. Specifically, the AG is the difference in concentration between the major plasma cation, **Na⁺,** and the major plasma anions, **Cl⁻** and HCO_3^-. When Cl^- and HCO_3^- concentrations are subtracted from the Na^+ concentration, the AG is normally approximately 8 to 12 mEq/L. The AG represents the sum of the concentrations of about 10 anions present in the plasma and includes proteins, lactate, citrate, phosphates, sulfates, and so on:

$$AG = Na^+ - (Cl^- + HCO_3^-)$$

Plate 5.20 illustrates a normal AG on the left and the AG in acidosis arising from an acid load (middle diagram) or bicarbonate loss (right diagram). Note that **gaining acid increases the AG,** a result of the decrease in plasma HCO_3^- (which was used to buffer the increase in acid).

In contrast, when HCO_3^- is lost from the body through diarrhea or renal tubular acidosis, it is replaced by an increase in Cl^-, and the **AG is normal** (far right diagram). Therefore the AG can help determine whether the metabolic acidosis is due to acid gain or base loss, but the specific cause of the acid load or base loss would remain to be determined (see Plate 5.19).

REVIEW ANSWERS

A. Acidosis

B. Decreases, utilization to buffer the additional acid

C. Base loss, the Cl^- concentration increases as HCO_3^- is lost (in urine or feces)

Plate 5.20   **Renal Physiology**

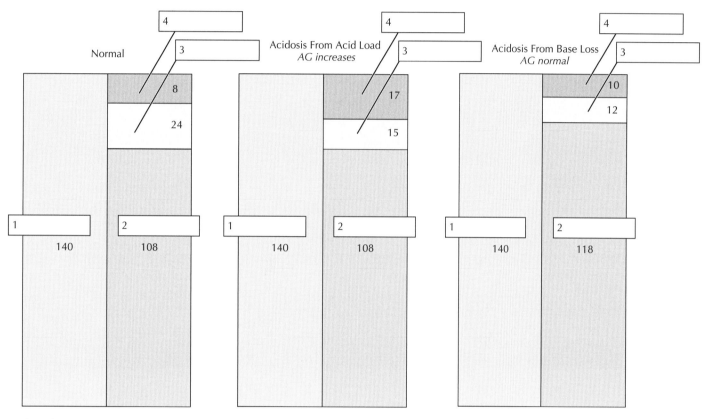

Normal

Acidosis From Acid Load
AG increases

Acidosis From Base Loss
AG normal

Electrolyte concentrations are in mEq/L

REVIEW QUESTIONS

A. The anion gap is used to determine the possible cause of metabolic _____.

B. When the anion gap increases because of excess acid, plasma HCO_3^- _____ because of _____.

C. The anion gap is normal during acidosis caused by _____ because _____.

Chapter 6 Gastrointestinal Physiology

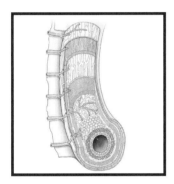
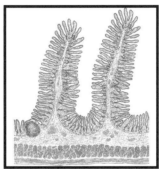
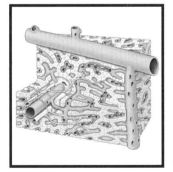
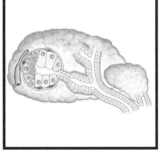

The gastrointestinal (GI) tract can be viewed as one long tube with an input (mouth) and output (anus), with specialized areas for direct input from associated organs (i.e., the liver, gallbladder, and pancreas) and absorption of nutrients. Plate 6.1 illustrates the GI tract. The structures and their general functions are listed in sequence below:

1. **Mouth:** Mechanical breakdown and mixing of food with salivary secretions
2. **Salivary glands:** Secretion of lubricants and enzymes to initiate digestion of **starches** and **lipids**
3. **Esophagus:** Transport of food from mouth to stomach
4. **Stomach:** Chemical breakdown of food by acid and enzymes, producing **chyme**
5. **Small intestine**, made of three sections:
   - **Duodenum:** About 1 ft in length; secretions from the liver, gallbladder, and exocrine pancreas enter the duodenal lumen near the stomach
   - **Jejunum:** About 10 ft in length; site of enzymatic digestion of nutrients and absorption of most nutrients
   - **Ileum:** About 12 ft in length; continued absorption of nutrients including vitamin B_{12}; site of bile recycling
6. **Liver:** Secretion of bile into duodenal lumen, metabolism of nutrients
7. **Gallbladder:** Storage of bile and secretion into the duodenum
8. **Pancreas:** Secretion of buffers and digestive enzymes into the duodenal lumen; secretion of endocrine hormones into blood
9. **Large intestine (colon):** Absorption of sodium and water, which dehydrates the undigested chyme to form feces

The musculature of the GI tract is **smooth muscle,** except in the **mouth, upper esophagus,** and **external anal sphincter,** where **skeletal muscle is found.** Thus, there is voluntary control of input (chewing, swallowing) and output (defecation). The remainder of the tract has longitudinal and circular bands of smooth muscle necessary for propulsion and mixing of the chyme.

A vast network of blood vessels supplies the oxygen, nutrients, and hormones that support digestion, absorption, propulsion, and metabolism within the GI tract. In addition, efficient absorption of nutrients through the intestinal cells requires high blood flow to ensure that there is a gradient for nutrient entry into the bloodstream.

The main **functions** of the GI tract are the following:

- **Digestion** of nutrients by specific enzymes
- **Absorption** of nutrients into the intestinal cells **(enterocytes)**
- **Propulsion** of chyme through the tract
- **Secretion** of mucus, buffers, acid, and enzymes into the lumen of the GI tract
- **Storage** of chyme in the stomach (for mixing with digestive juices) and colon (for dehydration to form feces)
- **Elimination** of waste material as feces
- **Production of endocrine hormones** that act on the GI tract and other tissues

COLOR the following parts of the GI tract:

- [ ] 1. Mouth
- [ ] 2. Salivary glands
- [ ] 3. Esophagus
- [ ] 4. Stomach
- [ ] 5. Small intestine
- [ ] 6. Liver
- [ ] 7. Gallbladder
- [ ] 8. Pancreas
- [ ] 9. Large intestine (colon)

REVIEW ANSWERS

A. Duodenum, jejunum, and ileum

B. The duodenum

C. The jejunum

D. Smooth, skeletal

Plate 6.1 | **Gastrointestinal Physiology**

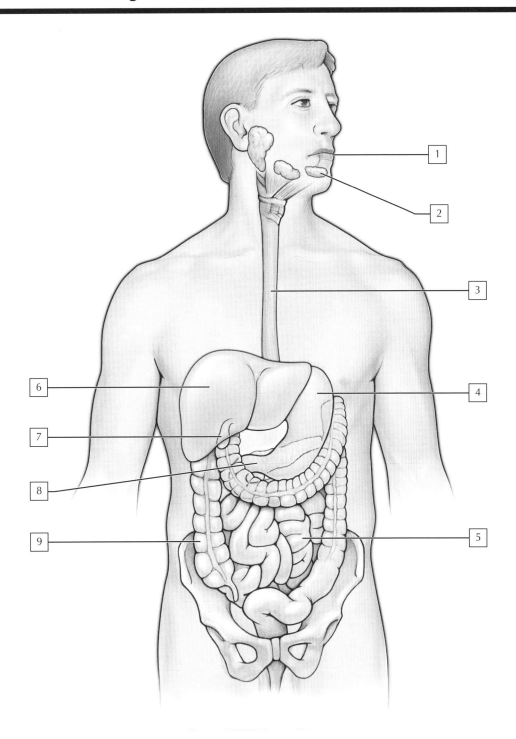

REVIEW QUESTIONS

A. What are the three anatomical sections of the small intestine?

B. Where do the secretions from the liver, pancreas, and gallbladder enter the lumen of the GI tract?

C. The majority of nutrient absorption occurs in which segment of the small intestine?

D. Musculature in the GI tract is _____ muscle, except in the mouth, upper esophagus, and external anal sphincter, where it is _____ muscle.

The **enteric nervous system (ENS)** is intrinsic to the GI tract and is made up of the myenteric and submucosal nerve plexuses. The ENS can function independently based on input from mechanoreceptors, chemoreceptors, and osmoreceptors located in the luminal epithelium of the tract. The ENS also receives input from the central nervous system, autonomic nervous system, and hormones, which help fine-tune and regulate the ENS. Without autonomic innervation, the ENS would still function but in a less coordinated manner.

The **myenteric plexus** (also called Auerbach's plexus) is located between the **circular** and **longitudinal muscle** layers. Stimulation of this plexus regulates the contraction and relaxation of the musculature, producing **motility and mixing** of the luminal contents. The **submucosal plexus** (also called Meissner's plexus) is located between the circular muscle and submucosa and regulates local fluid secretions.

Regulation by the **autonomic nervous system (ANS)** is primarily through the **parasympathetic nervous system (PNS)**, which promotes secretion and motility in the GI tract. The majority of the actions occur in response to **vagal** stimulation. In contrast, stimulation by the **sympathetic nervous system (SNS)** slows secretion and motility of the GI tract.

Sensory input to the **central nervous system (CNS)** provides the initial stimulus for secretion of saliva and gastric acid and is integral to many GI reflexes. Thus, simply smelling or seeing food can initiate the central response. The CNS acts through the PNS and SNS. As stated previously, the actions of the ANS and CNS increase the efficiency of the system.

COLOR and **LABEL** the exposed layers of the:

☐ 1. Longitudinal muscle

☐ 2. Circular muscle

COLOR and **LABEL** the plexuses of the ENS, noting their relationship to the muscle layers:

☐ 3. Submucosal plexus

☐ 4. Myenteric plexus

REVIEW ANSWERS

A. Enteric nervous system (ENS)

B. True

C. The myenteric and submucosal plexuses

D. Motility (and mixing)

E. Sensory input to the CNS (and subsequent modulation of PNS and SNS activity)

Plate 6.2
Gastrointestinal Physiology

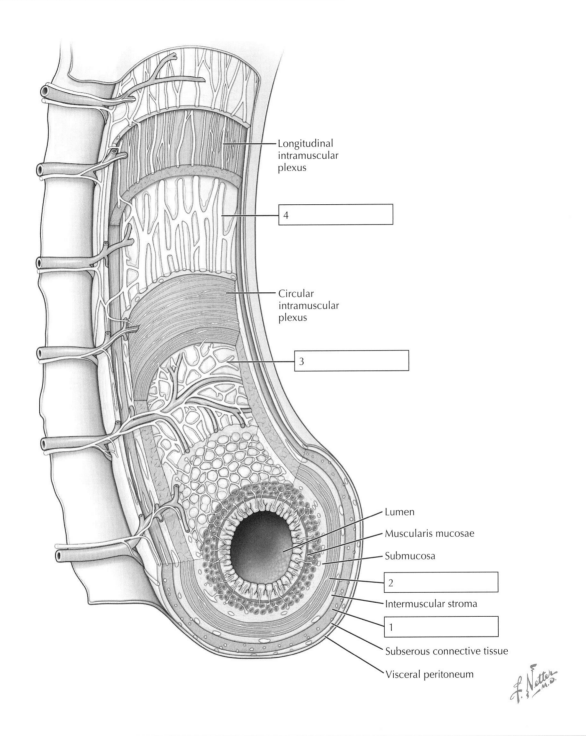

Longitudinal intramuscular plexus

4

Circular intramuscular plexus

3

Lumen
Muscularis mucosae
Submucosa
2
Intermuscular stroma
1
Subserous connective tissue
Visceral peritoneum

REVIEW QUESTIONS

A. The intrinsic nervous system of the GI tract is the _____.

B. True or False: The ENS can function without input from the CNS or ANS.

C. What two nerve plexuses make up the ENS?

D. Stimulation of the myenteric plexus regulates _____.

E. The initial stimulus for salivary and gastric secretions occurs through _____ nervous system.

Endocrine cells in the gastric and intestinal epithelia synthesize and release a variety of hormones into the bloodstream. The hormones act on other areas of the body, such as the brain, liver, and pancreas, in addition to the stomach and intestines. These hormones regulate GI function, as well as hunger, satiety, and insulin secretion. The major hormones secreted by the GI tract are listed below, and their role in GI function is discussed further in Plates 6.9 to 6.11.

Hormones synthesized by the stomach include the following:

1. **Gastrin:** Secreted in response to carbohydrates, proteins, and fats in chyme; stimulates gastric acid secretion as well as motility in the lower GI tract (ileum and colon)
2. **Histamine:** Secreted in response to gastrin and the vagus nerve during feeding; acts on adjacent parietal cells to stimulate acid secretion
3. **Ghrelin:** Secreted during the interdigestive period (between meals); acts on the brain to stimulate hunger (an **orexigenic** action)

Hormones synthesized in the small intestine include the following:

1. **Gastrin** (from **duodenum**): Secreted in response to carbohydrates, proteins, and fats in chyme; stimulates gastric acid secretion as well as motility in the lower GI tract (ileum and colon)
2. **Secretin** (from duodenum): Secreted in response to acidic chyme; stimulates secretion of intestinal and pancreatic buffers
3. **Cholecystokinin** (from duodenum): Secreted in response to fats, carbohydrates, and proteins; stimulates secretion of pancreatic enzymes and bile
4. **Glucose-dependent insulinotropic peptide (GIP)** (from duodenum): Secreted in response to carbohydrates and fats in the chyme; stimulates pancreatic insulin release
5. **Motilin** (from duodenum): Secreted during fasting between meals (interdigestion); stimulates phase 3 contractions of the **migrating myoelectric complex** (**MMC;** see Plate 6.5)
6. **Glucagon-like peptide (GLP)-1** (mainly from the **jejunum**): Secreted in response to the presence of chyme in that area; acts on the brain to inhibit hunger (an **anorexic** action, in opposition to ghrelin)

REVIEW ANSWERS

A. Motilin

B. Ghrelin

C. GIP

D. Gastrin

E. Secretin. It stimulates pancreatic and intestinal buffer secretion.

COLOR and LABEL

☐ 1. Stomach
☐ 2. Duodenum
☐ 3. Proximal jejunum

WRITE the hormones that are secreted by the stomach:

☐ 4. Gastrin
☐ 5. Histamine
☐ 6. Ghrelin

WRITE the hormones that are secreted by the duodenum:

☐ 7. Gastrin
☐ 8. Secretin
☐ 9. Cholecystokinin
☐ 10. Glucose-dependent insulinotropic peptide (GIP)
☐ 11. Motilin

WRITE the hormone that is secreted by the jejunum:

☐ 12. Glucagon-like peptide (GLP)-1

Clinical Note

Although rare, **Zollinger-Ellison syndrome** is a disease in which endocrine tumors that secrete gastrin into the blood **(gastrinomas)** arise in the pancreas or duodenum. The abnormal and uncontrolled elevation in gastrin results in a continual secretion of acid by the gastric parietal cells and eventual ulcer formation. Symptoms of gastrinomas include malabsorption of nutrients (especially fats) and diarrhea with **steatorrhea** (excess fat in the feces). Treatment involves the removal of the gastrinoma and pharmacologic suppression of gastric acid until the ulcers can heal.

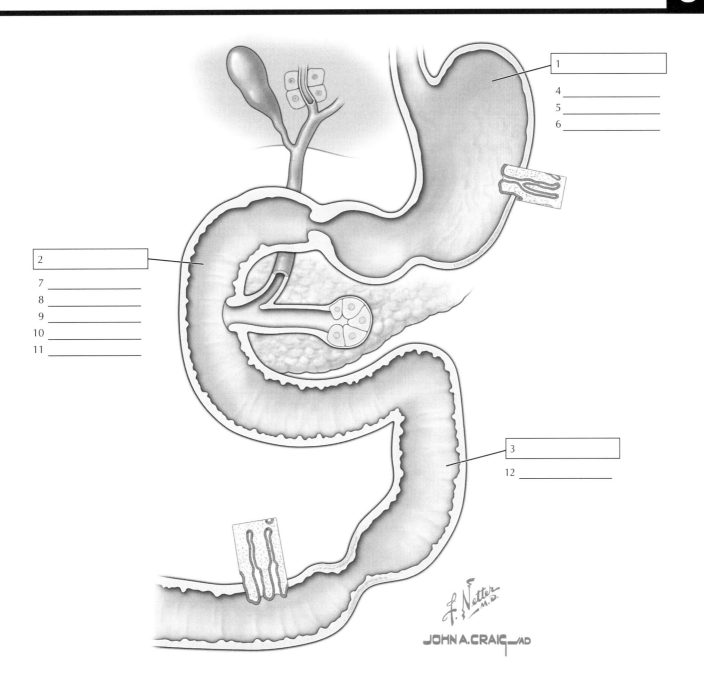

1 _____

4 _____
5 _____
6 _____

2 _____

7 _____
8 _____
9 _____
10 _____
11 _____

3 _____

12 _____

JOHN A.CRAIG—AD

REVIEW QUESTIONS

A. The GI hormone that is secreted when fasting between meals and stimulates phase 3 contractions of the MMC is _____.

B. The GI hormone that is secreted when fasting between meals and stimulates hunger is _____.

C. Which GI hormone can stimulate pancreatic insulin release?

D. Which GI hormone is released from both the stomach and the duodenum and stimulates gastric acid secretion?

E. Which duodenal hormone is secreted in response to acidic chyme? What does it do?

Mixing and propulsive movements in the GI tract are generated by unique types of mechanical activity in the smooth muscle, which are present from the esophagus through the rectum. Unlike other tissues, there are undulations in the **resting membrane potential (RMP)** known as **slow waves** (also called the **basic electrical rhythm** or basal electrical rhythm).

Under resting conditions, slow waves undulate between −70 and −80 millivolts (mV). However, if the slow waves are depolarized (i.e., made less negative) by nerve activity or circulating hormones, the amplitude of the waves may also increase, and when the peaks of the slow waves are elevated above **threshold of −40 mV,** the cells will generate one or more **action (or spike) potentials** on the top of the wave. The spike potentials are caused by the entry of **calcium** into the smooth muscle cells. The calcium then binds to calmodulin, initiating events leading to contraction of the smooth muscle.

Neurotransmitters such as **acetylcholine** and **substance P** released from **parasympathetic nerves** terminating on the myenteric plexus **depolarize** the slow waves, generating action potentials and causing contractions. Some GI hormones, such as **gastrin** and **cholecystokinin,** can also depolarize the slow waves, causing contractions. In addition, luminal mechanoreceptors (sensing **stretch**) or chemoreceptors (sensing composition of chyme) can signal the myenteric plexus to fire excitatory motor neurons, depolarizing the slow waves and causing contractions. The frequency of the spike potentials (and thus the magnitude of contraction) increases with greater depolarization.

In contrast, inhibitory motor neurons are present that are stimulated by **sympathetic nerves** and release **vasoactive intestinal peptide** and **nitric oxide,** which **hyperpolarize** (i.e., make more negative) the slow waves, relaxing the smooth muscle. The interplay between the excitatory and inhibitory motor neurons results in the different propulsive movements in the tract (see Plates 6.5 and 6.6).

TRACE and LABEL

☐ 1. Slow waves (i.e., resting membrane potential, upper line) as the waves are depolarized above the electrical threshold and produce spike potentials

☐ 2. Contractile force, noting the higher force generated with the greater depolarization of slow waves and additional spike potentials

REVIEW ANSWERS

A. Slow waves

B. Spike

C. Acetylcholine and substance P, contract

D. Vasoactive intestinal peptide and nitric oxide, relax

Plate 6.4   **Gastrointestinal Physiology**

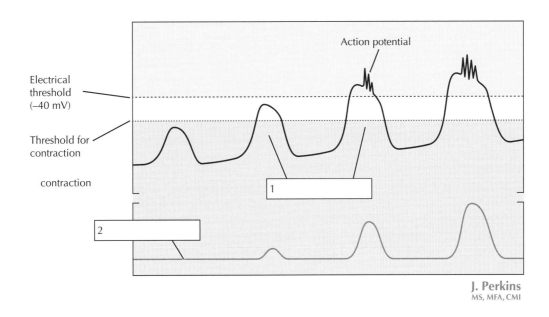

Action potential

Electrical threshold (–40 mV)

Threshold for contraction

contraction

1

2

J. Perkins
MS, MFA, CMI

REVIEW QUESTIONS

A. The resting membrane potential in the GI tract is unique because it is in the form of _____.

B. Depolarization of the resting membrane potential above –40 mV produces _____ potentials (the action potentials in the GI tract).

C. Neurotransmitters that can depolarize the slow waves include _____; they stimulate the smooth muscle to _____ (contract/relax).

D. Neurotransmitters that can hyperpolarize the slow waves include _____; they can cause the smooth muscle to _____ (contract/relax).

In the small intestine there are two types of propulsion: peristalsis and segmentation.

Peristalsis occurs by the simultaneous contraction of smooth muscle behind the bolus of chyme and relaxation of the muscle ahead of the bolus. This is accomplished by the stimulation of excitatory (behind bolus) and inhibitory (ahead of bolus) motor neurons. This results in chyme moving aborally (further down the tract). In the small intestines **peristaltic rushes** can occur when there is irritation or bacteria in an area, and the rapid movement quickly propels the irritant further down the tract (see arrow associated with 3 in Plate 6.5). Because this is a rapid action, much less absorption can occur, and **diarrhea** can result (see Clinical Note in Plate 6.6). **Reverse peristalsis** (seen in vomiting) can also occur, causing upper intestinal contents to move rapidly toward the stomach and mouth.

Segmentation forms **pockets of chyme** by constricting multiple segments of circular muscle (see 1 in Plate 6.5). However, unlike peristalsis, the circular muscle contracts in the middle of the bolus, spreading the chyme proximally and distally. These contractions occur rhythmically, moving in **waves** down a length of intestine. As the "pockets" move aborally, they simultaneously mix and propel the chyme.

Segmentation and peristalsis occur in adjacent segments of the small intestine throughout digestion and absorption. The overall process is orchestrated by the **myenteric nerve plexus,** with fine-tuning occurring through the autonomic nerves and hormones.

Unlike peristalsis and segmentation, which are active during feeding, the **MMC** is a "housekeeping" movement that is active 3 to 4 hours after eating, when most of the chyme is further down the small intestine. The MMC is active from mid-stomach through the ileum and sweeps remaining bacteria and undigested chyme out of the stomach and small intestine and into the colon. **Phase 3**, the main propulsive phase of the MMC, occurs when the hormone **motilin** (see Plate 6.3) is elevated in the blood; motilin initiates specific waves of peristaltic contractions that sweep the waste further down the tract. This action reduces the possibility of damage to the intestinal mucosa from waste.

COLOR and **LABEL** the areas of the small intestine that illustrate:

☐ 1. Rhythmic segmentation

☐ 2. Peristaltic wave

☐ 3. Peristaltic rush

Note that segmentation and peristalsis can occur in adjacent segments.

Clinical Note

Crohn's disease and **ulcerative colitis (UC)** are the most common inflammatory bowel diseases. Crohn's disease can occur anywhere in the tract (from mouth to anus) and is notable for lesions that can penetrate the entire bowel wall. **UC** is restricted to the **colon and rectum** and produces more superficial lesions. In each case, the inflammation damages sections of the tract, leading to malabsorption and increased motility, resulting in diarrhea. Treatment depends on severity of the disease and progresses from nonsteroidal anti-inflammatory drugs and steroids to biologics such as **tumor necrosis factor-α inhibitors**. Although there is no cure for Crohn's disease, unmanageable UC can be "cured" by surgical removal of the rectum and colon (the only area affected by UC) and re-forming a rectum from the lower ileum.

REVIEW ANSWERS

A. Segmentation

B. Peristalsis

C. Peristaltic rushes

D. Myenteric

Plate 6.5

Gastrointestinal Physiology

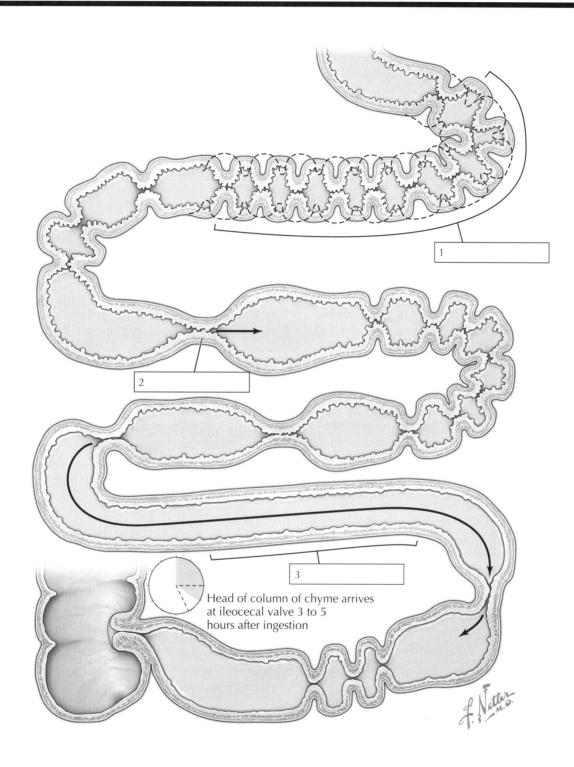

1

2

3

Head of column of chyme arrives
at ileocecal valve 3 to 5
hours after ingestion

A. The type of motility in the small intestine that forms "pockets" of chyme is called _____.

B. The type of motility that relaxes the smooth muscle in front of the bolus of chyme is called _____.

C. An irritant in the small intestine can cause _____, which rapidly move the chyme further down the intestines.

D. The _____ nerve plexus orchestrates the motility in the small intestines.

The colon also has specialized forms of motility: haustrations and mass movements. The muscle structure in the colon is different than in the small intestine: In addition to circular muscle, there are three bands of longitudinal muscle called the **taenia coli** that run the length of the organ (see 1 in Plate 6.6).

When the taenia coli contract, they form sacs called **haustrations (or haustra).** The haustrations will relax and then re-form a few minutes later, moving the chyme slowly toward the anus. This slower movement mixes the chyme, and absorption of sodium and water dehydrates the chyme, producing solid feces. Haustration is the predominant form of propulsion in the colon; however, several times a day mass movements will occur, interrupting this process.

Mass movements are **peristaltic** (with contraction behind the bolus of chyme/feces and relaxation ahead of the bolus), but the contractions and movement extend over a greater length than seen in the small intestine (see Plate 6.6). When mass movements are stimulated, the taenia coli relax, and strong contractions move the feces through the descending colon and eventually into the rectum, where a **defecation reflex** can be generated (see Plate 6.7). The mass movements are stimulated by **parasympathetic nerves** and the hormones **gastrin** and **cholecystokinin (CCK).** All of these stimuli are present during active digestion when chyme is present in the stomach and duodenum, and the stimulation of mass movements clears the lower GI tract of waste, in preparation for new waste coming down the tract. These neural and humoral mechanisms are part of the **gastrocolic reflex** (see Plate 6.7). Conversely, if the sympathetic nerves are stimulated, movement is inhibited, which is consistent with the overall actions of the sympathetic nervous system on the GI tract.

COLOR and LABEL

- ☐ 1. Bands of taenia coli
- ☐ 2. Area of haustra formation

Clinical Note

Diarrhea is the presence of loose, watery stools and has many different causes, including viruses, bacteria, irritants in the tract, inflammatory diseases (such as **inflammatory bowel diseases** and **irritable bowel syndrome**), or undigested carbohydrates (as seen in **lactose intolerance**). In each case the chyme moves through areas of the intestines rapidly, reducing the ability to absorb nutrients and water. The rapid movement of chyme into the rectum initiates the defecation reflex and expulsion of loose stool. Although most bouts of diarrhea are short lasting (2 to 3 days), they can be of longer duration in inflammatory diseases. Dehydration is a major problem arising from diarrhea, and hydration is necessary to maintain fluid and electrolyte homeostasis. Severe diarrhea, as observed in the bacterial infection **cholera,** can rapidly deplete the extracellular fluid, resulting in shock and death.

REVIEW ANSWERS

A. Haustration and mass movements

B. The haustra (sacs formed by segmental propulsion) are made by contraction of the taenia coli, whereas the pockets formed by segmentation are a result of contraction of bands of circular muscle.

C. Haustration is slow, allowing for final dehydration of chyme to form feces.

D. Mass movements are initiated by the parasympathetic nerves and the hormones gastrin and CCK, all of which are stimulated when there is chyme in the stomach and duodenum.

Plate 6.6　　　　　　　　　　　　　　　　　　　　　**Gastrointestinal Physiology**

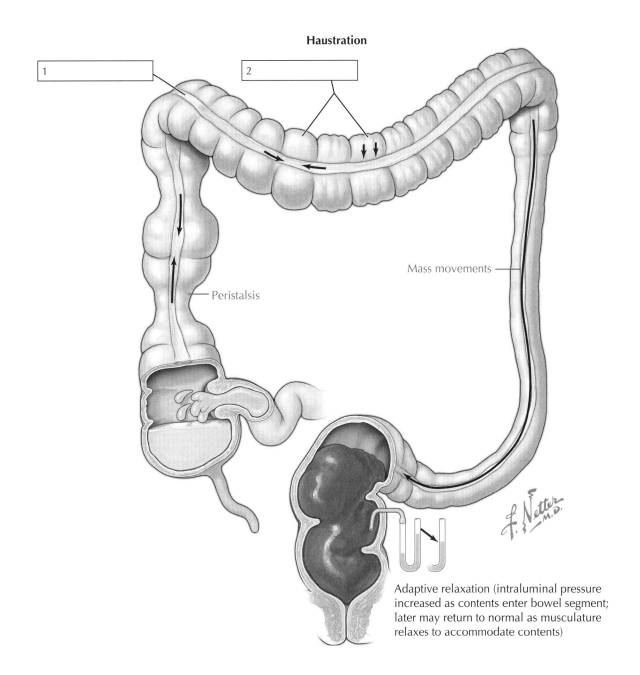

Haustration

1

2

Mass movements

Peristalsis

Adaptive relaxation (intraluminal pressure increased as contents enter bowel segment; later may return to normal as musculature relaxes to accommodate contents)

REVIEW QUESTIONS

A. What are the two types of propulsion in the colon?

B. What makes the sacs formed by haustration different from the segmentation found in the small intestine?

C. Is haustration a slow or fast movement?

D. What signals mass movements?

There are several reflexes in the GI tract that increase its efficiency in handling chyme and ridding the GI tract of waste. Two important reflexes are the **gastrocolic** and **defecation** reflexes.

During feeding, the presence of chyme in the stomach and duodenum initiates the **gastrocolic reflex,** which increases **colonic mass movements.** The mass movements are stimulated by the parasympathetic nerves (specifically the vagus and pelvic nerves) and the hormones gastrin and CCK. This stimulates colonic motility and moves the feces toward the rectum.

Luminal mechanoreceptors sense **rectal distension** and signal the ENS, rapidly initiating the **defecation reflex,** which is the involuntary **relaxation of the internal anal sphincter,** and a feeling of the **urge to defecate.** To prevent immediate defecation, we voluntarily constrict the **external anal sphincter.** If defecation does not occur, the rectum relaxes, and we relax the external anal sphincter until another movement pushes additional feces into the rectum and the defecation reflex recurs. At the appropriate time for defecation, we voluntarily relax the external anal sphincter and increase intraabdominal pressure, and feces are eliminated.

Although the gastrocolic reflex is already active in infants, the voluntary part of the defecation reflex takes time to fully develop in children and is usually intact by 2 to 4 years of age.

COLOR

☐ 1.   Area of the colon indicating a mass movement (part of the gastrocolic reflex)

☐ 2.   Rectum with feces; note that this stimulates the defecation reflex

Clinical Note

The ENS can be thought of as the central processing center that responds to a variety of signals; if the ENS is absent from an area in the tract, function is disrupted, and disease can ensue. An example of this is the congenital disorder **Hirschsprung disease,** which involves the absence of the ENS in the distal colon and rectum. The normal defecation reflex (urge to defecate and relaxation of the internal anal sphincter) does not occur. Because the internal anal sphincter does not relax, the feces back up, dilating the colon. Symptoms include little or no bowel movements and vomiting. Surgical removal of the aganglionic region typically restores the ability to defecate.

REVIEW ANSWERS

A.   Gastrocolic

B.   Defecation

C.   Parasympathetic nerves; gastrin, CCK

D.   External anal sphincter

Plate 6.7   **Gastrointestinal Physiology**

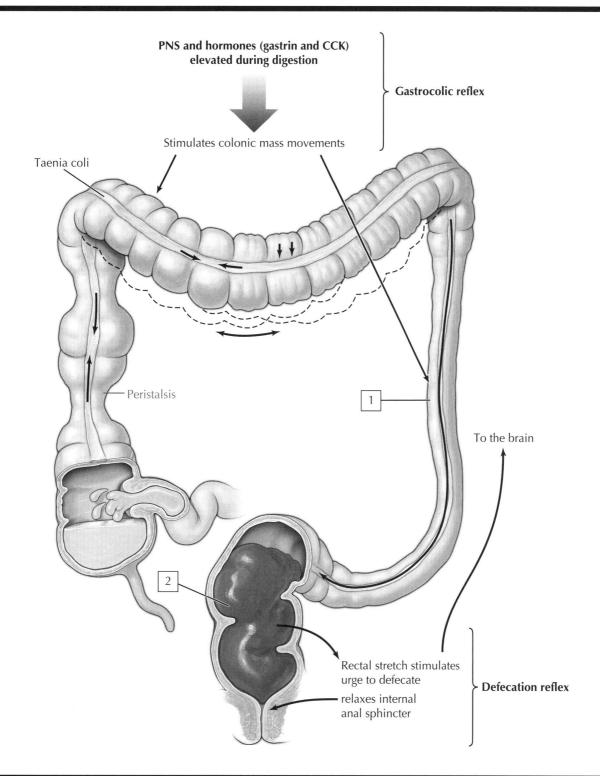

PNS and hormones (gastrin and CCK)
elevated during digestion

Stimulates colonic mass movements

Gastrocolic reflex

Taenia coli

1

Peristalsis

To the brain

2

Rectal stretch stimulates
urge to defecate

relaxes internal
anal sphincter

Defecation reflex

REVIEW QUESTIONS

A. Chyme in the stomach and duodenum can stimulate the _____ reflex.

B. Rectal distension will signal the _____ reflex.

C. Colonic mass movements are stimulated by the _____ nerves and the hormones _____ and _____.

D. When we feel the urge to defecate, we voluntarily contract the _____ sphincter.

Salivary secretions make foods easier to ingest (and digest) by lubricating, cooling, and adding digestive enzymes to the food. Approximately 1.5 L of **saliva** is secreted daily, primarily when food enters the mouth; the secretions are produced by the parotid, submandibular, and sublingual glands, which are under **parasympathetic control** through **cranial nerves VII (facial) and IX (glossopharyngeal).**

The **salivary glands** are **exocrine glands,** with the secretions draining through the **ducts** into the mouth. The glands are highly vascularized, and when the glands are stimulated, an ultrafiltrate of plasma (fluid and electrolytes) diffuses through the acinar cells into an **acinus** (see Plate 6.8) to form the **primary secretion.** This secretion is mixed with the additional products of the acinar cells (**mucins** and **α-amylase**) and then drains into the mouth. When the secretion enters the mouth, it mixes with **lingual lipase** (from Von Ebner's glands in the tongue) and **transcobalamin I (TC-I).** Thus, in addition to electrolytes, the saliva contains the following:

- Mucus, to lubricate the food as it moves through the esophagus
- α-Amylase, an enzyme that starts digestion of starch to produce smaller glucose polymers (maltose, isomaltose)
- Lingual lipase, an enzyme that starts digestion of lipids to produce diglycerides and free fatty acids
- TC-I, a protein that binds to the essential vitamin B_{12} and protects it from the acid environment in the stomach.

Salivation is **stimulated** by **parasympathetic nerves** (VII and IX) in response to various sensory inputs related to food and food intake (including esophageal distension and nausea). Salivation is **inhibited** by the **SNS** and hormones that promote water conservation (during dehydration). It is also reduced during sleep and by aging, as well as by certain drugs and chemotherapy.

COLOR

☐ 1.   Salivary gland

☐ 2.   Representative acini (made up of acinar cells)

FILL IN the following components of saliva:

☐ 3.   Mucus

☐ 4.   α-Amylase

☐ 5.   Lingual lipase

☐ 6.   Transcobalamin I (TC-I)

REVIEW ANSWERS

A.   Exocrine

B.   Parasympathetic nerves (specifically VII and IX)

C.   α-Amylase and lingual lipase

D.   A protein that protects vitamin B_{12} from acid in the stomach

Plate 6.8

Gastrointestinal Physiology

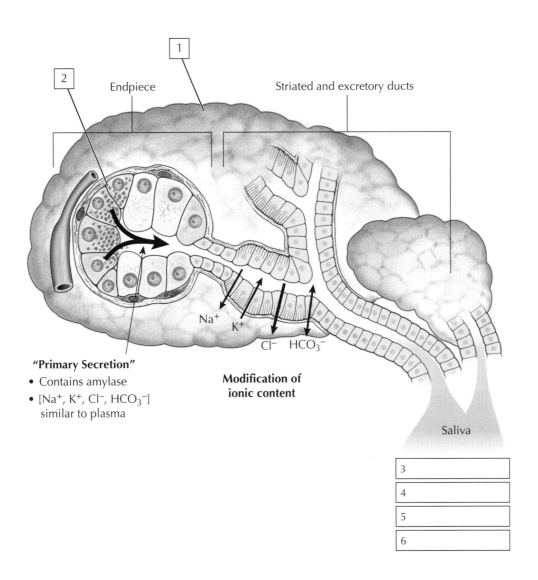

1 Striated and excretory ducts

2 Endpiece

Na⁺ K⁺

Cl⁻ HCO₃⁻

"Primary Secretion"
- Contains amylase
- [Na⁺, K⁺, Cl⁻, HCO₃⁻]
  similar to plasma

**Modification of
ionic content**

Saliva

3	
4	
5	
6	

A. The salivary glands are _____ glands, meaning their products are secreted through ducts to the outside or into the gastrointestinal tract.

B. The primary stimulus for salivation is through the _____ nerves.

C. What are the two digestive enzymes found in saliva?

D. What is transcobalamin I?

Gastric secretions facilitate digestion, lubricate the bolus of food, and protect the gastric mucosa. The mixing of gastric juices with food produces chyme. Secretions into the stomach lumen are initiated by **parasympathetic (vagal) nerves** when food enters the mouth. The presence of food in the stomach increases this action and stimulates more secretions that primarily serve to digest the food. Secretions into the gastric lumen include the following substances:

- **Hydrochloric acid (HCl)** is produced in **parietal cells** of the gastric glands and breaks up food, kills ingested bacteria, and converts inactive pepsinogens to pepsins (active proteases).
- **Intrinsic factor (IF)** is also produced in parietal cells and is an essential gastric secretion required for vitamin B_{12} absorption in the ileum (see Plate 6.18).
- **Pepsinogens** are produced in the **chief cells** of the gastric glands and are the inactive form of pepsins, which digest proteins; they are activated in the gastric lumen by low pH.
- **Gastric lipase** is also produced in the chief cells and is an enzyme that continues the process of lipid digestion initiated by lingual lipase.
- **Mucus** is produced in mucus neck cells of the gastric glands and traps bicarbonate in a thin layer on the surface epithelial cells, protecting the cells from HCl.

In addition to these exocrine secretions into the lumen, endocrine cells in the stomach produce and secrete hormones into the circulation, which then act on the GI tract. **Gastrin** is secreted into the blood by G cells in the antrum (narrow portion before the pyloric sphincter) and the duodenum, stimulates parietal cell HCl secretion, and increases motility in the lower GI tract (including mass movements). **Histamine** is produced in mast cells and acts in a paracrine manner to stimulate parietal cell HCl secretion. **Somatostatin** is produced in endocrine cells and acts in a paracrine manner to decrease HCl.

To produce the concentrated HCl in the stomach lumen, H^+ derived from CO_2 (see lower right inset in Plate 6.9), is actively pumped out of the parietal cells via the **luminal H^+/K^+ ATPases (proton pumps).** This is the **rate-limiting step** in the process, because HCl secretion depends on the number of proton pumps in the membrane. At the basolateral membrane, HCO_3^- is transported into the blood in exchange for Cl^-, and the Cl^- diffuses through luminal Cl^- channels down its electrochemical gradient. Insertion of proton pumps in the membranes is stimulated by the vagus nerve, histamine, and gastrin.

COLOR and LABEL

☐ 1. Parietal cells

☐ 2. Chief cells

☐ 3. Luminal proton pump

TRACE

☐ 4. Arrows from the gastric gland to the stomach lumen, illustrating secretion

Clinical Note

Gastroesophageal reflux disease (GERD, "indigestion") and **peptic ulcers** (ulcers of the esophagus, stomach, or duodenum) are prevalent GI problems, and drugs that target acid production are widely used. GERD results from the reflux of gastric acid through a weakened lower esophageal sphincter, causing gastric and esophageal pain and eventual ulcerations of the esophagus. Although acid is the ultimate cause, the majority of peptic ulcers are caused by the bacterium *Helicobacter pylori,* which disrupts the protective mucus layer over the epithelial cells, causing inflammation and erosion of the cells by gastric acid. Treatment of both GERD and peptic ulcer disease includes the use of drugs that block gastric acid secretion, including **H_2 receptor antagonists** and **proton pump inhibitors.** When ulcers are caused by *H. pylori*, treatment also includes antibiotics.

REVIEW ANSWERS

A. Chief cells

B. H^+/K^+ ATPase (proton pump) activity

C. Gastrin stimulates HCl production.

D. Parietal cells

Plate 6.9

Gastrointestinal Physiology

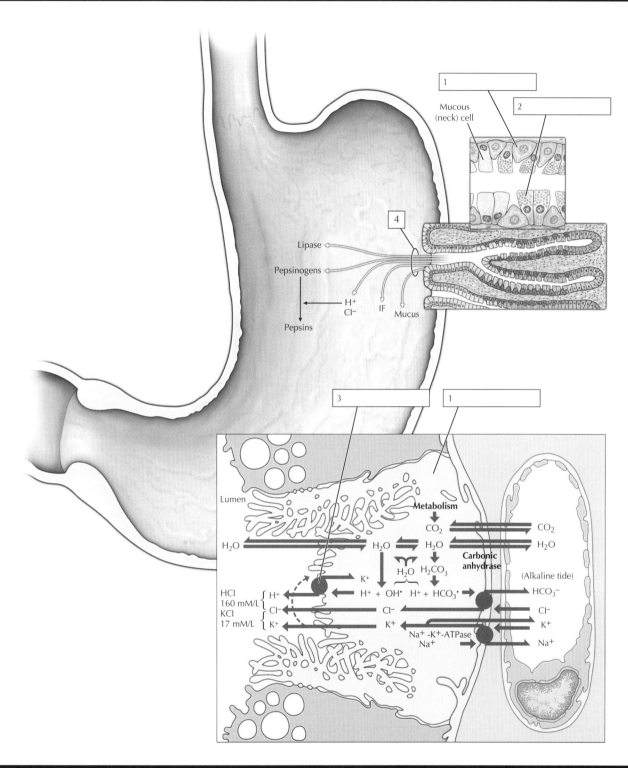

REVIEW QUESTIONS

A. What gastric cells secrete digestive enzymes?

B. What is the rate-limiting step in HCl production?

C. What does gastrin do to HCl production?

D. What cells secrete intrinsic factor into the stomach lumen?

Acinar cells secrete pancreating juice containing **enzymes**, HCO_3^- buffer, and electrolytes through ducts into the duodenum. Pancreatic **electrolyte and fluid** secretion is stimulated by the duodenal hormone **secretin,** which is released in response to acidic chyme. The bicarbonate buffer increases the pH of the chyme, allowing for optimal enzyme function.

Pancreatic **enzyme secretions** are stimulated by the duodenal hormone CCK, which is released into the blood in response to the presence of **fats** and carbohydrates in the chyme. Important pancreatic enzymes include the following:

- **Pancreatic proteases: Trypsin, chymotrypsin,** and **carboxypeptidase,** the major proteases, are stored and released as inactive **zymogens (trypsinogen, chymotrypsinogen,** and **procarboxypeptidase).** Storage of the proteases as zymogens protects the pancreas and ducts from digestion. When the zymogens enter the duodenum, **enterokinase** (in the duodenal brush border) cleaves trypsinogen to trypsin, and then trypsin can activate additional trypsinogen as well as the other proteases.
- **Pancreatic α-amylase:** Pancreatic α-amylase is activated by Cl^- and continues the digestion of starch to maltose and isomaltose.
- **Pancreatic lipase** and **co-lipase:** Pancreatic lipase hydrolyzes triglycerides to monoglycerides and free fatty acids; co-lipase is a cofactor in this process (see Plate 6.15). Other lipases convert cholesterol esters to cholesterol and fatty acid and phospholipids to lysophospholipids and fatty acid.

COLOR and LABEL

- ☐ 1. Pancreas
- ☐ 2. Acinus (and cells)
- ☐ 3. Pancreatic duct

FILL IN the nutrients that are digested by their associated pancreatic enzymes:

- ☐ 4. Starches
- ☐ 5. Fats
- ☐ 6. Proteins

REVIEW ANSWERS

A. Exocrine

B. Electrolyte solution that buffers the acidic chyme

C. Enzymes

D. Zymogens

Plate 6.10   **Gastrointestinal Physiology**

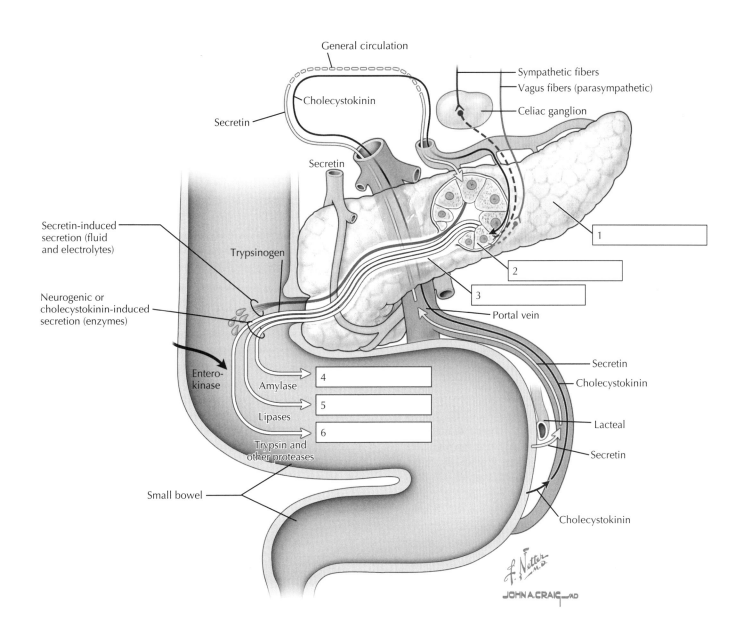

REVIEW QUESTIONS

A. Enzymes and electrolyte solutions are produced by the _____ pancreas.

B. The duodenal hormone secretin stimulates pancreatic secretion of _____.

C. The duodenal hormone cholecystokinin stimulates pancreatic secretion of _____.

D. Pancreatic proteases are produced and secreted as _____ to prevent digestion of the pancreas.

Secretions from the small intestine include electrolytes, mucus, enzymes, and hormones that facilitate digestion and absorption of the nutrients in the chyme. The anatomy of the small intestine makes it extremely efficient at digestion and absorption; the lumen of the small intestine is composed of circular folds, villi, and microvilli (forming the **brush border**), which dramatically increase the surface area to approximately 250 square meters. This **large surface area** is necessary for proper digestion and absorption, and loss of the villus lining (as seen in celiac disease) can cause serious maldigestion and malabsorption of nutrients.

The top half of the **brush border** is the site of membrane-bound enzymes (the brush border enzymes) necessary for final digestion of carbohydrates and proteins (see Plates 6.13 and 6.14) and the site of nutrient absorption. The bottom part of the villi forms the **crypts of Lieberkühn,** where secretion into the intestinal lumen occurs. Within the small intestine:

- **Brunner's glands,** located in the duodenum, secrete a **thick mucus,** which helps protect the early part of the small intestine from the acidic chyme leaving the stomach.
- **Paneth cells,** located deep in the crypts throughout the small intestine, are stimulated by secretin to **secrete ions and water,** which buffer the chyme. They also secrete **lysozyme, which has antimicrobial actions.**
- **Goblet cells,** found through the small intestine, secrete mucus.

Intestinal epithelial cells also contain cAMP-regulated **chloride channels** (the **cystic fibrosis transmembrane conductance regulator [CFTR]**) that secrete ions and water during digestion. In cystic fibrosis, a defect in the *CFTR* gene and the transporter can result in serious intestinal problems (as well as lung and pancreatic dysfunction).

In addition to the brush border digestive enzymes (covered in Plates 6.13 and 6.14), another important brush border enzyme is **enterokinase** (also known as enteropeptidase), which activates the pancreatic protease trypsinogen to trypsin.

COLOR

☐ 1. Brush border lining, noting the large increase in surface area for absorption

FILL IN the secretions from the Paneth cells:

☐ 2. Ions and water (buffer)

FILL IN the secretions from the Goblet cells:

☐ 3. Mucus

FILL IN the secretions from the CFTR-rich epithelial cells:

☐ 4. Ions and water (following Cl– secretion)

Clinical Note

The importance of an intact intestinal brush border is evident in persons with **celiac disease,** an **autoimmune** condition caused by a reaction to **gliadins** and **glutenins** found in **gluten-**containing foods such as wheat, rye, and barley. Chronic inflammation of the small intestine results in the **atrophy of the brush border,** severely limiting the area for absorption and decreasing brush border enzymes. The decreased digestion and absorption results in symptoms including diarrhea, weight loss, and anemia; in younger children it can cause growth delay. The only effective treatment is removal of gluten from the diet.

REVIEW ANSWERS

A. Folds, villi, and microvilli

B. Goblet cells

C. Paneth cells

D. A cAMP-regulated Cl– channel

Plate 6.11   **Gastrointestinal Physiology**

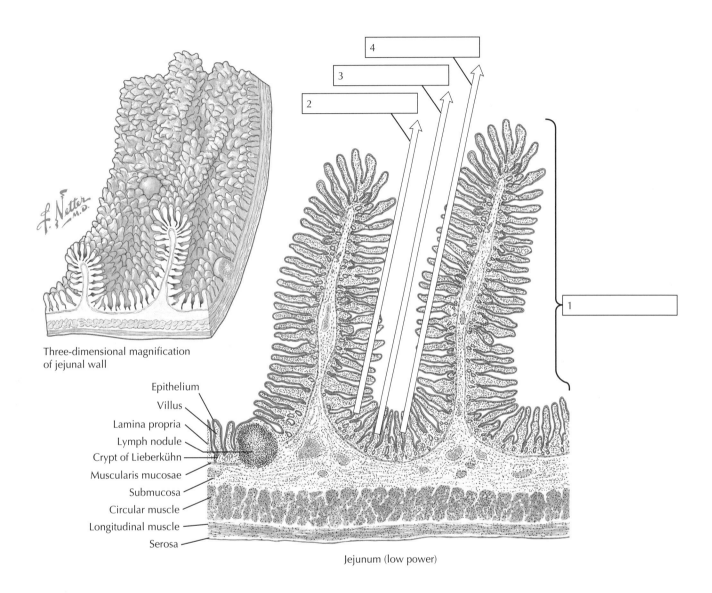

Three-dimensional magnification
of jejunal wall

Epithelium
Villus
Lamina propria
Lymph nodule
Crypt of Lieberkühn
Muscularis mucosae
Submucosa
Circular muscle
Longitudinal muscle
Serosa

Jejunum (low power)

REVIEW QUESTIONS

A. What increases the surface area in the small intestine?

B. Which cells secrete mucus throughout the small intestine?

C. Which cells in the crypts of Lieberkühn secrete ions and water to buffer chyme?

D. The CFTR is what kind of channel?

6 | Liver Function and Bile Secretion

The numerous important functions of the liver are expressed through its metabolic and secretory functions and depend on its unique vascular structure. Plate 6.12 illustrates its extensive vascularization, with liver **sinusoids** (capillary network) surrounding the **hepatocytes** (the functional liver cells). The liver receives approximately 25% of the cardiac output, including about 1 L/min from the portal veins draining the intestines; thus the liver filters and "processes" both portal and systemic blood. The basic functions of the organ include the following:

- **Carbohydrate, lipid, and protein metabolism:** The newly absorbed nutrients enter from the portal veins and are processed according to the needs of the body. For example, the liver produces albumin, fibrinogen, immunoglobulins, and binding proteins from amino acids and cholesterol, lipoproteins, and bile from lipids.
- **Cholesterol production and excretion:** The body requires cholesterol (for steroid hormone synthesis and cell membranes), and the liver can synthesize it at a high rate when the dietary intake is not sufficient. Cholesterol is also used to synthesize bile; thus when bile is excreted in the feces, cholesterol is removed from the body.
- **Detoxification:** Steroid hormones, drugs, and other chemicals are metabolized by the **hepatocytes.** Also, the liver contains reticuloendothelial cells, known as **Kupffer cells,** which are fixed macrophages on the endothelial lining of hepatic sinusoids. As blood passes through the liver, old and damaged erythrocytes undergo phagocytosis by these cells, and the iron and bilirubin are processed by the hepatocytes.
- **Vitamin and iron storage:** The liver stores several substances critical for normal body functions, including **vitamin B_{12}, folic acid, and iron.** Iron and B_{12} are necessary for red blood cell formation and maturation, respectively. The iron is bound to the protein **ferritin** for storage.

- **β-Oxidation of fatty acids:** The liver has a high capacity for β-oxidation to provide energy during the interdigestive period.
- **Endocrine function:** Hepatocytes produce and secrete hormones into the blood, including insulin-like growth factor-1, hepatocyte growth factor, and cytokines, as well as angiotensinogen, the precursor to angiotensin. It converts thyroxine to active triiodothyronine (see Plate 7.5) and participates in activation of vitamin D (see Plate 7.13).
- **Bile acid production and secretion:** Bile is necessary for efficient lipid absorption (see Plate 6.15), because lipids alone cannot efficiently pass through the water that bathes the enterocytes. **Bile acids** are synthesized in the hepatocytes, and the amphipathic character of the bile allows it to incorporate the digested lipids into **micelles** and transport the lipids through the water to the enterocytes, where the lipids can dissociate from the micelle and diffuse through the enterocyte membrane. Without bile, the bulk of the lipids would not be able to get near the enterocytes for absorption.

Because it performs a great variety of functions, from maintaining blood glucose levels and metabolizing all nutrients to detoxifying the blood, if the liver is seriously damaged, it can have profound effects on overall health.

COLOR and LABEL

- ☐ 1. Hepatocytes
- ☐ 2. Sinusoids, noting that the sinusoids surround the hepatocytes
- ☐ 3. Bile duct, note the bile ductules leading from the hepatocytes to the bile duct

REVIEW ANSWERS

A. Hepatocytes

B. Hepatocytes (drug and hormone metabolism), Kupffer cells (red blood cell phagocytosis)

C. Amphipathic

D. Albumin, fibrinogen, immunoglobulins; also angiotensinogen

Plate 6.12   **Gastrointestinal Physiology**

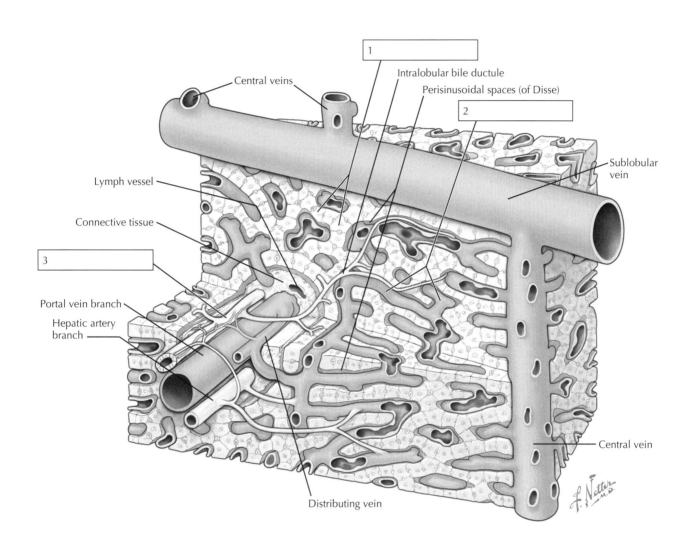

Central veins

1

Intralobular bile ductule

Perisinusoidal spaces (of Disse)

2

Sublobular vein

Lymph vessel

Connective tissue

3

Portal vein branch

Hepatic artery branch

Central vein

Distributing vein

REVIEW QUESTIONS

A. What are the functional liver cells called?

B. Detoxification by the liver occurs in the _____, and _____ phagocytose old red blood cells.

C. Bile acids are conjugated with taurine or glycine to make them more _____.

D. The liver makes plasma proteins including _____, _____, and _____.

In general terms, for all nutrients in our diet, about 25% to 30% of digestion occurs pre-duodenally (by enzymes in the mouth and/or stomach), and the remaining 70% to 75% of digestion occurs in the small intestine. As previously stated, the presence of food in the stomach and duodenum activates the PNS and hormones, which stimulate gastric, pancreatic, liver, and intestinal secretions involved in digestion and absorption of nutrients.

Much of the **carbohydrate** in our diet is in the form of **starches, sucrose** (table sugar), and **lactose** (milk sugar). Starch is a large, branched long-chain **polysaccharide** synthesized by plants, with the glucose moieties within the molecule bound together by **α-1,4 glycosidic linkages**. **Sucrose** and **lactose** are **disaccharides** made from the **monosaccharides** glucose and **fructose** (sucrose) and **glucose** and **galactose** (lactose), respectively. Although we ingest the polysaccharides and disaccharides, we can only absorb **monosaccharides.**

Digestion of carbohydrates begins in the mouth and continues through the small intestines:

- In the **mouth, salivary α-amylase** initiates starch digestion, breaking the α-1,4 glycosidic linkages and creating the disaccharide **maltose** (and some **isomaltose**). The amylase is activated by chloride ions in the saliva and inactivated in the stomach as the chyme becomes more acidic.
- In the **small intestine, pancreatic α-amylase** continues the digestion of starch, forming more maltose and isomaltose.
- Final digestion of starch and disaccharides to **monosaccharides** occurs at the **brush border of the small intestine.** As the chyme contacts the villous brush border, specific **brush border saccharidases** perform the final digestion.
  - **Maltase** digests maltose to two glucose molecules.
  - **Isomaltase** digests isomaltose to two glucose molecules.
  - **Sucrase** digests sucrose to glucose and fructose.
  - **Lactase** digests lactose to glucose and galactose.

The **monosaccharides** are rapidly transported into the enterocytes, with glucose and galactose transported by **SGLT-1** cotransporters (secondary active transport); fructose has its own transport protein, glucose transporter (**GLUT**)-5 (facilitated transport). The monosaccharides leave the enterocytes through facilitated GLUT-2 transporters, diffuse into the capillary, and are transported through the portal system to the liver for processing and storage or release into the systemic circulation. It is important to recognize that glucose transport in the GI tract (including the liver) is **insulin independent.** Carbohydrates are easily digested and quickly absorbed.

COLOR and LABEL the arrows indicating digestion of starches by:

☐ 1. Salivary α-amylase

☐ 2. Pancreatic α-amylase

COLOR and LABEL the arrows to indicate the enzymes responsible for digesting the disaccharides:

☐ 3. Maltase

☐ 4. Sucrase

☐ 5. Lactase

TRACE the arrows from the final products through the enterocyte and into the portal vein:

☐ 6. Glucose

☐ 7. Fructose

☐ 8. Galactose

Clinical Note

Carbohydrate digestion is extremely efficient; however, there is a high incidence of **lactase deficiency** in certain populations, including Asians, Africans, and African Americans. In affected persons, the **lactase** enzyme decreases through adolescence, and symptoms usually start in the late teens or early 20s. As undigested lactose continues down the intestine and into the colon, bacterial action produces gas (and cramping), and the osmotic action of the undigested carbohydrate can produce diarrhea. Treatment is either avoiding dairy products or the use of oral lactase pills before eating dairy products.

REVIEW ANSWERS

A. Salivary α-amylase and pancreatic α-amylase

B. Sucrose and lactose

C. Digest the maltose, isomaltose, sucrose, and lactose to monosaccharides

D. Via sodium-glucose cotransporters (SGLT-1)

E. No, sodium-glucose transport in the GI tract does not require insulin.

Plate 6.13   **Gastrointestinal Physiology**

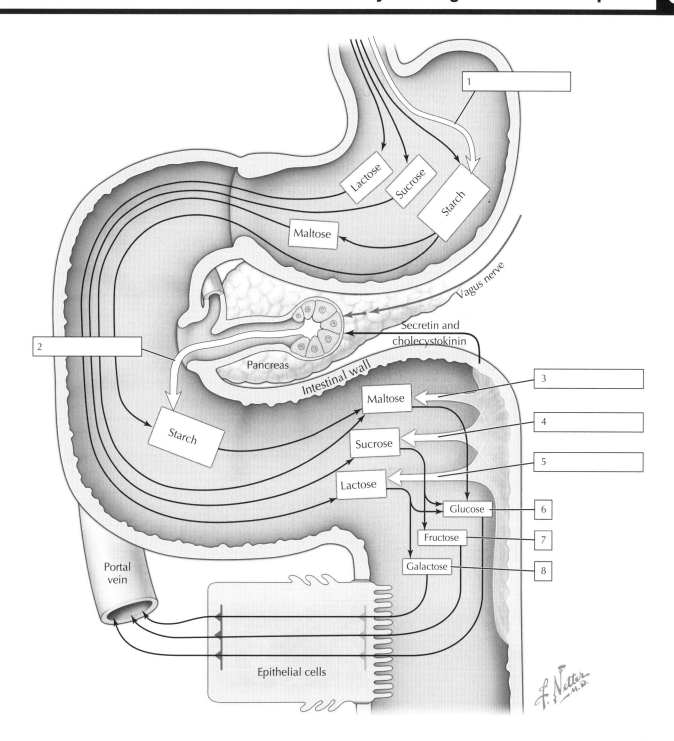

A. What enzymes digest starches to maltose and isomaltose?

B. Which of our dietary carbohydrates are disaccharides?

C. What do the brush border enzymes do?

D. How is glucose transported into enterocytes?

E. Is glucose transport in the GI tract insulin dependent?

6 Protein Digestion and Absorption

Dietary **protein digestion** begins in the stomach and continues in the small intestine:

- In the **stomach, pepsinogens** are secreted from the **gastric chief cells** and are activated by stomach acid to pepsins (endopeptidases, similar to pancreatic trypsin and chymotrypsin). They digest proteins, creating oligopeptides, and are inactivated in the higher pH in the duodenum.
- In the **small intestine, pancreatic proteases** (Plate 6.10) continue digesting protein to **oligopeptides.** These proteases are also secreted as zymogens, and once in the duodenum the trypsinogen is activated to trypsin by the enzyme **enterokinase** (secreted by cells in the brush border membrane). The trypsin activates the other pancreatic proteases.
- In the **small intestine brush border,** a variety of **brush border peptidases** hydrolyze the oligopeptides to amino acids, dipeptides, and tripeptides, which can then be absorbed.
- In the **enterocytes, cytoplasmic peptidases** digest the dipeptides and tripeptides to amino acids.

In the small intestine, most of the proteins are absorbed into the enterocytes in dipeptide and tripeptide form via H^+ symporters that are specific for the peptides. Different Na^+-dependent transporters are present for basic, acidic, and neutral amino acids. Once inside the intestinal cells, cytoplasmic peptidases hydrolyze the dipeptides and tripeptides to amino acids, which leave the cells by facilitated transport into the capillaries.

TRACE

☐ 1. Arrow in the stomach indicating pepsinogen secretion from chief cells, noting activation of pepsinogen to pepsin by HCl

COLOR and **LABEL** the arrows corresponding to the pancreatic protease zymogens below, noting the activation to trypsin by enterokinase, and the subsequent activation of the other proteases:

☐ 2. Chymotrypsinogen

☐ 3. Trypsinogen

☐ 4. Procarboxypeptidase

TRACE

☐ 5. Arrow indicating brush border peptidases acting on the oligopeptides to produce dipeptides, tripeptides, and amino acids

COLOR and **LABEL** the line leaving the enterocyte:

☐ 6. Amino acids, noting that cytoplasmic peptidases hydrolyze the dipeptides and tripeptides

REVIEW ANSWERS

A. Pepsinogen

B. Zymogens

C. Brush border peptidases

D. Amino acids, dipeptides, and tripeptides

E. Cytoplasmic peptidases hydrolyze dipeptides and tripeptides to amino acids, which can then be transported out of the cell into the capillaries.

Plate 6.14   **Gastrointestinal Physiology**

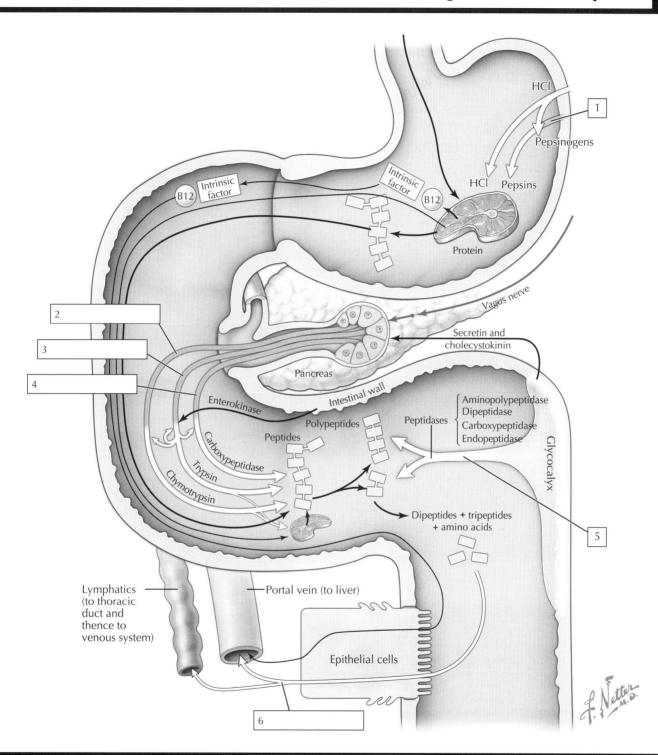

HCl

1

Pepsinogens

Intrinsic factor

HCl   Pepsins

B12   Intrinsic factor

B12

Protein

Vagus nerve

2

3

4

Secretin and cholecystokinin

Enterokinase

Pancreas

Intestinal wall

Aminopolypeptidase
Dipeptidase
Carboxypeptidase
Endopeptidase

Polypeptides   Peptidases

Peptides

Glycocalyx

Carboxypeptidase

Trypsin

Chymotrypsin

5

Dipeptides + tripeptides + amino acids

Lymphatics
(to thoracic
duct and
thence to
venous system)

Portal vein (to liver)

Epithelial cells

6

REVIEW QUESTIONS

A. What protease is secreted by gastric chief cells?

B. Proteases are stored and released as _____ and are activated in the lumen of the GI tract.

C. Digestion of oligopeptides to dipeptides, tripeptides, and amino acids occurs by the _____.

D. What constituents of proteins can be absorbed into the enterocytes?

E. What functions do cytoplasmic peptidases perform?

The bulk of ingested lipids are **triglycerides (TGs),** with the remainder being mainly **cholesterol esters** and **phospholipids.** Lipids are easily hydrolyzed to molecules that can be absorbed; however, their **hydrophobicity** does not allow easy access to the absorptive cells in the brush border of the small intestine. As a result, a complex mechanism exists utilizing **bile** to incorporate the digested lipids into **micelles** (Plate 6.12), which can efficiently move lipids through the unstirred water layer to the enterocytes.

Lipid digestion occurs in the following locations:

- In the **mouth, lingual lipase** is secreted from von Ebner's glands in the tongue into the saliva and begins the hydrolysis of TGs to diglycerides and free fatty acids (FFAs).
- In the **stomach, gastric lipase** is secreted from the chief cells and also hydrolyzes TGs to diglycerides and FFAs.
- In the **small intestine,** lipid digestion occurs through the action of various lipases that are secreted by the pancreatic acinar cells in response to CCK. However, as soon as lipid enters the small intestine it is surrounded by **bile** (Plate 6.12), and the **pancreatic lipase** cannot readily access the lipid for hydrolysis to occur. To facilitate the action of the lipase, **procolipase** is also secreted from the pancreas and is activated by trypsin to **colipase.** The colipase displaces the bile from the lipids, providing the lipase access to hydrolyze the TGs to monoglycerides and FFAs. These aggregates of bile and hydrolyzed lipids are called **micelles.**

In a micelle, the hydrophilic ends of the bile are oriented outward, allowing micelles to move through the unstirred water layer to the brush border, where lipids leave the micelle and diffuse through the cell membrane into the enterocyte. The bile remains in the lumen of the small intestine, until most is absorbed in the **terminal ileum** and "recycled" through the portal system back to the liver. It can then be re-secreted into the duodenum as long as chyme is present. Recycling of bile can occur 3 to 6 times per meal depending on the amount of lipids in the meal. With each cycle, about 10% of the bile is unabsorbed and is lost in the feces.

Once lipids diffuse into the enterocytes, TGs, cholesterol esters, and phospholipids are re-formed in the **smooth endoplasmic reticulum.** The lipids then form small lipid droplets called **chylomicrons.** The chylomicrons are exported from the enterocytes by exocytosis and enter the **lymph lacteals;** they are too large to enter capillaries. Thus, the chylomicrons enter the systemic blood with lymph through the thoracic ducts and travel through the systemic circulation to the liver for processing.

COLOR

☐ 1. Bile solution leaving bile duct and surrounding the lipids in the small intestine

TRACE

☐ 2. Pancreatic lipase from the pancreas to the bile emulsion and note that colipase is necessary for the pancreatic lipase to access the lipid

REVIEW ANSWERS

A. Triglycerides

B. Lingual lipase (mouth), gastric lipase (stomach), pancreatic lipase (small intestine)

C. Without the micelle, lipids would not be able to approach the cells. Bile incorporates digested lipids into a micelle, with the hydrophilic ends of the bile oriented outward, allowing the micelle to move through the water layer next to the enterocytes.

D. Lipids are lipophilic and diffuse through the cell membrane.

E. Colipase

Plate 6.15   **Gastrointestinal Physiology**

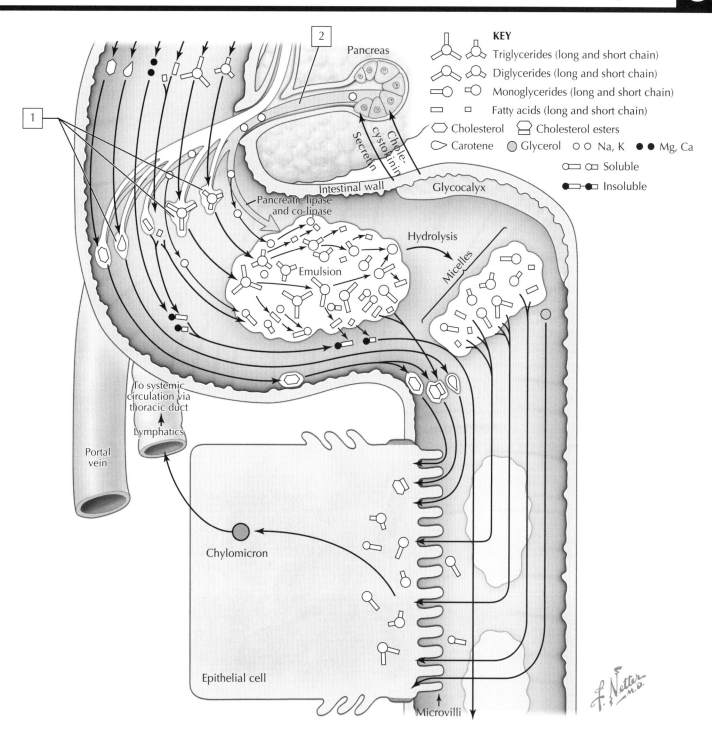

KEY

Triglycerides (long and short chain)
Diglycerides (long and short chain)
Monoglycerides (long and short chain)
Fatty acids (long and short chain)
Cholesterol   Cholesterol esters
Carotene   Glycerol   Na, K   Mg, Ca
Soluble
Insoluble

Pancreas

Chole-cystokinin
Secretin

Intestinal wall   Glycocalyx

Pancreatic lipase and co-lipase

Emulsion   Hydrolysis   Micelles

To systemic circulation via thoracic duct
Lymphatics
Portal vein

Chylomicron

Epithelial cell   Microvilli

REVIEW QUESTIONS

A. What is the main form of lipids in our diet?

B. What enzymes digest lipids?

C. Why is bile needed for efficient lipid absorption?

D. How do lipids enter the cells?

E. The pancreatic enzyme _____ displaces bile from lipids so that pancreatic lipase can access the lipids.

6 Electrolyte and Water Absorption

In addition to the 2+ liters of fluid ingested each day, 7 or more liters are added to the GI tract in various segments to facilitate digestion and absorption of the nutrients. Almost all of the fluid is absorbed as part of the process of nutrient and electrolyte absorption.

The large surface area of the small intestine makes digestion and absorption extremely efficient, and the majority of absorption occurs in the jejunum. There is also significant absorption of electrolytes and water in the ileum, and the last sodium and water absorption occurs in the colon as feces are produced. There are several mechanisms through which **sodium, chloride, and water** are absorbed in the different segments:

- In the **jejunum, sodium** absorption is a driving force for nutrient and water absorption. The basolateral Na^+/K^+ ATPase maintains the low intracellular Na^+ concentration necessary for the luminal Na^+ to enter the cells. Sodium absorption occurs with nutrients (e.g., via Na^+-glucose cotransporters) and through other sodium transporters **(Na^+/H^+ exchangers, NKCC-2 cotransporters;** see Part A in Plate 6.16). As the sodium is absorbed, the water follows the osmotic gradient. Chloride absorption occurs paracellularly following its electrochemical gradient.
- In the **ileum, sodium** and **water** absorption continues in similar manner as in the jejunum. **Chloride absorption** occurs via **HCO_3^-/Cl^- exchangers** (see Parts B and C); the chloride leaves through the basolateral membrane following the electrochemical gradient generated by sodium absorption. Sodium leaves the enterocytes via the Na^+/K^+ ATPase (water follows), and chloride leaves the cell via a chloride channel (facilitated transport).
- In the **colon, aldosterone** stimulates luminal sodium absorption through epithelial sodium channels (ENaC) and potassium *secretion* via luminal potassium channels. As water follows sodium, the chyme is dehydrated, producing feces. The colon usually absorbs ~400–500 mL of water per day (following sodium absorption), and water absorption can increase to ~1 L per day when aldosterone is elevated. As observed in the ileum, chloride is absorbed via HCO_3^-/Cl^- exchangers.

Although there is a large functional capacity in the GI tract (e.g., large surface area, excess transporters) to ensure absorption of all the nutrients and water, if a change occurs that increases the rate of flow of chyme or osmotic content of the chyme, absorption (especially of water and electrolytes) can decrease, resulting in **diarrhea.** For example, foods that irritate the intestinal lining, undigested carbohydrates (as occurs in lactose intolerance), or viruses can increase motility, moving the chyme rapidly through the intestines to the rectum, stimulating a defecation reflex. In contrast, if the progress of chyme through the colon is slowed or there is less fiber in the chyme (fiber holds water, keeping chyme moving), **constipation** can occur, limiting fecal movement and defecation. Chronic constipation is associated with colonic polyp formation and a greater incidence of colon cancer.

COLOR and **LABEL** the following luminal transporters, noting the variety of secondary-active sodium transporters in the jejunum and ileum, as well as the HCO_3^-/Cl^- exchangers in the ileum and colon:

☐ 1. Glucose or amino acid cotransport with sodium
☐ 2. NKCC-2 cotransporters
☐ 3. Na^+/H^+ exchangers
☐ 4. HCO_3^-/Cl^- exchangers

TRACE

☐ 5. Dotted arrows indicating Na^+ absorption through Na^+ channels (ENaC)
☐ 6. Dotted arrows indicating K^+ secretion through K^+ channels

---

REVIEW ANSWERS

A. Jejunum

B. Na^+-glucose cotransporters, Na^+-amino acid transporters, NKCC-2 cotransporters, and Na^+/H^+ exchangers

C. HCO_3^-/Cl^- exchanger

D. Through the chloride channels (facilitated transport)

Plate 6.16   **Gastrointestinal Physiology**

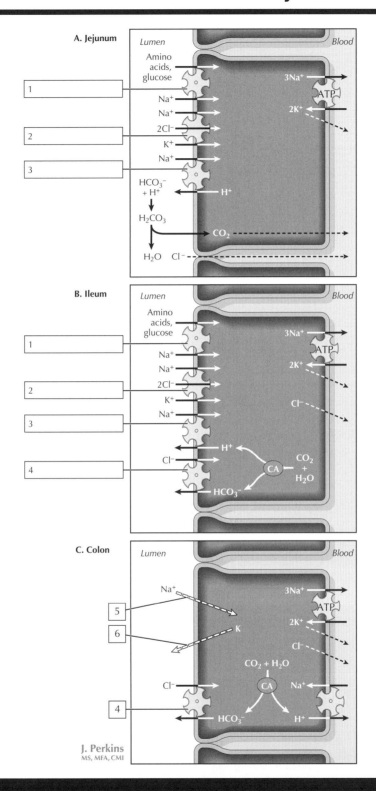

A. Jejunum

B. Ileum

C. Colon

J. Perkins
MS, MFA, CMI

REVIEW QUESTIONS

A. The majority of nutrient absorption occurs in the _____.

B. Name the luminal transporters that carry sodium into the enterocytes.

C. What transporter brings chloride into the enterocytes?

D. How does chloride leave the basolateral side of enterocytes?

Calcium and iron are typically absorbed in the early part of the small intestine, from the duodenum to about halfway through the jejunum. The slightly lower pH in the early part of the small intestine favors the reduced form of iron (Fe^{2+}) and keeps the divalent cations (e.g., Ca^{2+}, Fe^{2+}) from forming insoluble salts that are excreted in feces.

Calcium absorption is regulated by circulating **active vitamin D_3** (1,25-dihydrocholecalciferol), which increases **calcium channels** at the luminal membrane of the enterocytes, as well as the channel-associated cytosolic binding protein **calbindin.** The Ca^{2+} entering the cell is immediately bound to the calbindin, keeping the intracellular free Ca^{2+} levels very low (10^{-7} M), thus maintaining a gradient for Ca^{2+} entry into the cell and allowing Ca^{2+}-dependent messenger systems to function properly. The Ca^{2+} exits the basolateral side through active Ca^{2+} ATPase pumps and Na^+/Ca^{2+} exchangers (see Part A). The activity of the **Ca^{2+} ATPase** is also stimulated by vitamin D_3.

Iron is absorbed in the **ferrous (Fe^{2+})** form or in **heme** (Part B).

- When heme is absorbed, intracellular **heme oxygenase** frees Fe^{2+}, which is then bound to **ferritin** in the cell (for storage) or is transported into the blood, where it is bound to **transferrin.**
- The membrane also contains a **ferroreductase (FR),** which reduces Fe^{3+} to Fe^{2+} for absorption. In the case of **Fe^{2+}** absorption, luminal membranes in the jejunum have **divalent metal transport (DMT) proteins** that transport free Fe^{2+} into the cell, where it is bound to ferritin and stored or transported out of the cell via the iron-regulated transporter 1 (IREG-1) proteins and bound to transferrin.

In the **blood,** the **transferrin-bound iron** is transported to the liver and spleen for storage or to the **bone marrow** for hemoglobin and red blood synthesis. Iron absorption and transport are highly regulated; although it is critical for red blood cell production, a variety of binding proteins ensure that iron is never unbound, because it is highly toxic.

COLOR and **LABEL** in Part A:

- ☐ 1. Calcium channel
- ☐ 2. Calbindin using the same color as calcium channel to indicate that calbindin is associated with the channel

TRACE and **LABEL** in Part A:

- ☐ 3. Arrows from vitamin D_3 to the calcium channel and Ca^{2+} ATPase, reinforcing that circulating vitamin D_3 increases calcium channels and the calcium pumps

COLOR and **LABEL** in Part B:

- ☐ 4. Ferroreductase (FR), which reduces iron to the ferrous (Fe^{2+}) form
- ☐ 5. DMT-1 transporters, illustrating that the ferrous iron (Fe^{2+}) can be transported via the DMT-1 proteins
- ☐ 6. Basolateral IREG-1 protein, which transports the iron out of the cell

REVIEW ANSWERS

A. Active vitamin D_3

B. Calbindin

C. Calcium channels and associated calbindin, Ca^{2+} ATPase (calcium pump)

D. DMT-1 proteins, ferritin, IREG-1

Plate 6.17   **Gastrointestinal Physiology**

A. Ca²⁺

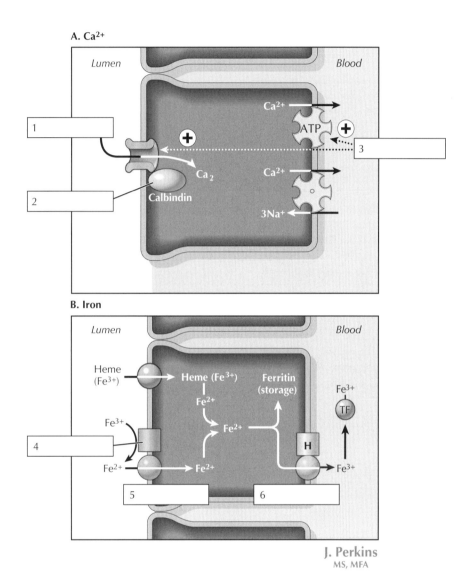

Lumen

Blood

1

Ca₂

Calbindin

2

Ca²⁺

ATP

+

+

Ca²⁺

3

Ca²⁺

3Na⁺

B. Iron

Lumen

Blood

Heme
(Fe³⁺)

Heme (Fe³⁺)

Ferritin
(storage)

Fe³⁺

TF

Fe²⁺

Fe³⁺

Fe²⁺

4

H

Fe²⁺

Fe²⁺

Fe³⁺

5

6

J. Perkins
MS, MFA

REVIEW QUESTIONS

A. Calcium absorption is regulated by the circulating hormone _____.

B. The calcium transporter on the luminal membrane is associated with cytosolic _____, which binds the calcium as it enters the cell.

C. Vitamin D₃ increases the luminal _____ and the basolateral _____.

D. Ferrous (Fe²⁺) iron enters the cells via _____ and can be stored in the enterocytes as _____ or exit the cell through _____ proteins.

---

6 Vitamin B$_{12}$ Absorption

Most vitamins are readily absorbed through **cotransport with sodium** (vitamin C, thiamin [B$_1$], riboflavin [B$_2$], biotin) or **passive diffusion,** as seen with pyridoxine (B$_6$) and the fat-soluble vitamins A, D, E, and K (which are usually associated with micelles, to cross the unstirred water layer and access the enterocytes).

Vitamin **B$_{12}$** (cobalamin) is an anomaly in several ways, including its absorption via **facilitated diffusion.** It is associated with animal proteins (meat, fish, dairy), and it must be freed from the proteins and then protected from digestion until it is absorbed in the terminal ileum. This process requires several steps:

- The glycoprotein **TC-I** is secreted into the saliva.
- In the stomach, **HCl** and **IF** are secreted by the gastric parietal cells. The acid frees B$_{12}$ from the ingested protein, and the **TC-**I (from saliva) binds to the B$_{12}$, protecting it from degradation by the acidic environment in the stomach.
- In the duodenum, the TC-I is cleaved from the B$_{12}$-TC-I complex by trypsin (secreted from the pancreas), and the **IF binds to B$_{12}$.**
- The **B$_{12}$-IF complex dimerizes** (Plate 6.18), protecting the B$_{12}$ from catalysis by intestinal bacteria. The dimer continues down the small intestine to the distal end of the ileum, where it binds to a transport protein and enters the cell. Within the cell the B$_{12}$ binds to cytosolic **transcobalamin II (TC-II),** exits the cell into the blood in that form, and is transported to the liver for storage (or to bone marrow, where it promotes red blood cell maturation).

Clinical Note

B$_{12}$ is a **co-factor in DNA synthesis** and is important in the metabolism of fatty acids and amino acids, the synthesis of myelin, and the maturation of red blood cells. B$_{12}$ deficiency can have potentially serious and irreversible pathophysiologic effects on the brain and nervous system and can result in **pernicious anemia.** One cause of B$_{12}$ deficiency is the prolonged use of **gastric acid blockers,** such as proton pump inhibitors and H$_2$ receptor antagonists, which reduce acid and IF secretion. The reduction in acid secretion limits the amount of B$_{12}$ that is freed from the ingested proteins, and with less IF present for dimerization and protection, absorption is decreased. Treatment is with intravenous, intramuscular, or intranasal dosing of B$_{12}$ every few weeks, depending on individual need.

REVIEW ANSWERS

A. Facilitated

B. Transcobalamin I (TC-I)

C. Intrinsic factor (IF)

D. Transcobalamin II (TC-II)

Plate 6.18　　　　　**Gastrointestinal Physiology**

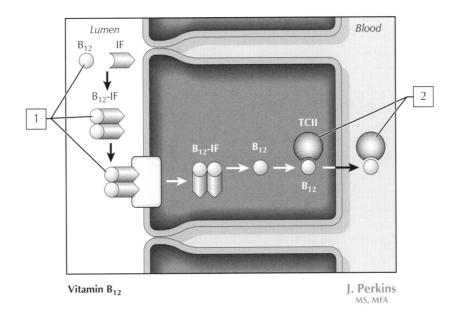

Vitamin B$_{12}$

J. Perkins
MS, MFA

A. Vitamin B$_{12}$ enters the cells via _____ diffusion.

B. The glycoprotein that binds to B$_{12}$ in the stomach and protects it from the low pH is _____.

C. What is the factor that is secreted by the gastric parietal cells and protects B$_{12}$ from intestinal bacteria?

D. Within the enterocyte, B$_{12}$ binds to _____.

Chapter 7   Endocrine Physiology

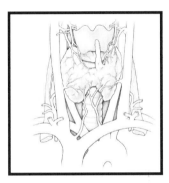
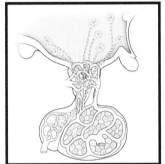
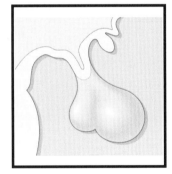
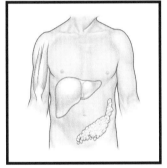

Hormones are substances secreted by a gland or tissue into the blood and bind to receptors that are on other tissues, where they affect specific physiologic processes. Plate 7.1 illustrates the organization of the endocrine system, including hormones discussed in Chapters 3, 5, and 6. Chemically, hormones are **peptides** (e.g., insulin and growth hormone), **steroids** (e.g., estrogen, testosterone, and cortisol), or **amines** or their derivatives (e.g., epinephrine, thyroxine [T_4], and triiodothyronine [T_3]). **Neurohormones** are a subclass of hormones secreted by neurons (e.g., vasopressin and oxytocin).

When hormones reach their target tissues, they bind to **membrane** or **nuclear receptors,** initiating a chain of events that results in the physiologic effects of the hormone. Most peptide hormones and catecholamines bind to membrane receptors linked to G-proteins, which stimulate or inhibit intracellular second messenger systems. **Steroid hormones** (e.g., testosterone, estradiol, progesterone), **thyroid hormone,** and **active vitamin D** are lipophilic and enter the target cell, where they bind to nuclear receptors (or cytoplasmic receptors, which translocate to the nucleus) and initiate gene transcription (thyroid hormone requires a carrier to pass through the cell membrane). The RNA produced is translated to synthesize proteins that regulate biochemical and physiologic processes.

COLOR and **LABEL** the important tissues and glands, noting the hormones that are released from these sites:

☐ 1. Hypothalamus
☐ 2. Pituitary gland
☐ 3. Parathyroid glands
☐ 4. Heart
☐ 5. Adrenal glands
☐ 6. Kidneys
☐ 7. Adipose tissue
☐ 8. Testes
☐ 9. Ovaries
☐ 10. Pancreatic islet cells
☐ 11. Digestive (gastrointestinal) tract
☐ 12. Thymus
☐ 13. Thyroid gland
☐ 14. Pineal gland

REVIEW ANSWERS

A. Peptides, steroids, and amines

B. Neurohormones

C. Membrane receptors and nuclear receptors

D. Lipophilic hormones such as steroid hormones, thyroid hormone, and vitamin D

Plate 7.1

Endocrine Physiology

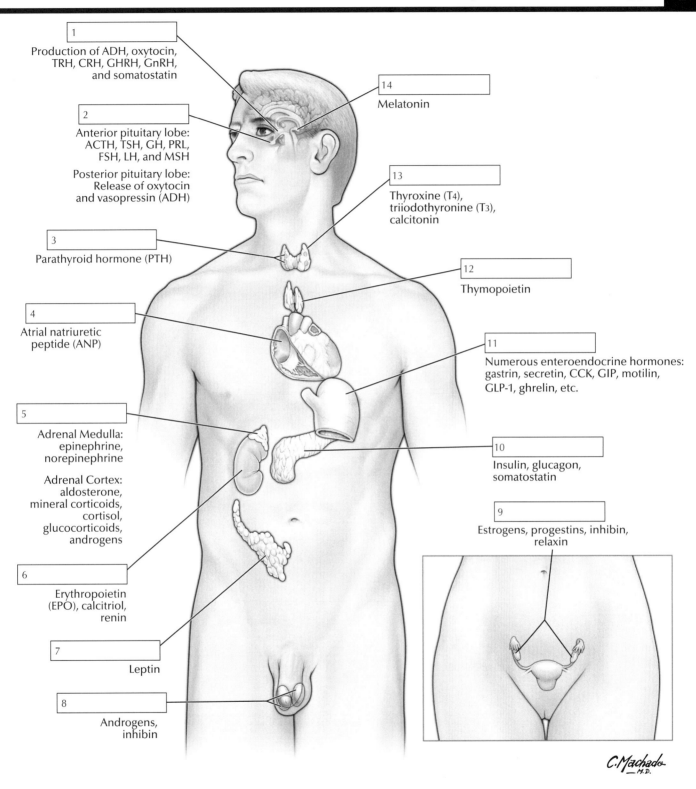

1 Production of ADH, oxytocin, TRH, CRH, GHRH, GnRH, and somatostatin

14 Melatonin

2 Anterior pituitary lobe: ACTH, TSH, GH, PRL, FSH, LH, and MSH

Posterior pituitary lobe: Release of oxytocin and vasopressin (ADH)

13 Thyroxine (T4), triiodothyronine (T3), calcitonin

3 Parathyroid hormone (PTH)

12 Thymopoietin

4 Atrial natriuretic peptide (ANP)

11 Numerous enteroendocrine hormones: gastrin, secretin, CCK, GIP, motilin, GLP-1, ghrelin, etc.

5 Adrenal Medulla: epinephrine, norepinephrine

Adrenal Cortex: aldosterone, mineral corticoids, cortisol, glucocorticoids, androgens

10 Insulin, glucagon, somatostatin

9 Estrogens, progestins, inhibin, relaxin

6 Erythropoietin (EPO), calcitriol, renin

7 Leptin

8 Androgens, inhibin

C. Machado
_M.D._

REVIEW QUESTIONS

A. What are the three chemical forms of hormones?

B. Hormones that are secreted from nerves are called _____.

C. What types of receptors do hormones bind to?

D. What types of hormones bind to nuclear receptors?

The hypothalamus and pituitary gland regulate the function of much of the endocrine system. The **hypothalamus** is connected by the pituitary stalk to the **pituitary gland.** The pituitary gland consists of two lobes, the **anterior pituitary** and the **posterior pituitary.**

The posterior pituitary is directly attached to the hypothalamus by the stalk, which contains axons originating in the hypothalamic nuclei that synthesize **antidiuretic hormone (ADH;** also known as **vasopressin)** and **oxytocin.** The ADH and oxytocin are carried by axonal transport and stored in vesicles within the posterior pituitary.

- ADH is released in response to hyperosmolar plasma or hypovolemia. The primary action of ADH is on the renal collecting ducts, to stimulate solute-free water reabsorption, limiting urinary fluid loss (see Plates 5.13, 5.14, and 5.16).
- Oxytocin is released in response to breastfeeding or cervical and vaginal stimulation. It causes the **expulsion of milk** from mammary glands of the breasts and **uterine contractions.**

The anterior pituitary is connected to the hypothalamus by vessels of the **hypophyseal portal circulation.** This circulation carries **hypothalamic releasing hormones** through the **portal veins** directly to cells in the anterior pituitary. The releasing hormones regulate the synthesis and secretion of pituitary tropic hormones. You will learn more about these hormones and their effects in later plates.

HYPOTHALAMIC-RELEASING HORMONE	ANTERIOR PITUITARY HORMONE	ACTION OF PITUITARY HORMONE
Thyrotropin-releasing hormone (TRH)	Thyroid-stimulating hormone (TSH)	Thyroid hormone (TH) synthesis and release by the thyroid gland
Corticotropin-releasing hormone (CRH)	Adrenocorticotropic hormone (ACTH)	Synthesis of adrenal steroids
Gonadotropin-releasing hormone (GnRH)	Luteinizing hormone (LH) and follicle-stimulating hormone (FSH)	Steroidogenesis and gametogenesis by the testes and ovaries
Thyrotropin-releasing hormone (TRH)	Prolactin (PRL) (control of PRL is mainly through inhibition by dopamine)	Milk production by the breasts
Growth hormone–releasing hormone (GHRH)	Growth hormone (GH)	Synthesis of insulin-like growth factors (IGFs) by the liver and other target tissues

COLOR the features of hormonal release from the pituitary gland:

- ☐ 1. Supraoptic and paraventricular neurons and their axons, noting the peptides that are secreted
- ☐ 2. Hypophyseal portal veins in the anterior pituitary
- ☐ 3. GH (arrow) targeting the liver
- ☐ 4. TSH (arrow) targeting the thyroid gland
- ☐ 5. ACTH (arrow) targeting the adrenal cortex
- ☐ 6. FSH (arrows) targeting the testis and ovary
- ☐ 7. LH (arrows) targeting the testis and ovary
- ☐ 8. Prolactin (arrow) targeting the breast
- ☐ 9. Release of insulin-like growth factors (IGFs) by the liver

REVIEW ANSWERS

A. ADH (antidiuretic hormone) and oxytocin

B. Hypophyseal portal circulation, anterior

C. LH, FSH

D. ACTH

Plate 7.2   **Endocrine Physiology**

Pituitary Function

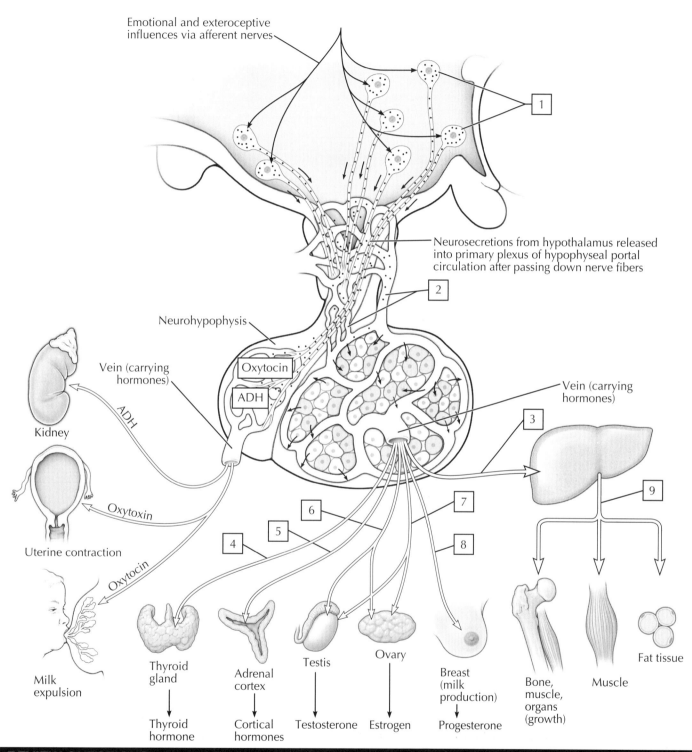

Emotional and exteroceptive influences via afferent nerves

1

Neurosecretions from hypothalamus released into primary plexus of hypophyseal portal circulation after passing down nerve fibers

2

Neurohypophysis

Vein (carrying hormones)

Oxytocin

ADH

Vein (carrying hormones)

3

Kidney

ADH

9

Oxytoxin

Uterine contraction

7

6

5

4

8

Oxytocin

Milk expulsion

Thyroid gland

Adrenal cortex

Testis

Ovary

Breast (milk production)

Bone, muscle, organs (growth)

Muscle

Fat tissue

Thyroid hormone

Cortical hormones

Testosterone

Estrogen

Progesterone

REVIEW QUESTIONS

A. Hypothalamic neurons carry what two peptide hormones to the posterior pituitary gland?

B. Hypothalamic releasing hormones are secreted into the _____, which perfuses the _____ pituitary gland.

C. Gonadotropin-releasing hormone stimulates synthesis and release of _____ and _____.

D. Corticotropin-releasing hormone stimulates synthesis and release of _____.

Feedback systems regulate blood hormone levels and thereby their physiologic effects. Some hormones have cyclic variations, which are important in regulating complex processes such as menstrual cycles and diurnal cycles in activity levels.

Typical control of hormone secretion is through **negative feedback,** whereby increased blood levels of a hormone inhibit its synthesis, maintaining normal levels. For example, synthesis and release of pituitary **GH** (a 191–amino acid polypeptide) are stimulated by hypothalamic **GHRH.** GH acts on the liver and other target tissues to produce **IGF** (also called somatomedin), which has growth and anabolic effects on a variety of tissues (see Plate 7.3). At the same time, GH and IGF inhibit hypothalamic GHRH and pituitary GH (see Plate 7.3). In addition, GH secretion by the anterior pituitary is inhibited by the hypothalamic hormone **somatostatin** (not illustrated).

In endocrine systems consisting of hypothalamus, pituitary, and a target endocrine gland, feedback loops are mainly classified as follows:

- **Long-loop feedback,** in which hypothalamic and pituitary hormones in an endocrine axis are inhibited by the target gland hormone (as in the case of IGF inhibiting GHRH and GH)
- **Short-loop feedback,** whereby an anterior pituitary hormone inhibits the release of its associated hypothalamic hormone (as in the case of inhibition of GHRH by GH)
- **Ultra-short-loop feedback,** in which secretion of a hypothalamic hormone is inhibited by that same hormone (as in the case of GHRH inhibiting further GHRH secretion)

The multiple feedback systems allow for the fine-tuning of hormone levels and participate in the generation of the cyclic variations observed in levels of many hormones, including GH.

COLOR

☐ 1. Arrows from the hypothalamus to GHRH, pituitary GH, and the end tissues to reinforce the pathways stimulating hormone production

☐ 2. Arrows to indicate the inhibitory effects of GH and IGF on GHRH and GH, and GHRH on further GHRH secretion (ultra-short-loop feedback)

Clinical Note

GH promotes growth in the young and has anabolic effects in adults, with these normal actions maintained by the feedback systems. However, certain conditions can override the feedback systems and can result in pathophysiology. An example of this is the hypersecretion of GH seen in GH-secreting adenomas. The adenoma is not sensitive to negative feedback, so the GH continues to be secreted. In adults, over time, this hypersecretion results in **acromegaly,** a condition characterized by thickening of the soft tissue of the feet and hands and growth of the brow ridges and jaw, but not long bones. In adolescents whose growth plates have not yet fused, pituitary tumors hypersecreting GH can enhance long bone growth, causing **gigantism.**

REVIEW ANSWERS

A. Negative

B. IGF

C. Long-loop

D. Short-loop

Plate 7.3 | **Endocrine Physiology**

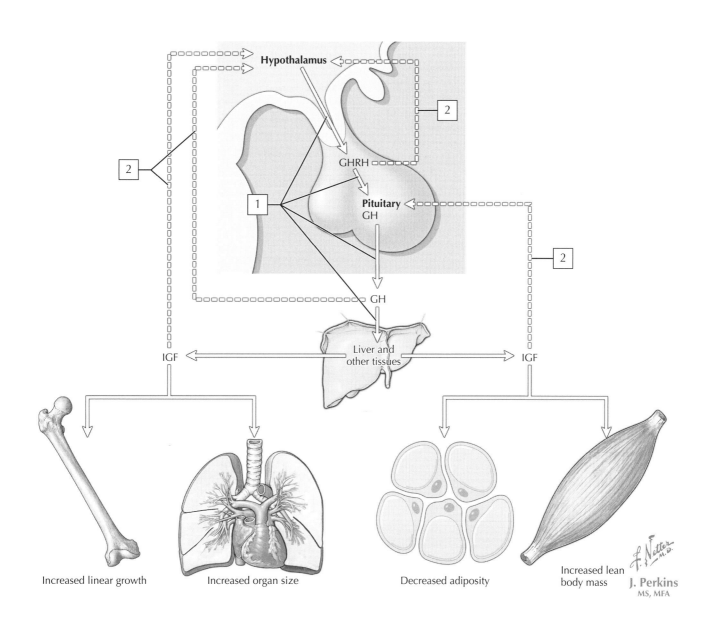

Hypothalamus

GHRH

Pituitary
GH

GH

Liver and
other tissues

IGF

IGF

Increased linear growth   Increased organ size   Decreased adiposity   Increased lean
body mass

J. Perkins
MS, MFA

REVIEW QUESTIONS

A. Regulation of blood hormone levels typically occurs through _____ feedback systems.

B. What hormone inhibits both GHRH and GH?

C. What type of negative feedback loop is illustrated by the inhibition of GHRH by IGF?

D. What type of negative feedback loop is illustrated by the inhibition of GHRH by GH?

TH has biologic actions in every organ in the body and are critical to proper fetal, postnatal, and pubertal growth and development. Because TH is important in regulating basal metabolic rate, thyroid excess and deficiency in adults affect a wide range of physiologic processes and can produce or contribute to various diseases.

The **thyroid gland** is a shield-shaped gland located on the anterior side of the **trachea.** As illustrated in Plate 7.4, the gland is composed of right and left lobes and an isthmus. As with all endocrine glands it is **highly vascularized** to supply nutrients for hormone synthesis and blood flow for hormone transport. The functional units of the gland are the **follicular cells,** which synthesize and store the TH, which is synthesized in two forms, T_4 and T_3. The synthesis of TH is under the control of pituitary **TSH** (Plate 7.2), which is under negative feedback control by the TH (Plate 7.5).

Clinical Note

The term "goiter" refers to an enlarged thyroid gland, which can visibly expand the front of the neck by centimeters. Goiters are slow growing and can take years to develop. They can occur in both hypothyroid (e.g., iodine deficiency) and hyperthyroid (e.g., TSH-secreting tumor) conditions. In each case, the elevation in TSH stimulates growth of the thyroid gland.

REVIEW ANSWERS

A. Anterior

B. Follicular

C. Thyroxine (T_4) and triiodothyronine (T_3)

D. Thyroid-stimulating hormone (TSH)

Plate 7.4   **Endocrine Physiology**

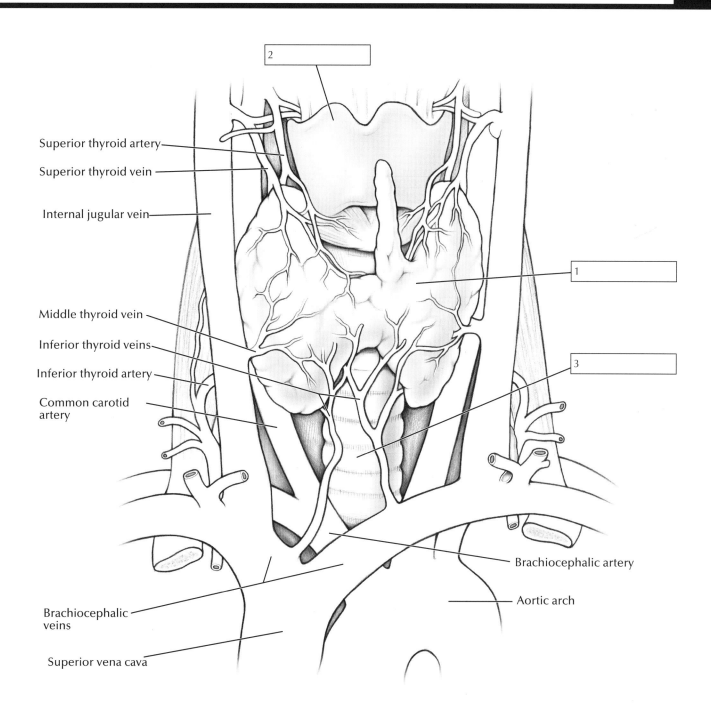

Superior thyroid artery

Superior thyroid vein

Internal jugular vein

Middle thyroid vein

Inferior thyroid veins

Inferior thyroid artery

Common carotid artery

Brachiocephalic veins

Superior vena cava

Brachiocephalic artery

Aortic arch

REVIEW QUESTIONS

A.   The thyroid gland is located on the (anterior or posterior) side of the trachea.

B.   The functional units of the gland are the _____ cells.

C.   What forms of thyroid hormone are secreted into the blood?

D.   What pituitary hormone stimulates the production and secretion of TH?

The thyroid gland synthesizes two main forms of TH, T_3 and T_4 (see Plate 7.4). About 20 times more T_4 is produced than T_3, but T_4 is less potent and is converted to T_3 by target cells before acting. **Pituitary TSH** regulates the synthesis and release of the TH, and as noted in the upper diagram of Plate 7.5, secreted T_3 and T_4 (after conversion to T_3) feed back to suppress TSH and TRH secretion by the pituitary and hypothalamus, respectively.

Binding of TSH to its receptors on the thyroid gland stimulates cAMP, which acts at each step in TH synthesis within the follicular cells (numbers shown on Plate 7.5):

1. **Thyroglobulin (Tg) molecules** are produced in the endoplasmic reticulum, packaged in vesicles by the Golgi apparatus, and exocytosed into the lumen of the follicle.
2. **Iodide (I^-)** enters the follicular cell via basolateral Na^+-I^- cotransporters, the **I^--trap.** The iodide exits the cell into the follicular lumen via I^-/Cl^- antiporters.
3. In the follicular lumen, I^- is oxidized to iodine by **thyroid peroxidase,** and the iodine attaches to the tyrosine residues of Tg.
4. Binding of one iodine will form **monoiodotyrosine (MIT)** and binding of two iodine moieties will form **diiodotyrosine (DIT).** This reaction is termed **organification.** Thyroid peroxidase also catalyzes the binding of DIT to another DIT, forming **T4.** Some DIT will also bind to MIT, forming **T3.** These products remain linked to the Tg.
5. The mature Tg containing MIT, DIT, T_4, and T_3 is endocytosed back into the follicular cell and can be stored as colloid (for several weeks) until it is secreted.
6. **Proteolysis** of the **colloid** (Tg) is stimulated by TSH and releases the constituent molecules. MIT and DIT reenter the synthetic pool, and T_3 and T_4 exit via the basolateral membrane into the blood.

In the blood, most of the T_3 and T_4 is bound to proteins, including albumin and **thyroxine-binding globulin.** The thyroxine-binding protein acts as a plasma reservoir for T_4, because T_4 is only active when it is released from the plasma proteins, enters the target cells, and undergoes **deiodination** to T_3. There is a high affinity for binding proteins to T_3 and T_4, leaving little "free" circulating T_3 and T_4, but the **free hormone** is the physiologically and clinically relevant fraction.

REVIEW ANSWERS

A. Iodine

B. Na^+- I^- cotransporter (the I^- trap)

C. MIT, monoiodotyrosine

D. DIT, diiodotyrosine

E. T_3, triiodothyronine

F. T_4, thyroxine

LABEL the important steps in TH synthesis:

☐ 1. Thyroglobulin (Tg) molecules, produced in the endoplasmic reticulum, are exocytosed into the lumen of the follicle

☐ 2. Basolateral I^- trap, transporting iodide into the follicular cell (I^- is then transported into the lumen of the follicle)

☐ 3. Thyroid peroxidase oxidizes iodide to iodine

☐ 4. Organification, whereby binding of one iodine to tyrosine on Tg forms MIT, and binding of two iodine molecules forms DIT; formation of T_3 (MIT + DIT) and T_4 (DIT + DIT)

☐ 5. Endocytosis of mature Tg into cell for storage

☐ 6. Proteolysis of Tg is stimulated by TSH, releasing T_3 and T_4 into the blood; MIT and DIT are recycled

LABEL

☐ 7. Pituitary TSH

☐ 8. Hypothalamic TRH

TRACE

☐ 9. Secretion of T_3 and T_4 into the blood, and their feedback path to inhibit pituitary TSH and hypothalamic TRH

Plate 7.5

Endocrine Physiology

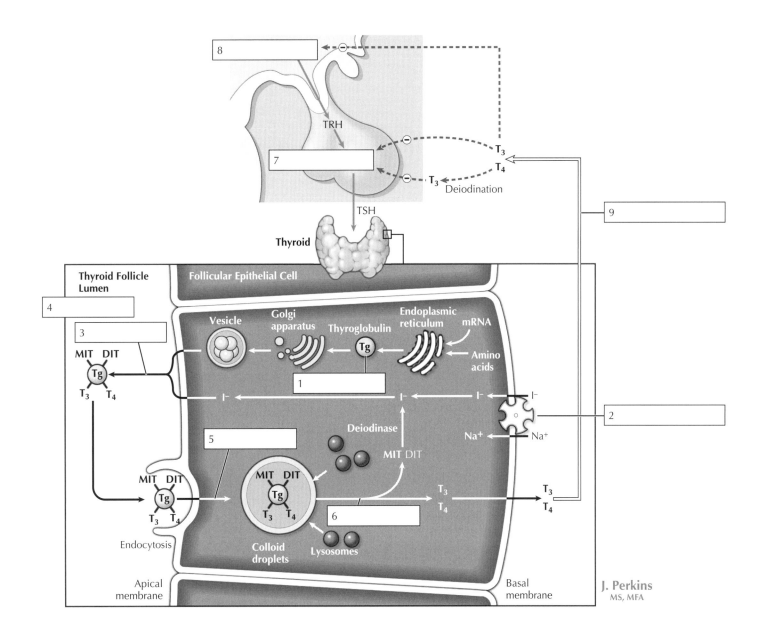

TRH

8 ⊖

7

⊖ T₃
T₄

⊖ T₃
Deiodination

TSH

9

Thyroid

Thyroid Follicle Lumen

Follicular Epithelial Cell

4

3

MIT DIT
Tg
T₃   T₄

Vesicle   **Golgi apparatus**   **Thyroglobulin**   **Endoplasmic reticulum**   mRNA

Tg

Amino acids

1

I⁻ ← I⁻ ← I⁻ ← I⁻

Na⁺ ← Na⁺

2

5

Deiodinase
MIT DIT

MIT DIT
Tg
T₃ T₄

MIT DIT
Tg
T₃ T₄

6

T₃
T₄

T₃
T₄

Endocytosis

Colloid droplets   **Lysosomes**

Apical membrane

Basal membrane

J. Perkins
MS, MFA

REVIEW QUESTIONS

A. Mature thyroglobulin is rich in _____.

B. Iodide (I⁻) enters the follicular cell through the _____ cotransporter.

C. Binding of one iodine molecule to a tyrosine residue on Tg will form _____.

D. Binding of two iodine molecules to a tyrosine residue on Tg will form _____.

E. Which form of TH is more biologically active?

F. Which form of TH is produced in greater quantities?

Circulating free T_3 and T_4 enter target cells through facilitated diffusion, and within the cells, the T_4 is deiodinated to T_3 by **5′-deiodinase**, and the T_3 then binds to the **nuclear TH receptor.** This forms a complex with the **TH response element** and stimulates gene transcription (top panel of Plate 7.6). The TH response elements are found in a variety of genes, including the GH receptor gene, cardiac and sarcoplasmic reticulum Ca^{2+} ATPase genes, and genes that encode Na^+/K^+ ATPase subunits. Thus TH can control diverse functions.

In general, low to normal levels of TH have anabolic effects and lead to synthesis of other hormones, and high levels of TH have catabolic effects, causing breakdown of proteins and hormones.

TH affects virtually all systems, typically **increasing metabolism** and **growth processes.** Within cells, TH increases production of proteins, as well as other hormones, increases Na^+/K^+ ATPase and other enzymes, and increases the number of mitochondria, elevating O_2 consumption. These actions of TH are seen in the following structures and systems:

- **Bones and tissues,** contributing to normal growth and development and bone cell proliferation
- **Brain and nervous system,** contributing to normal growth and development
- **Lungs,** increasing ventilation
- **Heart,** increasing cardiac output
- **Kidneys,** increasing renal function
- **Metabolism,** stimulating food intake; increasing lipolysis in adipose cells, thus releasing free fatty acids into circulation and decreasing adipose tissue; decreasing muscle mass; increasing body temperature

Because TH has major effects on metabolism and growth, disruptions in its normal rate and process of secretion can have dramatic consequences.

COLOR

- ☐ 1. Arrows from the T_3 and T_4 in the blood, into the cell, noting the deiodination of T_4 before binding to the nuclear receptor
- ☐ 2. Bones and tissues, where TH contributes to normal growth and development and bone cell proliferation
- ☐ 3. Brain and nervous system, where TH contributes to normal growth and development
- ☐ 4. Lungs, increasing ventilation (arrows indicate the effects of TH)
- ☐ 5. Heart, increasing cardiac output (arrows indicate the effects of TH)
- ☐ 6. Kidneys, increasing renal function (arrows indicate the effects of TH)

Clinical Note

Hypothyroidism, or low production of TH, can result from dietary iodine deficiency, as well as **Hashimoto thyroiditis.** The latter is an autoimmune disease in which antibodies to Tg or thyroid peroxidase reduce TH synthesis and secretion and eventually destroy the gland. Untreated hypothyroidism in children can result in **cretinism,** which is associated with stunted growth, mental retardation, impaired motor neuron function, and constipation. In adults, hypothyroidism results in **myxedema,** which is associated with fat deposition, nonpitting edema, cold intolerance, constipation, hypotension, fatigue, and depression. In each case the low circulating TH level results in high levels of circulating TSH. Hypothyroidism is treated with synthetic T_4. **Hyperthyroidism,** or elevated levels of TH, can result from **Graves disease,** an autoimmune disease that produces **thyroid-stimulating antibodies,** which bind to the TSH receptors on the thyroid gland, producing the same biologic actions as TSH. The elevated TH feeds back to suppress endogenous TSH, but the antibodies continue to stimulate TH secretion. Thus Graves disease is characterized by elevated TH but reduced TSH. **Exophthalmus** (protruding eyes) can be a symptom of Graves disease and is caused by deposition of glycoproteins and water behind the eyes. Drugs such as methimazole can be used to suppress TH synthesis and secretion; if poorly controlled by drugs, ablation of the thyroid by radioactive iodine or thyroidectomy can be performed, followed by T_4 replacement.

REVIEW ANSWERS

- **A.** Triiodothyronine, T_3
- **B.** Nuclear
- **C.** 5′-Deiodinase
- **D.** Metabolism, growth

Plate 7.6 **Endocrine Physiology**

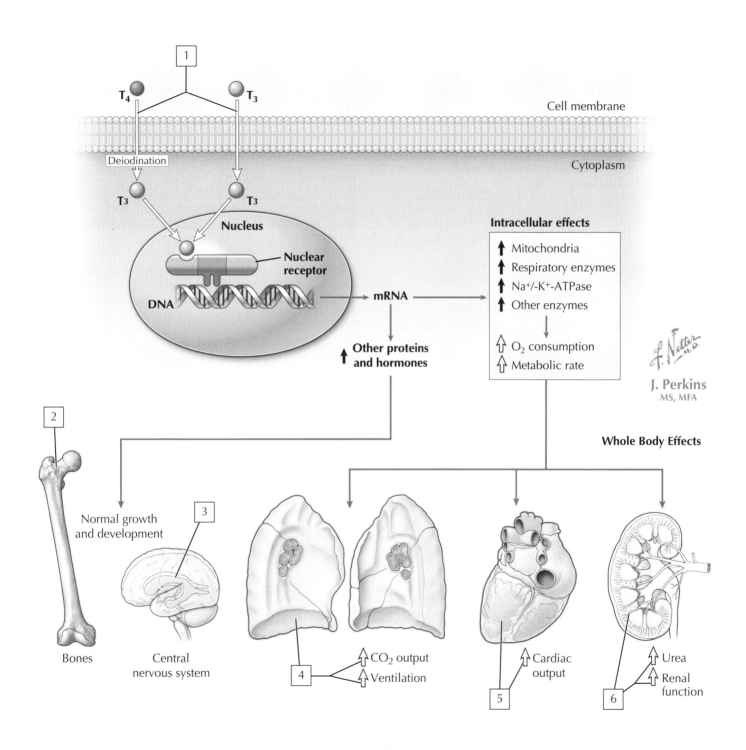

T₄ T₃

Cell membrane

Deiodination

Cytoplasm

T₃ T₃

Nucleus

Nuclear receptor

DNA

mRNA

Intracellular effects

↑ Mitochondria
↑ Respiratory enzymes
↑ Na⁺/-K⁺-ATPase
↑ Other enzymes

⇧ O_2 consumption
⇧ Metabolic rate

J. Netter
M.D.

J. Perkins
MS, MFA

↑ Other proteins and hormones

Whole Body Effects

Normal growth and development

Bones Central nervous system

⇧ CO_2 output
⇧ Ventilation

⇧ Cardiac output

⇧ Urea
⇧ Renal function

A. The active form of thyroid hormone is _____.

B. TH binds to a _____ receptor in the cell.

C. When thyroxine enters the cell, it is deiodinated by _____.

D. In general, TH affects _____ and _____ in almost all cells.

The paired **adrenal glands** are located above the kidneys in the retroperitoneal space. They consist of an outer cortex and inner medulla, which produce steroid hormones and catecholamines, respectively (the medulla acts functionally as part of the sympathetic nervous system, releasing catecholamines into the bloodstream during sympathetic nervous system stimulation). The adrenal cortex consists of three histological layers:

- The outer **zona glomerulosa,** which produces the mineralocorticoid hormone **aldosterone**
- The middle **zona fasciculata,** which synthesizes the glucocorticoid hormone **cortisol**
- The inner **zona reticularis,** which synthesizes androgens, mainly **dehydroepiandrosterone (DHEA)** and **androstenedione**

The biosynthetic pathways for adrenal steroids are illustrated. All of the steroid products are synthesized from **cholesterol,** derived either from dietary sources or synthesized de novo. Although the specific pathways for synthesis of the various adrenal steroids are illustrated here together, the main products differ between zones. For example, the enzymatic pathway in the zona glomerulosa favors synthesis of the mineralocorticoid aldosterone, whereas specific enzymes that synthesize cortisol are found in the zona fasciculata (see bulleted list above).

In Plate 7.7, note the regulation of steroid synthesis in the adrenal by the hypothalamic-pituitary-adrenal (HPA) axis. This axis is affected by various physiologic states, including **stress** (which activates this axis) and **sleep/wake cycles.** The paraventricular nucleus of the hypothalamus produces the 41–amino acid peptide hormone **corticotropin-releasing hormone (CRH),** which is carried by the hypothalamic-hypophyseal portal system to the anterior pituitary, where it stimulates **corticotrophs** to synthesize and release **ACTH.** ACTH stimulates the conversion of cholesterol to **pregnenolone** in the adrenal cortex. The increase in pregnenolone results in more cortisol synthesis in the zona fasciculata and more androgen synthesis in the zona reticularis (although other factors also affect androgen production). In the zona glomerulosa, ACTH has a **permissive effect** on aldosterone production; although ACTH is necessary for aldosterone synthesis, the synthesis is under primary control by other factors.

Thus the **predominant effect of HPA axis** activation is synthesis and release of **cortisol.** Of note, under the control of CRH, ACTH is released in a pulsatile fashion, with peak secretion in the morning before awakening. Stress of various types (e.g., hyperglycemia, heavy exercise, pain, trauma, and infection) has a major role in activation of the axis, with release of cortisol. Negative feedback of the HPA axis occurs via long-loop feedback by cortisol on the pituitary and hypothalamus and short-loop feedback by ACTH on CRH release.

TRACE the arrows in the HPA pathway, from stimulation of CRH to pregnenolone synthesis, noting that factors stimulating CRH include:

☐ 1. Sleep/wake cycle
☐ 2. Anxiety
☐ 3. Stress

TRACE the arrows in the negative feedback pathways in the HPA axis (red):

☐ 4. From ACTH to the hypothalamus and from cortisol to both the hypothalamus and the anterior pituitary

TRACE the pathways from pregnenolone that lead to synthesis of:

☐ 5. Aldosterone
☐ 6. Androgens (DHEA and androstenedione)
☐ 7. Cortisol

REVIEW ANSWERS

A. Cortisol

B. DHEA (dehydroepiandrosterone), androstenedione

C. Pregnenolone

D. Cortisol

Plate 7.7　　　　　　　　　　　　　　　　　　**Endocrine Physiology**

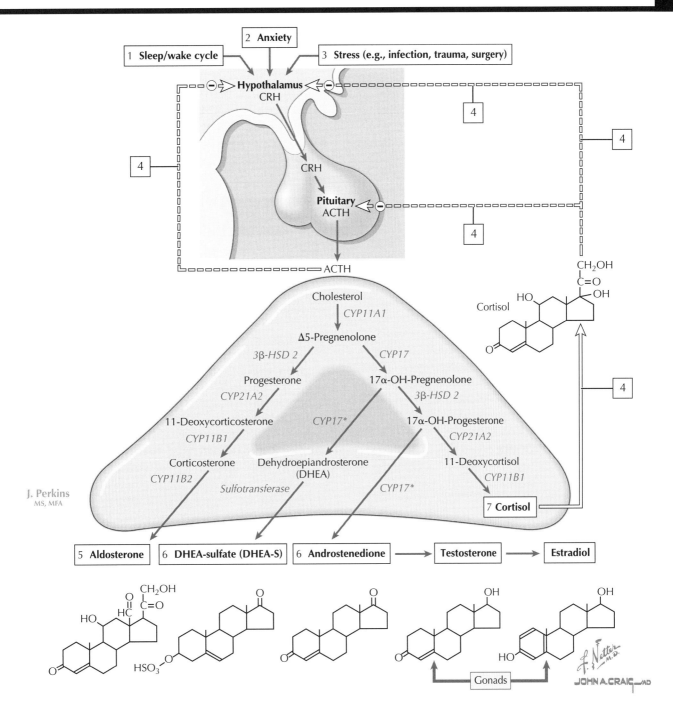

REVIEW QUESTIONS

A. ACTH release by the anterior pituitary has the predominant effect of stimulating synthesis of the steroid _____ .

B. The zona reticularis produces the male sex hormones _____ and _____.

C. ACTH action on the adrenal cortex results in the conversion of cholesterol to _____, the common precursor in the synthesis of mineralocorticoids, glucocorticoids, and androgens.

D. _____ produces negative feedback on both the pituitary release of ACTH and hypothalamic release of CRH.

Cortisol is secreted by the **zona fasciculata** of the adrenal cortex in response to HPA axis activation (see Plate 7.7). As a steroid hormone, it is lipid soluble and diffuses through cell membranes, binding to specific cytoplasmic receptors in target cells. The receptor-steroid complex enters the cell nucleus and affects the transcription of specific genes. Cortisol is called a **glucocorticoid** because of its action in raising blood glucose levels (**corticosterone,** another product of the steroid synthetic pathways, shares this effect). Cortisol has a wide range of other actions; in many cases, they are **permissive,** meaning that cortisol does not directly promote the action but is required for that effect to occur in response to another hormone. For example, cortisol stimulates the synthesis of hormones involved in **gluconeogenesis,** but that process is directly stimulated by other hormones such as **glucagon** and **epinephrine.**

The wide array of actions of cortisol can be loosely categorized as metabolic, immunosuppressive, and anti-inflammatory effects; at normal physiologic levels, the effects are mainly metabolic actions and permissive effects for the actions of other hormones. The immunosuppressive and anti-inflammatory effects are present when cortisol or another glucocorticoid is present in excess or used as a drug. The general metabolic effects are the following:

- **Stimulation of gluconeogenesis**
- **Catabolism of proteins**
- **Lipolysis**
- **Inhibition of insulin-stimulated glucose uptake** by muscle and adipose tissue (called a "diabetogenic effect," because plasma glucose will be elevated)

In Plate 7.8, the effects of excess cortisol secretion and effects of cortisol at **pharmacologic** levels are illustrated. Cortisol may be produced in excess during **chronic stress** or in **Cushing syndrome.** Pharmacologically, cortisol and related drugs can be useful in suppressing inflammatory and allergic reactions and treating asthma in some cases.

ACTH stimulates the **zona reticularis to synthesize** adrenal androgens (see Plate 7.7), although other factors are involved in this stimulation. The androgens **DHEA** and **androstenedione** contribute to pubertal changes in boys and girls but have a more important role in this regard in females, because they are the only normal significant source of androgen. Effects of the adrenal androgens in females include development of pubic hair, hypertrophy of sebaceous glands (producing acne), and stimulation of libido.

TRACE the arrows (different colors) to indicate effects that are:

☐ 1. Anti-inflammatory

☐ 2. Antiallergic/anti-immune

☐ 3. Metabolic

Clinical Note

Cushing syndrome is a disorder associated with prolonged exposure to excess cortisol (hypercortisolism) or other glucocorticoids. It can be caused by excess secretion of ACTH by the anterior pituitary (in **Cushing disease**), an ectopic ACTH-secreting tumor, an adenoma or carcinoma of the adrenal cortex producing excess cortisol, or exposure to exogenous glucocorticoids. Regardless of the etiology, clinical findings in hypercortisolism may include the following:

- Rounded, "moon" face with red cheeks
- Fat deposition on neck and shoulders forming a "buffalo hump" and pendulous abdomen
- Thinning of arms and legs
- Thinning of skin with red striae
- Osteoporosis
- Hypokalemia and alkalosis
- Poor wound healing
- Hypertension

Diagnosis and treatment involve identification of the cause and treatment to reduce hypercortisolism.

REVIEW ANSWERS

A. Inflammatory and immunologic, allergic diseases

B. Resorption

C. Inhibits insulin stimulated glucose uptake by muscle and fat, thereby elevating plasma glucose

D. Dehydroepiandrosterone, androstenedione

Plate 7.8　　　　　　　　　　　　　　　　　　　　　**Endocrine Physiology**

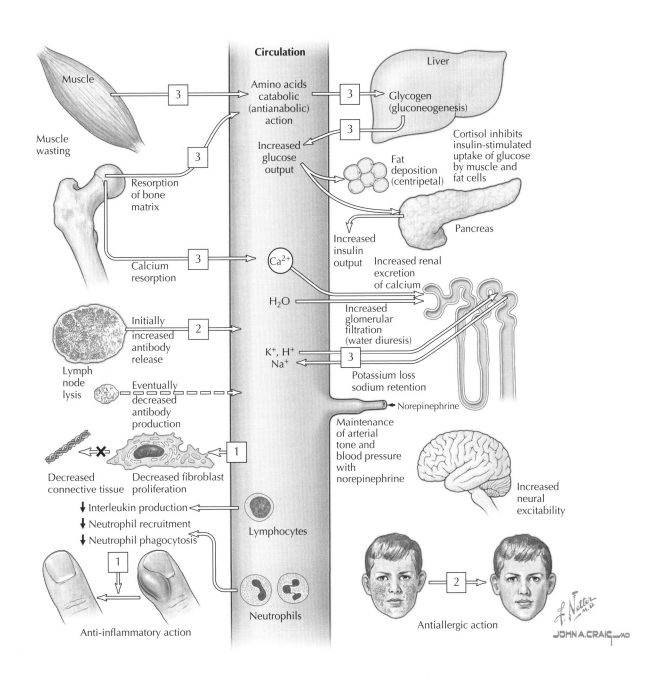

REVIEW QUESTIONS

A. Cortisol and synthetic glucocorticoids may be used as drugs to treat diseases in two categories, _____ and _____.

B. Excess cortisol may cause _____ of bone.

C. Cortisol is referred to as "diabetogenic" because it _____.

D. The two steroid hormones made by the adrenal cortex that promote development of pubertal secondary sexual characteristics, particularly in girls, are _____ and _____.

Aldosterone is an important regulator of extracellular fluid volume and K^+ homeostasis (Chapter 5). To summarize, aldosterone, by acting on the late distal tubules of the kidney, stimulates:

- Na^+ reabsorption and, consequently, water retention and expansion of extracellular fluid volume
- K^+ excretion
- H^+ excretion

Note that aldosterone also affects colonic handling of Na^+ and K^+ (Chapter 6).

ACTH stimulates the conversion of cholesterol to pregnenolone, the first step in the synthesis of steroid hormones (see Plate 7.7). Within the **zona glomerulosa,** the subsequent synthesis of aldosterone through the pathway is affected by these important factors:

- **Hyperkalemia** (elevated plasma K^+) increases aldosterone secretion, promoting renal K^+ excretion, thus reducing plasma K^+.
- **Angiotensin II** stimulates aldosterone secretion by the adrenal cortex. Stimuli for angiotensin II synthesis include reduced blood volume, and aldosterone raises extracellular fluid (and blood) volume by promoting Na^+ (and therefore water) retention.
- **Atrial natriuretic peptide (ANP)** is released by cardiac myocytes when blood volume is elevated. ANP inhibits adrenocortical aldosterone synthesis, thereby reducing blood volume, and has direct natriuretic and diuretic effects on the kidney.

The physiologic control of aldosterone secretion by these various factors is illustrated in Plate 7.9, along with the actions of aldosterone on the nephron, intestine (colon), and other tissues.

COLOR

- [ ] 1. Kidney, noting it secretes renin that stimulates aldosterone secretion
- [ ] 2. Heart, noting it secretes ANP that inhibits aldosterone secretion
- [ ] 3. Adrenal gland, the source of aldosterone

TRACE the arrows associated with:

- [ ] 4. Stimulation of aldosterone synthesis and secretion
- [ ] 5. Inhibition of aldosterone secretion
- [ ] 6. Actions of aldosterone in the colon and distal nephron to increase sodium (and water) reabsorption

Clinical Note

Addison disease is an uncommon endocrine disease in which the adrenal synthesis of steroids fails as a result of autoimmune disease, tubercular destruction of the gland, or rare genetic disorders. As is usually the case for endocrine disorders, many of the effects of deficiency of the hormones can be predicted based on the effects of those hormones in normal physiology. Thus, in Addison disease, signs and symptoms include the following:

- Poor stress tolerance
- Hypoglycemia
- Weight loss and fatigue
- Low blood pressure
- Salt appetite
- Hyperpigmentation of skin (resulting from ACTH excess and its effects on skin)

A severe deficiency of adrenal hormones will precipitate an **Addisonian crisis,** which must be treated as a medical emergency. Signs and symptoms include vomiting and diarrhea, low blood pressure, fainting, loss of consciousness, convulsions, and hypoglycemia. Patients with this disease require long-term replacement therapy with glucocorticoids and sometimes also mineralocorticoids.

REVIEW ANSWERS

A. Na^+, water

B. K^+ (and also H^+ in the nephron)

C. ANP

D. Angiotensin II

Plate 7.9   **Endocrine Physiology**

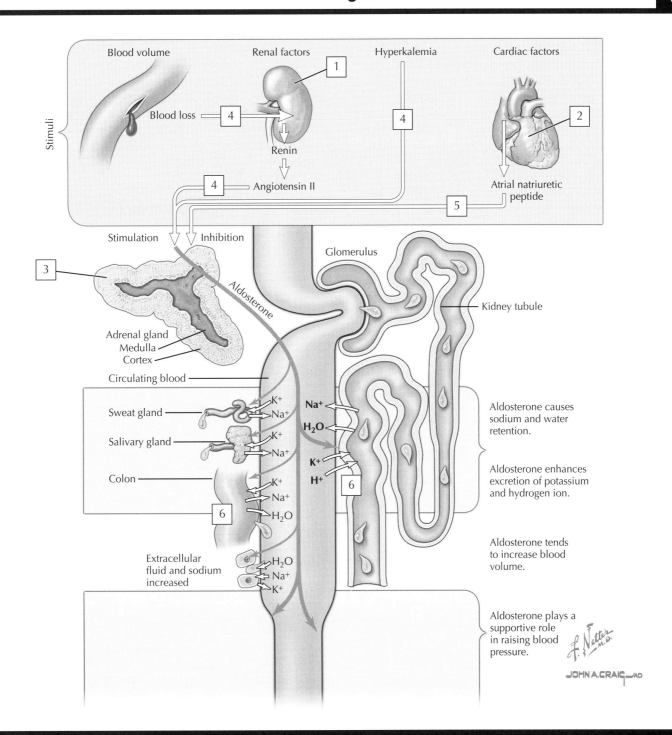

REVIEW QUESTIONS

A. Aldosterone acts at the colon and distal nephron to promote reabsorption or retention of _____ and
_____.

B. Aldosterone acts at the colon and nephron to promote excretion of _____.

C. Aldosterone synthesis and secretion by the zona glomerulosa of the adrenal cortex are inhibited by what peptide hormone produced by the heart?

D. Aldosterone synthesis and secretion by the adrenal cortex are stimulated by what peptide product of the renin-angiotensin-aldosterone system?

The primary role of the pancreatic hormones is to regulate glucose in the blood (fasting blood glucose is 70 to 90 mg%). When blood glucose levels rise during feeding, insulin release promotes entry of glucose into cells as well as glucose storage (the hypoglycemic effect of insulin). When blood glucose levels fall with fasting, glucagon mobilizes glucose by causing glucose synthesis (gluconeogenesis) and release from stores (the hyperglycemic effect of glucagon). The overall balance is achieved by the integration of glucose metabolic activity primarily within liver, muscle, and adipose tissues as well as regulation of glucose uptake by various tissues, which are orchestrated by the pancreatic hormones.

The endocrine portion of the pancreas consists of the **islets of Langerhans,** which contain three key cell types involved in glucose regulation:

- **α Cells** produce **glucagon,** which mobilizes glucose stores *into the blood*
- **β Cells** produce **insulin,** which stimulates glucose transport *into the cells*
- **δ Cells** produce **somatostatin,** which inhibits the secretion of both insulin and glucagon (to modulate responses)

As seen in Plate 7.10, there are many more insulin-producing β cells than α and δ cells.

Major control of blood glucose levels occurs through the production, secretion, and action of insulin, which is a 51–amino acid peptide hormone formed in the β cells from a prohormone. The prohormone contains the **A and B chains** (linked by disulfide bridges) of the active insulin molecule and a connecting **C-peptide** (Part C). The C-peptide is cleaved from the proinsulin to form active insulin, and the resulting insulin and C-peptide are packaged in **secretory granules** within the β cells.

When blood glucose levels increase, glucose enters the β cells through **GLUT2** (insulin-independent) transporters, which stimulates secretion of the insulin and C-peptide into the blood through a Ca^{2+}-dependent mechanism. In addition to a rise in blood glucose, insulin secretion is stimulated by **gut peptides** (e.g., GIP, see Plate 6.3), **increased amino acids and fatty acids in the blood,** and locally released **acetylcholine.** A common theme is that all of these elements reflect the fed state as a stimulus for insulin release.

COLOR and LABEL

☐ 1. Acini

☐ 2. Islet cells

☐ 3. α Cells

☐ 4. β Cells, noting the greater number of insulin-producing β cells in the islets than α cells or δ cells

☐ 5. δ Cells

☐ 6. A chain of the proinsulin molecule

☐ 7. B chain of the proinsulin molecule, noting that the C-peptide is cleaved to produce the active insulin

Clinical Note

Because both insulin and C-peptide fragments are secreted when the granule contents are released from the β cells, the amount of C-peptide in the blood is a reflection of insulin production. This is used clinically to determine the level of endogenous insulin secretion in patients with diabetes who receive insulin injections.

REVIEW ANSWERS

A. α, β, δ cells

B. A, B, C-peptide

C. C-peptide

D. Insulin, C-peptide

Plate 7.10   **Endocrine Physiology**

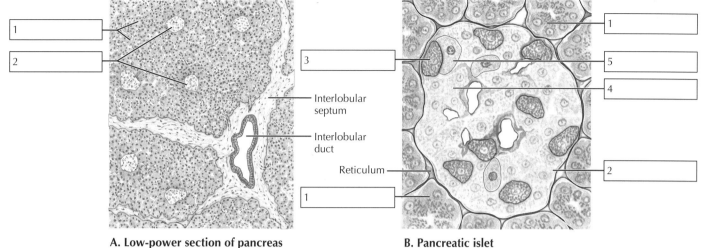

1

2

3

Interlobular
septum

Interlobular
duct

Reticulum

1

A. Low-power section of pancreas

1

5

4

2

B. Pancreatic islet

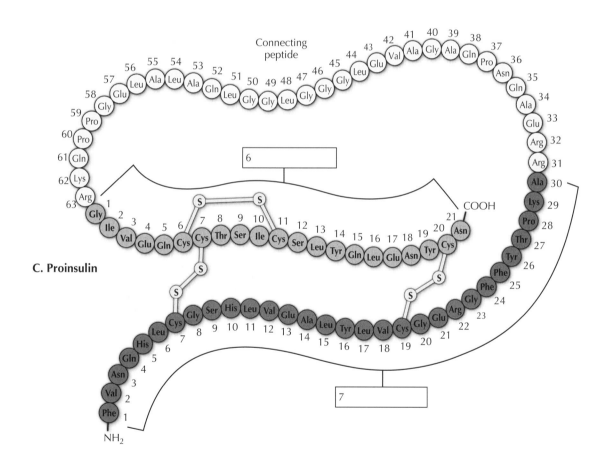

Connecting
peptide

C. Proinsulin

6

7

COOH

NH₂

A. The major endocrine cell types in the islets of Langerhans are _____, _____, and _____.

B. The proinsulin molecule is composed of the ____ chain, ____ chain, and _____.

C. The active insulin molecule is made by cleaving proinsulin to remove the _____.

D. Secretory granules in the β cells contain both _____ and _____.

Endocrine Pancreas: Actions of Insulin

Insulin is considered a **"fuel storage" hormone** and, overall, insulin promotes **entry of glucose into cells, synthesis of glycogen stores,** and **reduced lipolysis,** ensuring that nutrients are stored and thus available to tissues between meals. The insulin receptor is expressed on most tissues, but **liver, muscle,** and **adipose tissue** are major target tissues. When insulin binds to its receptor, it causes **hypoglycemic effects** by the following actions:

- **Increasing GLUT4** transporters (insulin-dependent) in membranes, allowing efficient glucose entry into cells
- **Increasing glycogen** synthesis from excess glucose for storage
- **Inhibiting glycogenolysis** and thus the release of glucose from glycogen stores
- **Inhibiting hepatic gluconeogenesis** (synthesis of new glucose from noncarbohydrate molecules)

All of these factors contribute to the rapid reduction of the blood glucose concentration when insulin is released by the pancreas. Insulin also affects lipid metabolism by **inhibiting hormone-sensitive lipase** in adipose tissue (reducing circulating free fatty acids) and **inhibiting oxidation of fatty acids.**

COLOR and **LABEL** the organs listed below, noting the mechanisms whereby insulin promotes "fuel storage" in these tissues:

- ☐ 1. Muscle
- ☐ 2. Liver
- ☐ 3. Adipose tissue

Clinical Note

Diabetes mellitus is a disease of impaired insulin function that results in hyperglycemia. **Type 1 diabetes** is insulin-dependent diabetes, which is caused by the **progressive destruction of the pancreatic β cells** by autoimmune attack, eventually resulting in minimal insulin secretion and hyperglycemia. This usually occurs before 20 years of age. The condition needs careful monitoring and is treated by insulin injections throughout life. **Type 2 diabetes,** or non-insulin-dependent diabetes, is a form of insulin resistance that results from a **reduction in insulin receptors** on target tissues. This type of diabetes has a hereditary component, which can be exacerbated by obesity. Although insulin and drugs that increase its secretion (sulfonylureas and meglitinides) or the sensitivity of tissues to insulin (thiazolidinediones) are used to treat non-insulin-dependent diabetes, reduction in weight and increased exercise can also help control the hyperglycemia.

Uncontrolled hyperglycemia can result in polyuria (caused by the osmotic effect of glucose in the nephron), polydipsia (to compensate for the urinary fluid losses), polyphagia (because glucose has difficulty entering tissues, hunger is stimulated), and metabolic acidosis (from keto acids). Long-term uncontrolled or poorly controlled diabetes is associated with retinopathy and blindness, nephropathy and renal failure, hypertension and cardiovascular disease, cerebrovascular disease, and peripheral vascular disease.

REVIEW ANSWERS

A. Entry, synthesis, reduced

B. Hypoglycemic effect

C. GLUT4 (an insulin-dependent transporter)

D. Inhibits hormone-sensitive lipase in adipose tissue and oxidation of fatty acids

---

Plate 7.11　　　　　　　　　　　　　　　　　　　　**Endocrine Physiology**

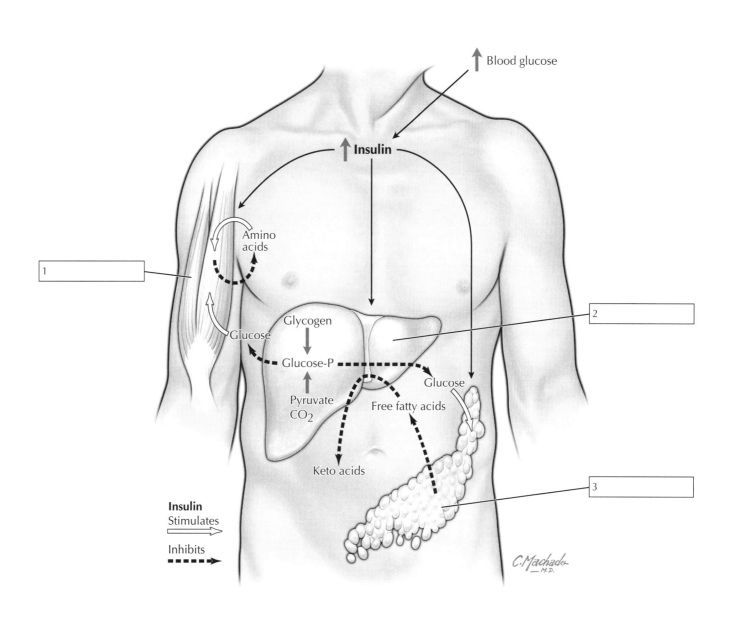

Blood glucose

Insulin

Amino acids

1

Glucose

Glycogen

Glucose-P

2

Pyruvate CO₂

Glucose

Free fatty acids

Keto acids

3

Insulin
Stimulates

Inhibits

C. Machado
— M.D.

REVIEW QUESTIONS

A. Insulin promotes _____ of glucose into cells, _____ of glycogen stores, and _____ lipolysis.

B. Binding of insulin to its receptor has what effect on blood glucose levels?

C. Insulin increases what type of glucose transporters?

D. What effect does insulin have on lipid metabolism?

Glucagon is a 29–amino acid peptide hormone produced in the α cells and is secreted primarily in response to **low blood glucose levels.** Its secretion is inhibited by high levels of glucose and fatty acids in the blood. In opposition to insulin, glucagon promotes the use of **cellular energy stores** through the release of glucose into the blood. Glucagon affects the activity of various enzymes that contribute to its hyperglycemic effect, mainly in the liver:

- **Inhibiting hepatic glycolysis**
- **Increasing hepatic gluconeogenesis**
- **Increasing glycogenolysis,** thus breaking down glycogen stores and causing release of glucose into the blood

Through these effects, glucagon produces a rapid increase in blood glucose levels. In addition, glucagon increases β-oxidation of fatty acids. In normal fasting between meals, a balance exists between the mobilization of glucose by glucagon and the replenishment of cellular glucose by insulin. However, with prolonged fasting the glucagon effect predominates, and after depletion of glycogen stores, rates of gluconeogenesis and fatty acid oxidation are high, the latter producing ketone bodies that contribute to the acid load of the body (see Plate 5.19).

Somatostatin is a 14–amino acid peptide produced in the δ cells, which acts in a **paracrine** manner on the islets to suppress *both* insulin and glucagon. This adds one more level of control in the modulation of blood glucose levels.

COLOR and LABEL

☐ 1. Muscle
☐ 2. Liver
☐ 3. Adipose tissue

TRACE

☐ 4. Arrows indicating the "fuel mobilization" actions of glucagon to break down glycogen, proteins, and lipids, thus releasing glucose, amino acids, fatty acids, and keto acids into the blood to serve the metabolic demand

REVIEW ANSWERS

A. α

B. Low

C. Stimulates

D. Somatostatin

Plate 7.12

Endocrine Physiology

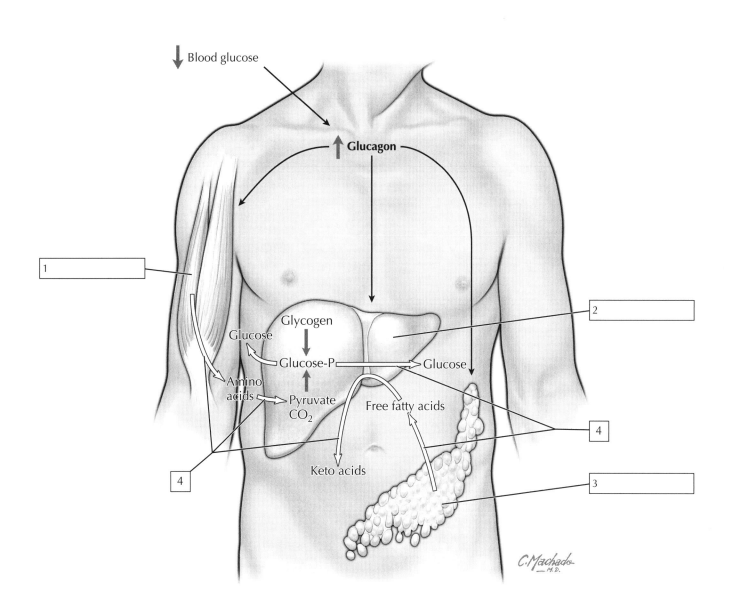

Blood glucose

Glucagon

1

2

Glycogen

Glucose

Glucose-P

Glucose

Amino acids

Pyruvate
CO_2

Free fatty acids

Keto acids

4

4

3

C. Machado
_M.D._

REVIEW QUESTIONS

A. Glucagon is synthesized in the _____ cells of the pancreatic islets.

B. Glucagon is released in response to _____ blood glucose levels.

C. Binding of glucagon to its receptor _____ glycogenolysis.

D. The hormone _____ suppresses both insulin and glucagon secretion.

Calcium in the blood exists as free Ca^{2+} (60%) and protein-bound calcium (40%). Free calcium ion concentration in blood is tightly controlled at approximately 9 mg/dL. This control reflects the importance of Ca^{2+} to a wide array of processes, including muscle contraction, bone mineralization, nerve impulse transmission, and cell secretory processes, with aberrations in plasma levels (hyper- or hypocalcemia) having potentially severe consequences.

The **major sites of calcium regulation** are intestines, kidneys, and bone. The typical adult ingests ~1000 mg of calcium daily and absorbs about one-fourth of this calcium. Intestinal Ca^{2+} absorption is facilitated by the **active form of vitamin D, 1,25-dihydroxycholecalciferol,** also called **calcitriol.** Intestinal absorption of calcium is balanced mainly by renal excretion to maintain homeostasis (losses from sweat and other pathways are minor). In the kidney, 98% of filtered Ca^{2+} is reabsorbed, in part because of the action of **parathyroid hormone (PTH).** Around 99% of body calcium is stored in bone, with significant unmineralized Ca^{2+} stored in the **osteoid** portion of bone. Ca^{2+} in osteoid is available for use in bone mineralization and can also re-enter the plasma. Much of the acute regulation of plasma Ca^{2+} is accomplished by the actions of PTH, which stimulates bone resorption, adding Ca^{2+} to plasma. Active vitamin D is necessary for the continual process of bone remodeling; it increases availability of calcium for deposition in bone and, at the same time, it increases the number of osteoclasts, which resorb bone.

The actions of PTH and the active form of vitamin D are illustrated. PTH is the most important hormone in the regulation of plasma Ca^{2+}. Synthesized by the **chief cells** of the parathyroid gland, the peptide is released at an elevated rate when plasma Ca^{2+} falls. It acts at the bone and kidney to raise plasma Ca^{2+}:

- At the kidney, it increases distal tubule Ca^{2+} reabsorption while inhibiting phosphate reabsorption and, as a result, rapidly restores plasma Ca^{2+}.
- At the kidney, PTH also stimulates formation of the active form of vitamin D (1,25-dihydroxycholecalciferol, or calcitriol).
- At the bone, PTH increases bone resorption through **osteocytic osteolysis,** resulting in release of Ca^{2+} into the bloodstream.

Prolonged elevation of PTH produces proliferation of osteoclasts as well, further demineralizing and breaking down bone. Overall, PTH produces bone demineralization and release of Ca^{2+} and phosphate into plasma. Plasma Ca^{2+} will be elevated, but plasma phosphate is somewhat reduced because of increased renal excretion.

Vitamin D (cholecalciferol) is structurally a modified steroid that functions as a hormone; it is synthesized from a precursor molecule in the skin in response to ultraviolet light in sunlight or is ingested in the diet. It is converted to 25-hydroxycholecalciferol in the liver and subsequently to 1,25-dihydroycholecalciferol in the kidneys. This active form of vitamin D is carried in the blood bound to plasma proteins. When plasma Ca^{2+} falls, PTH rises and stimulates formation of active vitamin D by the kidney. Active vitamin D increases intestinal Ca^{2+} absorption (see Plate 6.17). It also promotes bone remodeling by increasing the number of osteoclasts and is necessary for proper balance between bone mineralization and resorption.

Calcitonin, a peptide hormone produced by parafollicular cells of the thyroid, is released when plasma Ca^{2+} is elevated. Although it increases phosphate and Ca^{2+} excretion by the kidney and reduces bone resorption by reducing osteoclastic activity in animals, its physiologic relevance in humans is not clear.

TRACE the arrows using different colors:

1. ☐ Pathways for production of active vitamin D_3 (1,25-dihydrocholecalciferol)
2. ☐ Pathways for the actions of 1,25-dihydroxycholecalciferol
3. ☐ Pathways for actions of PTH
4. ☐ Stimulatory actions of low plasma Ca^{2+} levels (as illustrated in the center of the diagram) on PTH release and active vitamin D_3 synthesis in the kidneys
5. ☐ Inhibitory actions of high plasma Ca^{2+} levels on PTH and active vitamin D_3 synthesis, and inhibitory effect of high phosphate level on active vitamin D synthesis (as illustrated in the center of the diagram)

REVIEW ANSWERS

A. 1,25-Dihydrocholecalciferol (calcitriol)

B. Ca^{2+}, phosphate

C. Hydroxylation of 25-hydroxycholecalciferol to form 1,25-dihydroxycholecalciferol

D. Osteocytic osteolysis

E. Osteoclasts

Clinical Note

Osteoporosis, a disease characterized by loss of density and increased fragility of bone, is the most common cause of fractures in elderly people. Measures for prevention and treatment include regular exercise, adequate calcium intake, supplementation of vitamin D, and various medications. Postmenopausal women are more susceptible to osteoporosis because of low estrogen levels; other endocrine states associated with osteoporosis include hyperthyroidism and hyperparathyroidism.

Plate 7.13

Endocrine Physiology

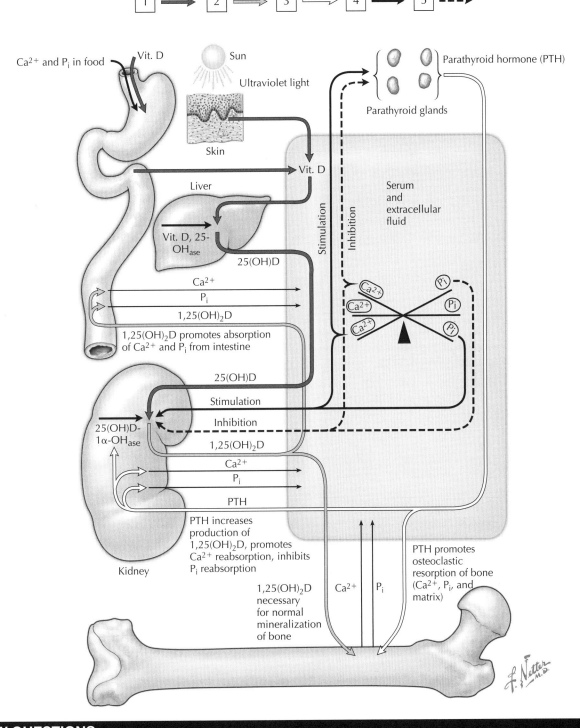

1 → 2 ⇒ 3 ⇒ 4 → 5 ---→

Ca^{2+} and P_i in food

Vit. D

Sun

Ultraviolet light

Skin

Vit. D

Liver

Vit. D, 25-OH_{ase}

25(OH)D

Ca^{2+}

P_i

1,25(OH)$_2$D

1,25(OH)$_2$D promotes absorption of Ca^{2+} and P_i from intestine

25(OH)D

Stimulation

Inhibition

25(OH)D-1α-OH_{ase}

1,25(OH)$_2$D

Ca^{2+}

P_i

PTH

PTH increases production of 1,25(OH)$_2$D, promotes Ca^{2+} reabsorption, inhibits P_i reabsorption

Kidney

Parathyroid hormone (PTH)

Parathyroid glands

Serum and extracellular fluid

Stimulation

Inhibition

Ca^{2+} P_i
Ca^{2+} P_i
Ca^{2+} P_i

1,25(OH)$_2$D necessary for normal mineralization of bone

Ca^{2+} P_i

PTH promotes osteoclastic resorption of bone (Ca^{2+}, P_i, and matrix)

REVIEW QUESTIONS

A. The active form of vitamin D is _____.

B. In the kidneys, PTH stimulates reabsorption of _____ and inhibits reabsorption of _____.

C. A third action of PTH at the kidney is stimulation of _____.

D. In the acute regulation of plasma Ca^{2+}, PTH increases bone resorption through the process of _____, resulting in release of Ca^{2+} into the bloodstream.

E. Prolonged elevation of PTH produces proliferation of _____, further demineralizing bone.

An individual's sex can be defined in terms of genetic sex (XX female genotype vs. XY male genotype), gonads (presence of testes vs. ovaries), and phenotype (external appearance of "femaleness" vs. "maleness"). After 5 weeks of fetal development, gonadal development begins as illustrated. In a male fetus, the undifferentiated gonads develop into testes under control of the Y chromosome **SRY gene** (full development of testes involves several other genes as well). Within 8 to 9 weeks of development, **Leydig cells** of the testes begin to secrete the male sex steroid **testosterone.** In the absence of the SRY gene and the Y chromosome and in the presence of two X chromosomes, **ovaries** begin development at week 9. Germ cells within the ovaries develop into **oogonia,** which proliferate and enter meiosis to become **primary oocytes.** Primary oocytes are then arrested in this stage until activated during sexual cycles after puberty. The developing ovary produces the female steroid hormone, **estrogen.**

Before the initiation of this gonadal development, two pairs of ducts develop in both sexes: the **wolffian (or mesonephric) ducts** and the **müllerian ducts.** The wolffian ducts develop into **male structures** under the control of testosterone (see Plate 7.14); meanwhile, the **Sertoli cells** of the fetal testes secrete the glycoprotein hormone **müllerian inhibitory factor,** which causes regression of the müllerian ducts. In the absence of testes and their hormones, the wolffian ducts regress and the müllerian ducts persist and form the **female structures** (Plate 7.14).

External genitalia are also undifferentiated early in development, until 9 to 10 weeks of gestation. In the absence of androgens, female genitalia develop. In males, testosterone secreted by the testes is converted to **dihydrotestosterone (DHT)** by the primitive genital structures, and DHT stimulates male genital development.

One or 2 years before onset of puberty, the adrenal **zona reticularis** begins to produce the androgens **DHEA** and **androstenedione** (see Plate 7.7), resulting in appearance of pubic and axillary hair, acne and oiliness of skin, and adult body odor. The actual onset of puberty is associated with maturation of the hypothalamus and anterior pituitary gland. Secretion of the decapeptide **GnRH** by the hypothalamus increases and becomes pulsatile in pattern, as the hypothalamus becomes less sensitive to negative feedback by sex steroids. As a result, pituitary secretion of the **gonadotropins (FSH and LH)** begins. These gonadotropins stimulate further gonadal maturation and sex steroid synthesis (estrogen and progesterone in women and testosterone in men). Control of the hypothalamic-pituitary-gonadal hormone systems is presented in Plate 7.15. The changes that occur physiologically and anatomically as a result of various hormone actions include the following:

- Gonadal maturation and sex steroid synthesis and release under the influence of gonadotropins
- Maturation of other sex organs and genitalia under the influence of mainly estradiol in females and testosterone in males
- Development of secondary sexual characteristics, including distribution of body and facial hair, breast development, and changes in body fat distribution, muscle development, and pitch of voice, under the influence of steroids (mainly estrogen in females and testosterone in males)
- The growth spurt, largely caused by estrogen, which eventually promotes closure of epiphyseal plates in bones and thus the end of the growth in height

COLOR

- [ ] 1. Wolffian bodies
- [ ] 2. Wolffian ducts
- [ ] 3. Müllerian ducts
- [ ] 4. Bladder
- [ ] 5. Urogenital sinus
- [ ] 6. Structures derived from the müllerian ducts (same color as 3)
- [ ] 7. Structures derived from the wolffian ducts (same color as 2)

REVIEW ANSWERS

A. SRY, Y

B. Testosterone, dihydrotestosterone

C. Müllerian ducts

D. Adrenal androgens (dehydroepiandrosterone and androstenedione)

Plate 7.14　　　　　　　　　　　　　　　　　　　　　　**Endocrine Physiology**

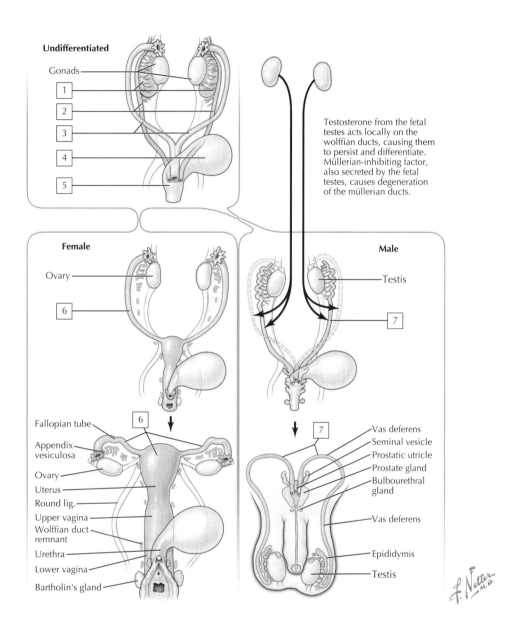

Undifferentiated

Gonads

1

2

3

4

5

Testosterone from the fetal testes acts locally on the wolffian ducts, causing them to persist and differentiate. Müllerian-inhibiting factor, also secreted by the fetal testes, causes degeneration of the müllerian ducts.

Female

Ovary

6

Male

Testis

7

Fallopian tube

6

Appendix vesiculosa

Ovary

Uterus

Round lig.

Upper vagina

Wolffian duct remnant

Urethra

Lower vagina

Bartholin's gland

7

Vas deferens
Seminal vesicle
Prostatic utricle
Prostate gland
Bulbourethral gland

Vas deferens

Epididymis

Testis

A. In the presence of the gene _____ on the _____ chromosome, undifferentiated gonads become testes.

B. Development of male genitalia is mainly due to the effects of the secretion of _____, which is converted to _____ before having this effect.

C. The fallopian tubes, ovaries, and uterus are formed from the _____.

D. Early development of secondary sexual characteristics such as appearance of pubic hair is caused by _____.

Late in puberty, girls experience **menarche,** the beginning of **menstrual cycles,** which continue until **menopause,** unless interrupted by pregnancy. The average cycle lasts 28 days and consists of three phases (Plate 7.15):

- The **follicular or proliferative phase** begins on the first day of menstruation, day 1 of the cycle. Menstruation typically lasts 3 to 5 days; meanwhile, several primordial follicles, under the influence of **FSH,** resume the maturation process that was halted in utero. **LH** stimulates **theca interna** cells in the developing follicles to synthesize **androgens,** which are converted by **granulosa cells** to **estradiol** under stimulation by FSH. Estradiol stimulates proliferation of the uterine **endometrium** (by this point, menses has finished), as well as growth of endometrial glands and spiral arteries, to support the possible implantation of a fertilized ovum in the uterine lining. Estradiol also promotes watery cervical mucus, which would allow entry of sperm into the uterus (and thus into the **fallopian tubes,** where fertilization occurs). Eventually, one of the developing follicles becomes a **mature follicle** or **graafian follicle.** During this phase, the hypothalamus-pituitary-gonadal axis is controlled by negative feedback (see Plate 7.16).
- Toward the end of the follicular phase, estradiol rises to a high level and triggers **positive feedback** on gonadotropin secretion, initiating the **ovulatory phase.** The positive feedback results in the large surge in LH and lesser increase in FSH, which stimulates ovulation at approximately midcycle, releasing the ovum. The ovum is swept by ciliary action into the fallopian tube. Ovulation occurs in only one ovary, alternating from month to month between the ovaries. If only one ovary is present, that ovary ovulates each month.
- During the **luteal phase,** the ruptured follicle involutes to form a **corpus luteum.** Theca interna cells become **theca lutein cells** and granulosa cells become **granulosa lutein cells;** the theca interna cells continue to produce **androgens** and the granulosa lutein cells produce **progesterone, inhibin,** and, to a lesser extent, estradiol. The endocrine axis now reverts to negative feedback control (see Plate 7.16). Secretory and

proliferative changes in the endometrium continue under the control of progesterone. Thus this phase is also called the **secretory phase.** Cervical secretions become thicker, making entry of sperm into the uterus more difficult. For conception, fertilization of the ovum must occur within a day or two from ovulation and usually takes place in the fallopian tube. Unless fertilization and implantation into the endometrium occur, eventually steroid and inhibin levels fall, menses commence, and the proliferated endometrium sloughs off. If implantation takes place, a **placenta** is formed from embryonic and placental cells, and secretion of **human chorionic gonadotropin** "rescues" the corpus luteum from the regression. With continued progesterone and estradiol secretion by the corpus luteum, the proliferated endometrium and pregnancy are supported. Further endocrine changes are required as the pregnancy progresses.

COLOR

- [ ] 1. Ova in the developing and mature follicles
- [ ] 2. Corpus luteum (yellow with a red center indicating rupture of the mature follicle resulted in hemorrhage)
- [ ] 3. Spiral arteries of the endometrium during the cycle (red)
- [ ] 4. Veins and venous lakes of the endometrium (blue)

TRACE the graphs illustrating hormone levels, noting how these hormones fluctuate in relation to the changes taking place in the ovary and endometrium:

- [ ] 5. LH
- [ ] 6. FSH
- [ ] 7. Progesterone
- [ ] 8. Estrogen
- [ ] 9. Inhibin

REVIEW ANSWERS

A. Progesterone

B. LH, FSH, ovulation

C. Luteal phase

D. Menarche

Plate 7.15 **Endocrine Physiology**

Menstrual Cycle

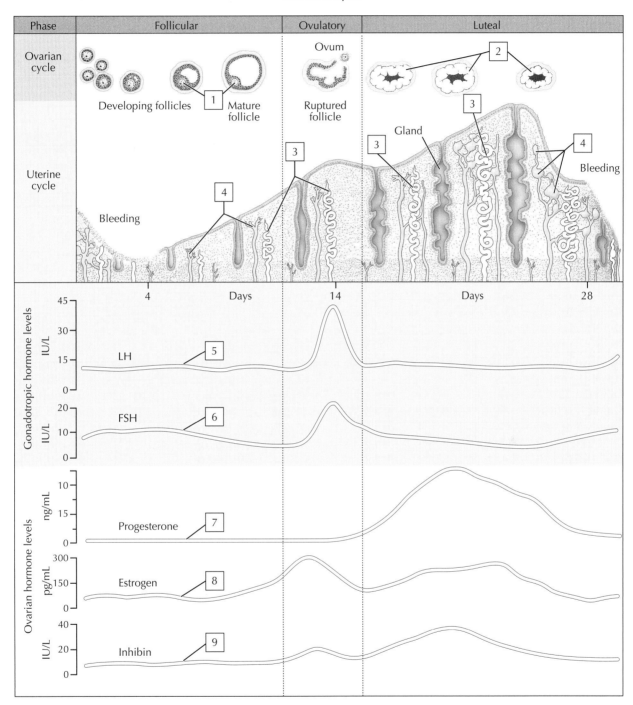

REVIEW QUESTIONS

A. Maintenance of the endometrium in the proliferated state is primarily the result of actions of _____.

B. Positive feedback by high levels of estradiol results in a surge in production of _____ and _____ and, consequently, _____ occurs.

C. The secretory phase of the menstrual cycle is synonymous with _____.

D. The time of life when a woman has her first menses is known as _____

In a reproductive-age woman, the endocrine system is ultimately regulated by the hypothalamus, where GnRH is synthesized by specialized **gonadotropin neurons** and released at the median eminence. GnRH diffuses into the **hypophysial portal system** and is carried to the **anterior pituitary gland** (see Part A and Plate 7.1). **Gonadotrophs** in the anterior pituitary respond to GnRH by releasing **LH** and **FSH.** Gonadotropin actions on the ovary result in follicular development and estrogen synthesis in the follicular phase of the cycle (Plate 7.16; also see Plate 7.15); **inhibin** synthesis and secretion by granulosa cells is also stimulated. During the follicular phase, estradiol and inhibin exert negative feedback on the axis, with estrogen inhibiting GnRH synthesis and release by the hypothalamus and gonadotropin (LH and FSH) release by the anterior pituitary gonadotrophs; inhibin suppresses FSH release by the gonadotrophs. Note that Part A is a composite diagram showing negative feedback systems that occur in either the follicular or luteal phase of the menstrual cycle.

Near midcycle, **estradiol levels** rise to levels that provoke **positive feedback** within this endocrine axis (Part B). Specifically, estradiol now further stimulates GnRH and gonadotropin secretion, and thus more estradiol, forming the positive feedback loop. LH and FSH levels peak as a result of this positive feedback, causing ovulation.

The luteal or secretory phase of the menstrual cycle begins with the involution of the ruptured follicle and the reversion of the system to the more common negative feedback-based endocrine axis (Part A). Note that under influence of the gonadotropins, progesterone levels rise greatly and estradiol rises to a lesser extent (see Plate 7.15). Both of the steroids exert negative feedback on GnRH and gonadotropin secretion; inhibin produced by the granulosa cells has a more specific effect of inhibiting FSH secretion.

TRACE

☐ 1. Arrows for negative feedback effects of hormones (red)

☐ 2. Arrows for stimulatory and positive feedback effects of hormones (green)

COLOR

☐ 3. Hypothalamus

☐ 4. Anterior pituitary

Clinical Note

Oral contraceptive pills are usually a combination of an estrogen and a progestin (progesterone-like drug). Women on oral contraceptive therapy usually take the drug combination daily for 21 days, followed by 7 days of placebo or no pill. Ovulation (and thus pregnancy) is prevented by inhibition of the hormonal axis by the exogenous steroids (similar to negative feedback); menstruation occurs when the steroids are withdrawn after 21 days. Drugs used for **emergency contraception** after unprotected sex (morning after pills or emergency contraceptives) may contain a combination of estrogen and progestin, progestin alone, or an anti-progestin and produce contraception usually by delaying or preventing ovulation (a result of effects of the exogenous hormone or drug on the endocrine axis).

REVIEW ANSWERS

A. FSH

B. Progesterone, estradiol

C. Estradiol

D. LH

Plate 7.16　　　　　　　　　　　　　**Endocrine Physiology**

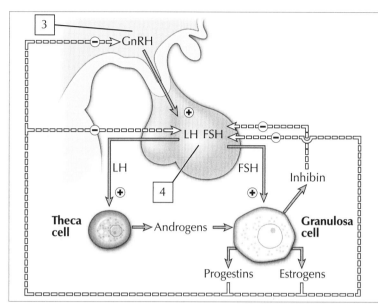

A. Negative feedback pathway

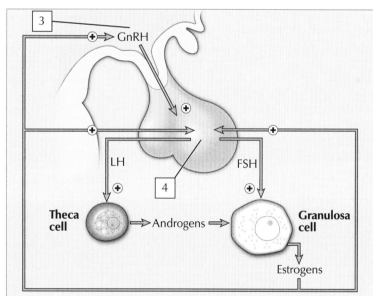

B. Positive feedback pathway at mid-cycle

J. Perkins
MS, MFA

REVIEW QUESTIONS

A. Inhibin exerts negative feedback on secretion of _____.

B. During the luteal phase of the menstrual cycle, negative feedback on GnRH is exerted by _____ and _____.

C. Positive feedback in the hypothalamic-pituitary-ovarian axis is exerted by high levels of the hormone _____.

D. At approximately midcycle, ovulation is provoked most directly by a surge in _____.

Analogous to ovaries in females, which produce mature ova and female steroids, the testes in males are the site of **spermatogenesis** and synthesize the male sex hormone **testosterone.** Spermatogenesis occurs within the convoluted **seminiferous tubules** of the testes, and **Leydig cells** between these tubules produce testosterone (Part A). In the lining of the tubules, differentiation from **spermatogonia** to **primary spermatocytes** to **secondary spermatocytes** to **sperm cells** occurs in close association with **Sertoli cells,** which support this process through the secretion of fluid and a variety of factors.

Spermatogenesis and steroidogenesis are ultimately regulated by the hypothalamus and anterior pituitary gland (Part C). As in females, GnRH is secreted by hypothalamic neurons and is carried to the anterior pituitary by the hypophysial portal circulation, where it stimulates gonadotrophic cells to synthesize and release LH and FSH. **LH** stimulates the synthesis of testosterone by Leydig cells, which binds to androgen-binding proteins on Sertoli cells in the seminiferous tubules; along with **FSH,** which also stimulates Sertoli cells, testosterone promotes spermatogenesis. Negative feedback in this endocrine axis is provided by testosterone inhibition of GnRH and gonadotropin secretion, along with inhibition of FSH secretion by inhibin (produced by Sertoli cells).

The role of androgens in pubertal development is covered in Plate 7.14. In addition to those effects, testosterone's nonreproductive effects include increased skeletal muscle mass, male pattern of hair distribution and baldness, and deepening of the voice. Whereas some effects of testosterone are direct, others depend on its conversion to DHT; for example, genital differentiation, prostate development and growth, male hair distribution, and baldness.

COLOR

- [ ] 1. Leydig cells
- [ ] 2. Seminiferous tubules
- [ ] 3. Secondary spermatocytes
- [ ] 4. Primary spermatocytes
- [ ] 5. Sertoli cell
- [ ] 6. Hypothalamus
- [ ] 7. Anterior pituitary

TRACE

- [ ] 8. Arrows for stimulatory effects of hormones (green)
- [ ] 9. Arrows for negative feedback effects of hormones (red)

Clinical Note

Testosterone and other naturally occurring and synthetic androgens have been used as **performance-enhancing drugs** and are now banned in most amateur and professional sports. Like endogenous testosterone, they promote skeletal muscle growth and muscle strength and are thus referred to as **anabolic** steroids. As such, these drugs have been abused at times by weightlifters, body builders, American football players, and baseball players, among other athletes. Of course, along with the anabolic actions, other androgen effects occur as well, including various physical and emotional changes. Masculinization in females is caused by anabolic steroids, and in both sexes, the presence of these drugs suppresses the endogenous endocrine axis, leading to infertility, atrophy of testes or ovaries, and other effects. Increased incidence of some cancers as well as heart disease and death may result.

REVIEW ANSWERS

A. GnRH, gonadotropins

B. Leydig cells, Sertoli cells

C. Inhibition of GnRH, gonadotropins, and testosterone secretion

D. DHT

Plate 7.17   **Endocrine Physiology**

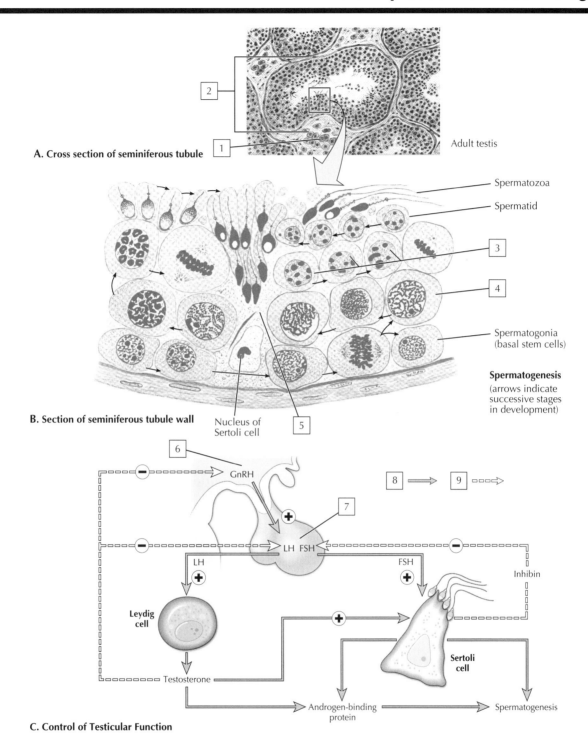

A. Cross section of seminiferous tubule

Adult testis

Spermatozoa

Spermatid

Spermatogonia
(basal stem cells)

Spermatogenesis
(arrows indicate
successive stages
in development)

B. Section of seminiferous tubule wall

Nucleus of
Sertoli cell

GnRH

LH FSH

LH

FSH

Inhibin

**Leydig
cell**

**Sertoli
cell**

Testosterone

Androgen-binding
protein

Spermatogenesis

C. Control of Testicular Function

REVIEW QUESTIONS

A. Testosterone inhibits the secretion of _____ and _____.

B. Testosterone synthesized by the _____ binds to androgen-binding proteins on the _____ in the seminiferous tubules.

C. The use of performance-enhancing drugs containing androgens has what effects on the male reproductive hormone axis?

D. Some of the actions of testosterone require its conversion to _____ by target cells.

Index

Note: Locators cited are plate numbers. Numbers in regular type indicate the discussion; **boldface** numbers indicate the art in the plate.

Index